HIDDEN TREASURE

THE NATIONAL LIBRARY OF MEDICINE

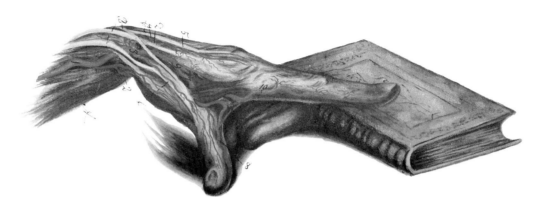

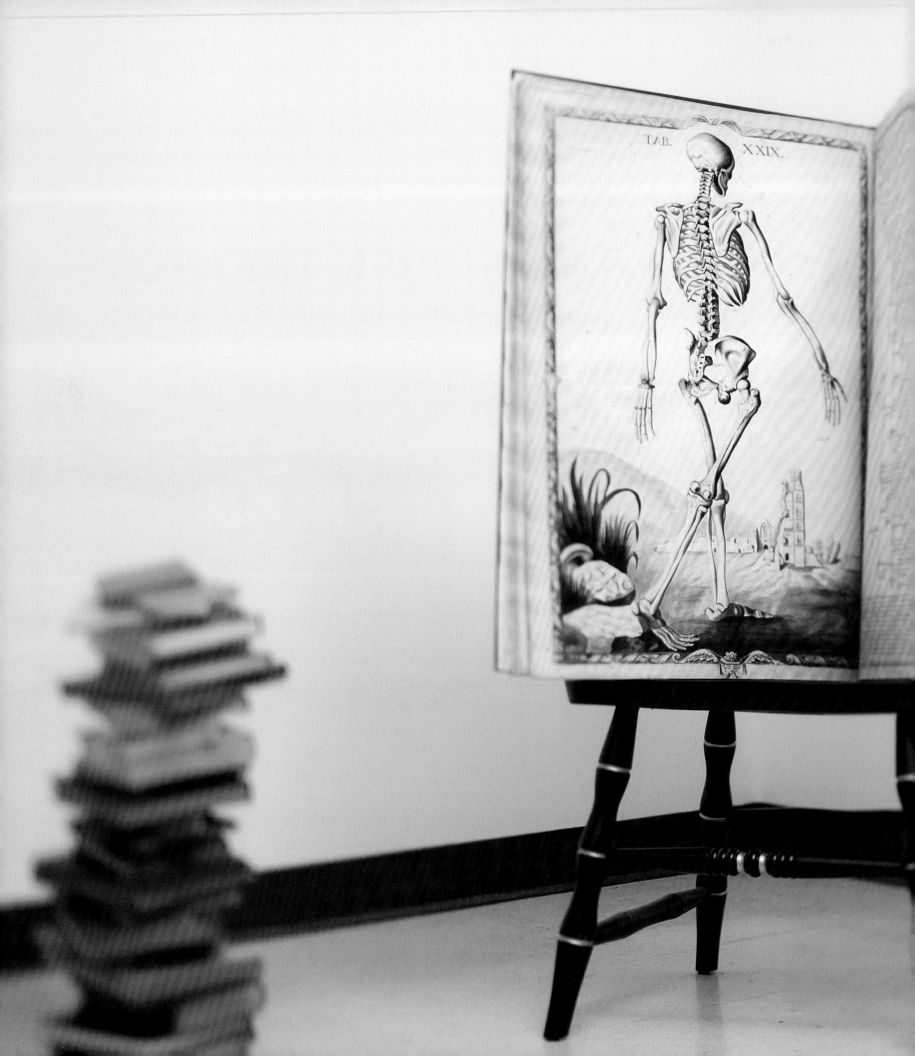

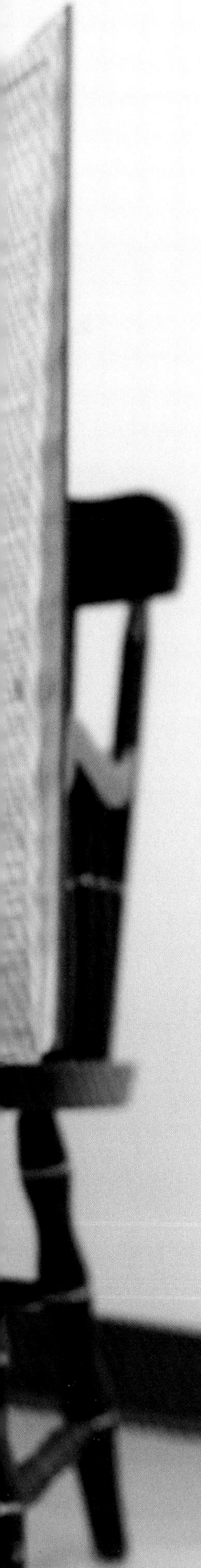

HIDDEN TREASURE

THE NATIONAL LIBRARY OF MEDICINE

EDITED BY

MICHAEL SAPPOL

DESIGNED BY

LAURA LINDGREN

PHOTOGRAPHY BY

ARNE SVENSON

NATIONAL LIBRARY OF MEDICINE   BETHESDA, MARYLAND
BLAST BOOKS   NEW YORK

CONTENTS

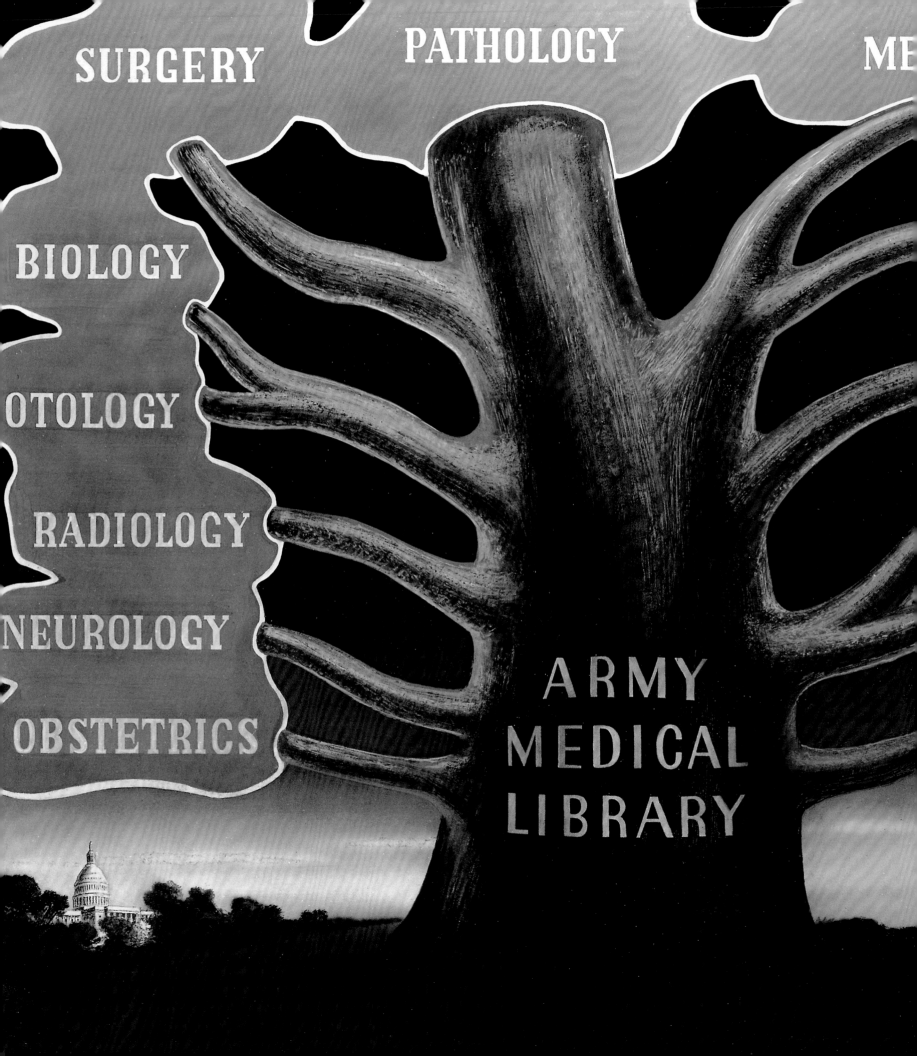

SURGERY

PATHOLOGY

ME

BIOLOGY

OTOLOGY

RADIOLOGY

NEUROLOGY

OBSTETRICS

ARMY
MEDICAL
LIBRARY

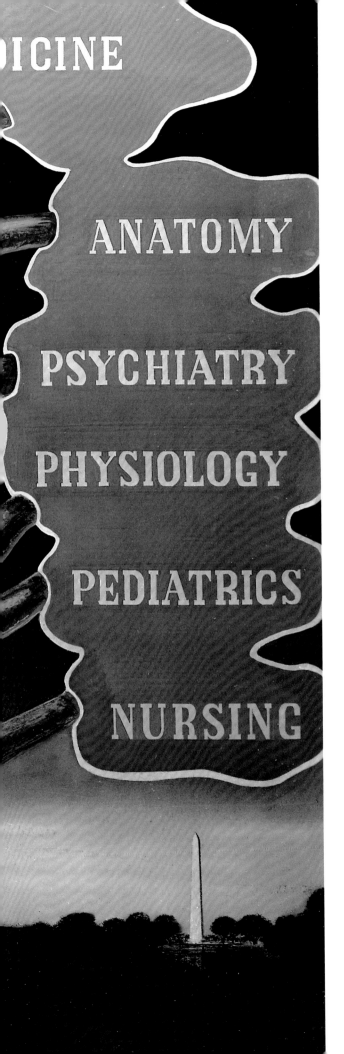

ICINE

ANATOMY

PSYCHIATRY

PHYSIOLOGY

PEDIATRICS

NURSING

FOREWORD: *The National Library of Medicine at 175*

The National Library of Medicine is now 175 years old. In 1836 it was a small collection of medical books on a single shelf in the Office of the Surgeon General of the Army. Today it is the world's largest biomedical library, with over 17 million items in more than 150 languages. For the past fifty years—since NLM created the Medline computer-based system for online retrieval of medical writings—we have increasingly become known for our automated Internet services to millions of users worldwide. In addition to writings, the Library now holds and distributes toxicologic, chemical, and genomic facts and teachings, and now even clinical trials records! We are proud of all this.

In contrast, this volume takes us closer to the beginnings of librarianship. Here in the History of Medicine Division of NLM, books, manuscripts, pamphlets, and prints of all sorts reside happily but somewhat anonymously within quiet, dark underground shelves. My friend and colleague the computer scientist Ed Feigenbaum once playfully described the Old Times as the period "when the books in the library could not talk to each other." In spite of all our efforts in artificial intelligence and computational linguistics, the books still need the help of a scholarly curator if they are to speak together—or to us. I am delighted that Dr. Michael Sappol has undertaken this effort and has recruited so talented a group of scholars for this task.

Lastly I take pleasure in echoing the enthusiasm for true, original, real books within our grasp, as Robert Darnton has said so well in *The Case for Books*. Here he notes that examination of multiple copies of the Shakespeare Folios is necessary because no two are alike. In science, too, speedy computer access to information is truly wonderful. Yet there are times—especially when we ask why or how a discovery or a belief arose—when we need to see and hold original intellectual works.

Dear Reader, please enjoy seeing and thinking about the Library's hidden treasures!

DONALD A. B. LINDBERG, MD
DIRECTOR, NATIONAL LIBRARY OF MEDICINE

The Army Medical Library (soon to be renamed the National Library of Medicine) as the tree of medical knowledge, with branches representing the major fields collected by the Library, ca. 1945. At the time, the Library was housed in a redbrick building on the National Mall, between the Capitol and the Washington Monument.

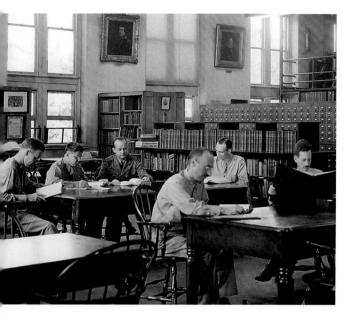

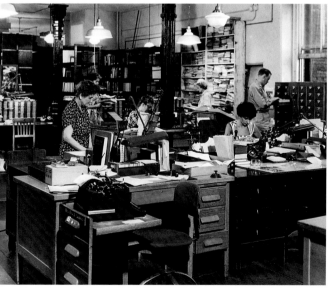

ABOVE, TOP: "Medical men use the library reading room" is the caption on this unidentified photograph, ca. 1940, when the Army Medical Library was on the National Mall.

ABOVE: View from behind a cataloging desk, ca. 1955.

In the past few decades libraries have been undergoing a transformation. According to Robert Darnton, the distinguished historian of print culture, in the 1950s, before the computer age, "knowledge came packaged between hard covers, and a great library seemed to contain all of it. To climb the steps of the New York Public Library, past the stone lions guarding its entrance and into the monumental reading room on the third floor, was to enter a world that included everything known. The knowledge came ordered into standard categories which could be pursued through a card catalog and into the pages of the books."

At the center of the university stood the library, Darnton continues, "the most important building, a temple set off by classical columns," where students congregated and read in silence, "no noise, no food, no disturbances." That is no longer the case today: "Reading rooms are nearly empty on some campuses.... To entice the students back, some librarians offer them armchairs for lounging and chatting, even drinks and snacks, never mind about the crumbs. Modern or postmodern students do most of their research at computers in their rooms."

It's no secret that nowadays we look for libraries on the Internet—without moving from our desks or laptops or mobile phones. And we find what we're looking for through search engines, which can execute near-instantaneous computerized word searches within both catalogues and texts, more and more of which have been digitized and posted on the Web. We read more and more on computers or Kindles or paper printouts. If we write an article or student paper or make a PowerPoint presentation, it in turn is often enough posted on the Web, where it can be added to the "universal library," which is not the collection of any one obsessed individual or any noble institution, but instead an aggregate, a library of libraries. Books, articles, paintings, sculptures—anything and everything seems to be reducible to digitized "information" that can be searched and packaged and repackaged and shared.

We're in a new and miraculous age. But there are still great libraries, in cities and on campuses, made of brick, sandstone, marble, and glass, containing physical objects, and especially enshrining the book: the Library of Congress, Bibliothèque Nationale de France, the British Library, the New York Public Library, the Wellcome Library, the great university libraries at Oxford, Harvard, Yale, Johns Hopkins, and elsewhere. And among them is the National Library of Medicine in Bethesda, the world's largest medical library, with its collection of over 17 million books, journals, manuscripts, prints, photographs, posters, motion pictures, sound recordings, and "ephemera" (pamphlets, matchbook covers, stereograph cards, etc.).

The NLM was established, with only a shelf of books, in 1836 as the Library of the Surgeon General's Office. In the late 1860s and '70s director John Shaw Billings, in the aftermath of the carnage of the American Civil War, took on the immensely ambitious task of collecting all of the world's medical knowledge in one place, and of collecting monuments and relics

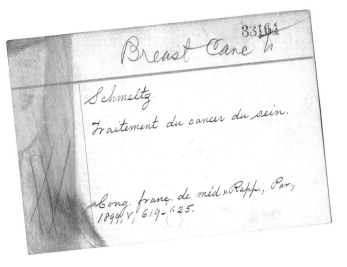

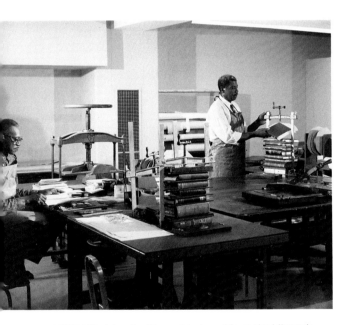

of the history of medicine and the health professions from antiquity to the present. Billings and his colleagues and successors built the library (later renamed the Army Medical Library, the Armed Forces Medical Library, and then the National Library of Medicine) into a great collection—and expected that in doing so it would play a vital role in the treatment of patients and the understanding and cure of disease.

The year 2011 marks the 175th anniversary of the National Library of Medicine. Today the Library is a global leader in information technology and distribution. It digitizes and digitally catalogues books and journals, develops databases and Internet "products," funds and implements vitally important telemedicine and bioinformatics projects, such as the Visible Human Project, and provides health information to the public and the health professions through MedlinePlus, PubMed, and ClinicalTrials.Gov. Its electronic services deliver trillions of bytes of vitally important data, every day, to millions of people. Scientists, scholars, educators, health professionals, and the general public in the United States and around the world search the Library's online resources, more than a billion times each year.

What is less known is that the Library also has a rich and various collection of handwritten, printed, and manufactured "things"—material objects—which originated in particular times and places, made by particular persons, and which have multiple meanings and histories of their own. The Library's mission has always been medical; it has always collected items of medical importance. But over the years, through happenstance or design, nonmedical items have also made their way into the collection. And some of what used to be vital medical material, even the cutting edge of medical knowledge, now seems more like precious evidence of something else, a resource for scholars tracing the history of medicine and health, but also the history of cities, race, factory production, sexuality, print technology, photography, feminism, motion pictures, the railroad, colonization, war, aesthetics, etc. So even though the Library, in its inception, was developed to be of use to the medical professions—and, in the last three decades or so, opened up to provide medical information to the global public—its collections pertain to nearly every aspect of human existence. They belong properly to everybody, not just those with particular medical interests.

In other words, the Library today—and its History of Medicine Division with its specially trained staff of historians, cataloguers, curators, and conservators—is the steward of a rich (and still growing) patrimony of historical objects. Primarily (but not exclusively), these are books and journals printed with ink on paper, with covers, bindings, illustrations, annotations, and marginalia, marked by former readers and by the Library staff itself. These are things that are not entirely reducible to "information," that are only partly susceptible to digitization. They have a feel and texture and smell and color; they are strong or brittle, clean or dusty; they have been taken from place to place, bought or sold or bartered or stolen or issued or given away as gifts. They have been treasured or neglected, defaced or mended, added to or pruned back. Each object has lived a "social life" (to use Arjun Appadurai's memorable phrase), sometimes several lives.

As in any vast collection, the individual objects are buried in the sheer mass of things, even if they glow with a particular wisdom or beauty or oddness or grotesquery or wit or sadness or horror. Despite more than a century and a half of classification and cataloguing and interpretation, they are largely obscure to the public and may even be obscure to the Library's cataloguers, librarians, curators, historians, and administrators. If we excavate them (and can figure out what to do with them), they once again speak to us, charm us, repulse us, amaze us, inform us, pleasure us. And teach us: even the most seemingly trivial or haphazard

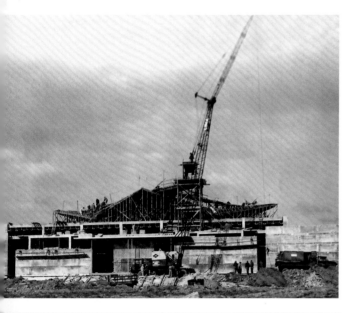

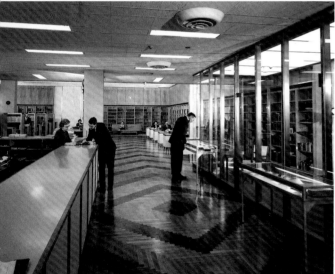

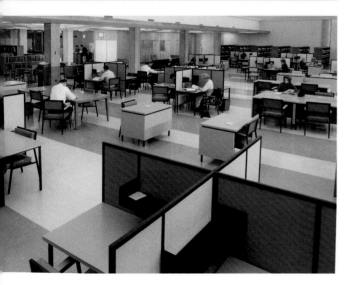

item in the Library's holdings is in some way connected to important issues, has played a key or symptomatic role in some important historical event or development.

The occasion of the Library's 175th anniversary has provided us with an excuse to troll the collection. We found items that are unique or rare, some of them unknown even to highly specialized scholars, and items that are known to the cognoscenti and which (in different copies) may also be buried in the collections of other libraries. Either way, they are hidden treasures. And here, in this volume, is a small selection of them.

There is one other hidden treasure: the Library itself. Its collection ranges in time from the eleventh century to the present and comes from nearly every region of the globe. The Library holds medieval manuscripts, rare first editions, silent films, paintings, photographs, lantern slides, original drawings, hospital records, and laboratory notebooks.

The Library is also something less tangible than its artifacts: its history. It is made up of the buildings where it has been housed—including Ford's Theatre (in the decades after the assassination of Abraham Lincoln) and from 1887 to 1962 a beautiful brick building on the Mall (in the spot the Smithsonian's Hirschhorn Museum presently occupies). And it is made up of the people who have staffed it and who diligently attended to the Herculean task of operating a great library: the people who guided it through key transitions; the people who acquired, shelved, catalogued, and described its holdings; the people who assisted patrons in finding a special article, monograph, print, or chapter and who reproduced the materials and sent them on their way through interlibrary loan and document delivery; and the people who cleaned the Library and guarded it from harm. It is also made up of a long and overlapping succession of technologies: the printing press and the computer, but also the pencil, microfilm, photostats, pneumatic tubes, typewriters, carbon paper, the Dictaphone, mimeograph machines, card catalogues, telephones, interoffice fax, and so on.

And the Library was shaped by a larger history. In the 1820s when Army Surgeon General Joseph Lovell (1788–1836) began collecting books, the United States was waging wars of expansion west and south of the Appalachian Mountains, and current medical literature was necessary to help keep the troops in fit condition by medical personnel. Scholarship and original research were not yet on the agenda; the Library served primarily as a subscription service, selecting a few of the best monographs and journals for military physicians and surgeons and sending them out to remote locations in the Republic.

In the aftermath of the Civil War, a cadre of army surgeons breathed new life into the Army Medical Museum and Library (the two were conjoined twins, separated only much later, in the twentieth century). Back then, the Library was staffed by military personnel, many of them veteran medical officers of the late war. Out of this group came John Shaw Billings (1838–1913), an army surgeon and bibliophile who had a vision of the Library as a vital repository for the military, the nation, and the world. He campaigned to acquire medical publications, especially all back and current issues of American medical journals, mostly by contacting physicians around the nation and persuading them to donate their collections to the Library, sometimes almost literally prying the books out of their hands. He also barraged Americans living overseas and foreign book dealers and publishers with pleas to send the Library materials from areas where they were located.

As Billings built up the collections, started the Library's *Index-Catalogue*, and began indexing articles on a regular basis, the Library became known as a refuge—or a place of

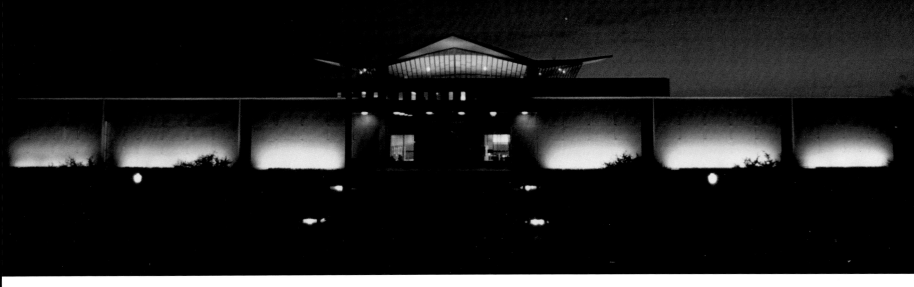

The glowing facade of the National Library of Medicine, Bethesda, 1972.

OPPOSITE, TOP: The new National Library of Medicine building, under construction, ca. 1960.

OPPOSITE, MIDDLE: The gleaming new reading room of the History of Medicine Division, National Institutes of Health, Bethesda campus, beckons from the entrance near the service desk (ca. 1963). Division Chief John B. Blake leans over the desk and speaks with a librarian.

OPPOSITE, BOTTOM: The National Library of Medicine's main reading room, with a Mondrian-influenced modernist design, soon after the Library reopened in its new Bethesda location in 1962.

exile—for older army personnel who could no longer withstand the rigors of field duty. Its nickname was "Botany Bay" (the prison colony founded by the British in Australia in the late 1700s). By 1906 only one Library staff member was under the age of forty; the average age of clerks was fifty-nine, most of them retirees from the Surgeon General's Office or the army. The first woman known to have asked for a position at the Library, in December 1903, was Kate Levy, a physician trained at Northwestern University who was interested in medical librarianship as a specialty. Billings was unwilling to make what he saw as a drastic change in the Library's culture. But labor shortages during World War I brought civilian women, some with training in library science, into the Library for the first time. By the late 1920s women and men worked in the Library in almost equal numbers. Later, women would come to predominate.

In 1941, when the United States entered the world war then raging, the Library was hit with a crisis—the need to protect the nation's medical knowledge from a potential attack on Washington by Hitler's Third Reich. The Library moved its rare holdings west to Cleveland, Ohio, where the curators of the historical collections, now named the History of Medicine Division, began a heroic initiative to conserve old and battered books, many of which had suffered damage in their overcrowded, damp, and dirty quarters in downtown Washington.

In the 1950s, upon its return from Cleveland, by authority of Congress the Library was detached from the Army Medical Museum, renamed the National Library of Medicine, and placed under the aegis of the U.S. Public Health Service. It moved to the campus of the National Institutes of Health in Bethesda in 1962, where it remains today as one of the Institutes, open and accessible to the public via Washington's Metro and, via the Internet, to patrons the world over. And where it continues to acquire, catalogue, and make available works famous and obscure—some of them hot off the presses (or the digital equivalent) and vital to current medical research into the nature of the human body and the treatment of disease and others vital to our understanding of times past, the world we have lost.

This book celebrates the legacy of the Library in its 175th year. In doing so, it reminds us that materials taken in by the Library today will be part of the historical collections of tomorrow.

—MICHAEL J. NORTH, JEFFREY S. REZNICK, AND MICHAEL SAPPOL

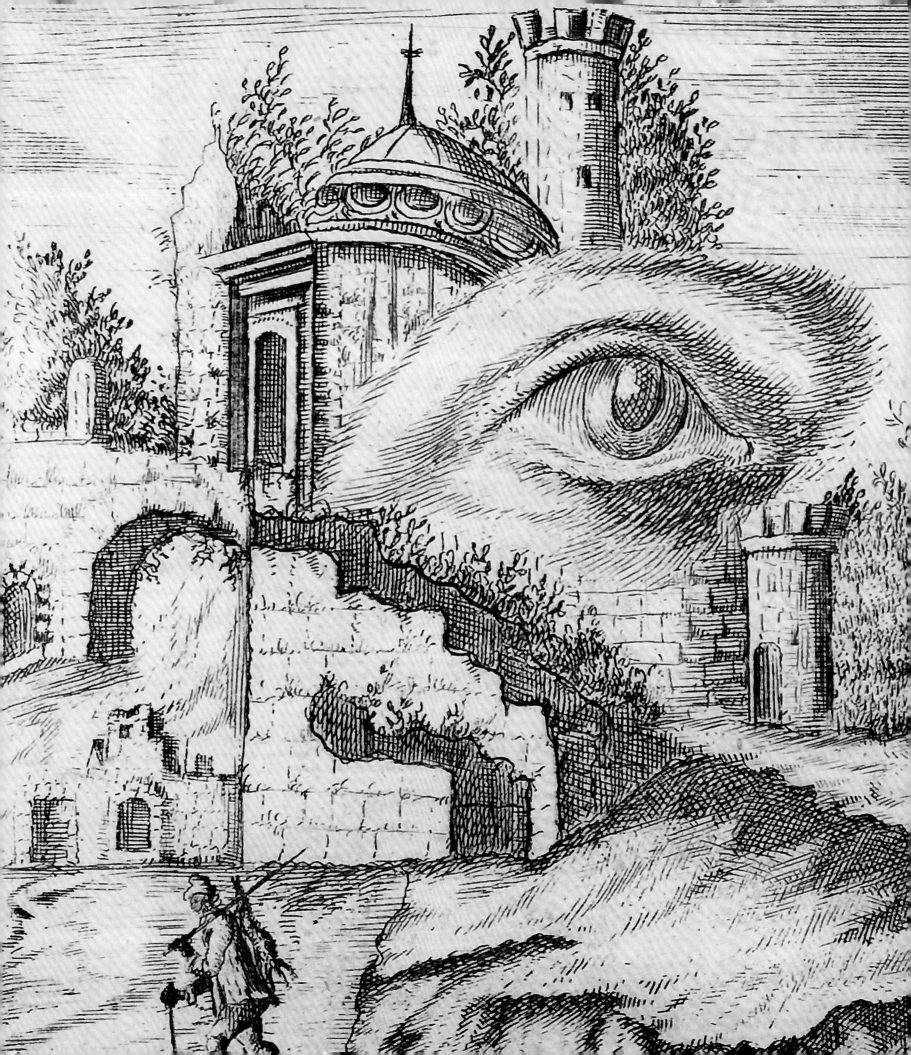

Commentaries on the Three Books of Aristotle's De anima According to the Teaching of Thomas Aquinas (ca. 1485)

Lambertus de Monte

Copulata super tres libros Aristotelis De anima iuxta doctrinam Thomae de Aquino. Cologne, Germany. Printed book on paper with manuscript marginalia; 105 folios; height 8¼ x 11⅜ in. (21.2 x 28.5 cm)

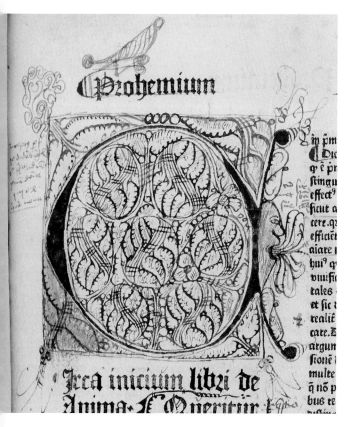

ABOVE AND OPPOSITE: Aristotelian ideas about the senses provided humorous inspiration for students. A waggish student drawing ridicules the size of the monastic nose. The same student also wrote a silly bilingual syllogism deriding his teacher's name, Frater Silvester Coci ("Silvester the Cook's Son"). The illuminations above and doodles on the next page show some of the book's many reader-titillating tongues. *Copulata,* "De anima," fols. 2a and 105b; "Phisicorum," fols. 57b and 58a

Jorge of Burgos, the scholar-villain of Umberto Eco's *The Name of the Rose,* damned Aristotle (384–322 BCE): "Every book by that man has destroyed a part of the learning that Christianity has accumulated over the centuries." With such a driving hatred Jorge embarked on a series of murders to suppress the philosopher's book on humor.

In the high and late Middle Ages the uncertainty generated by Aristotle's thought (unlike Plato's, which was more amenable to monotheism) began to undermine his status. By the end of the fifteenth century some scholars posed a concrete question: Should Aristotle, the great authority of antiquity and medieval scholasticism, be eternally damned or saved? That question struck Lambertus de Monte (1430/5–99) as specious. Lambertus was professor of arts and of theology, and then dean of theology, at the University of Cologne from 1455 to 1499. A devout Catholic, he fervently admired the works of St. Thomas Aquinas (1224/5–74), the great Parisian philosopher-theologian who "resurrected" Aristotle in the thirteenth century. So zealously did Aquinas favor Aristotle that Lambertus advocated his beatification.

Lambertus was born in modern-day Holland and studied under his uncle Gerhardus de Monte at the University of Cologne, receiving his master of arts degree in 1454 and doctorate of theology in 1473. He was a member of the Schola Coloniensis, whose medieval scholastic arguments were among the first to appear in printed books in the fifteenth century, but also among the first to be overturned by the newfangled humanists of the mid-sixteenth.

Copulata super tres libros Aristotelis De anima iuxta doctrinam Thomae de Aquino, the National Library of Medicine's book featured here, contains several of Lambertus's commentaries on Aquinas's interpretations of Aristotle's work, including one on the soul, *De anima.* A Dominican monastery in Frankfurt owned the volume in the sixteenth century. Pierre Duhem, the great French historian of medieval science, owned a similar copy. Unlike Duhem's copy, the NLM's is strewn with doodles and images, mostly in one of two brown-inked hands, of indeterminate age.

The ad hoc illustrations defacing the volume are compelling. Folio 105b (opposite) displays the bust of a tonsured monk. Surrounded by a profusion of banners describing actions of the soul in the body, the monk's visage also has pointers to the organs of the five senses. The visual trope, dating at least to the ninth century, proliferated in the thirteenth and beyond.

Illuminations of tongues, suggesting both the sense of taste and the organ of speech by which books were read aloud, humorously lick many of the tome's pages and echo *The Name of the Rose.* To kill his victims Father Jorge coated the folios of his Aristotelian manuscript with a poison that a reader would ingest by licking his finger on turning a page. The fictional tongue in cheek ensured that indulgence in Aristotelian ribaldry brought death. For us, as readers of this treasure, the provocative tongues bring humor and delight.

—WALTON O. SCHALICK

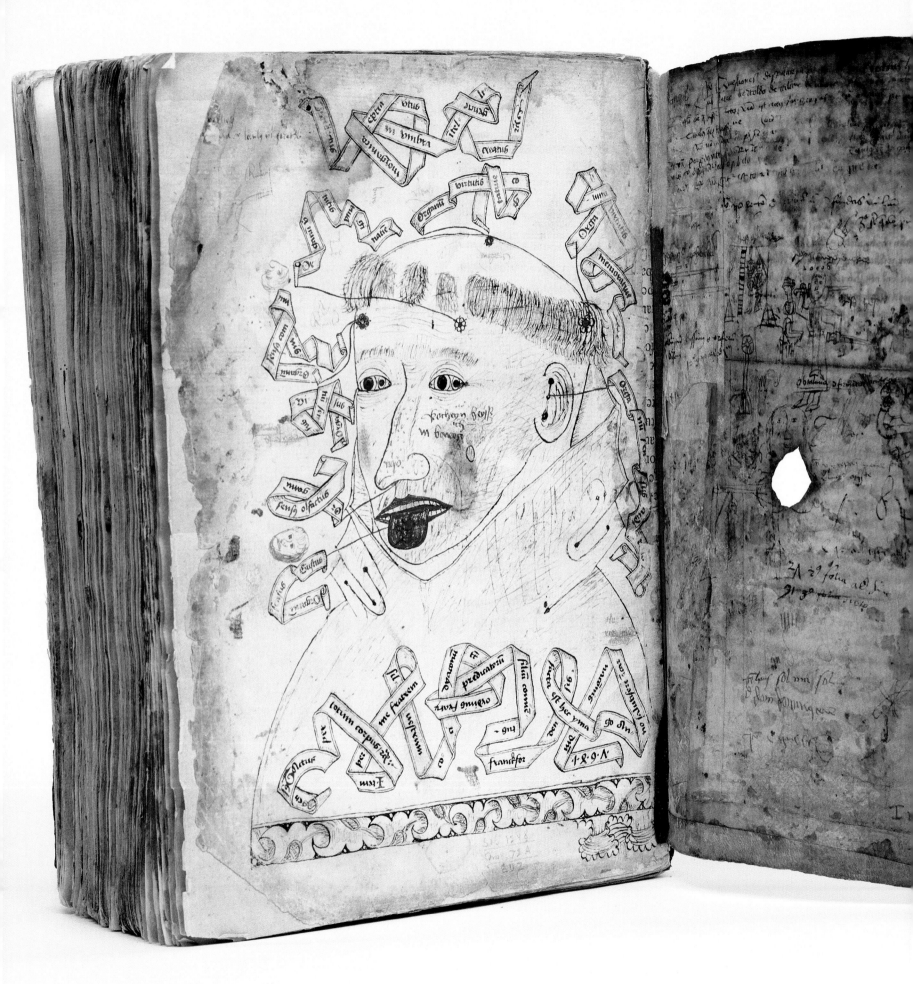

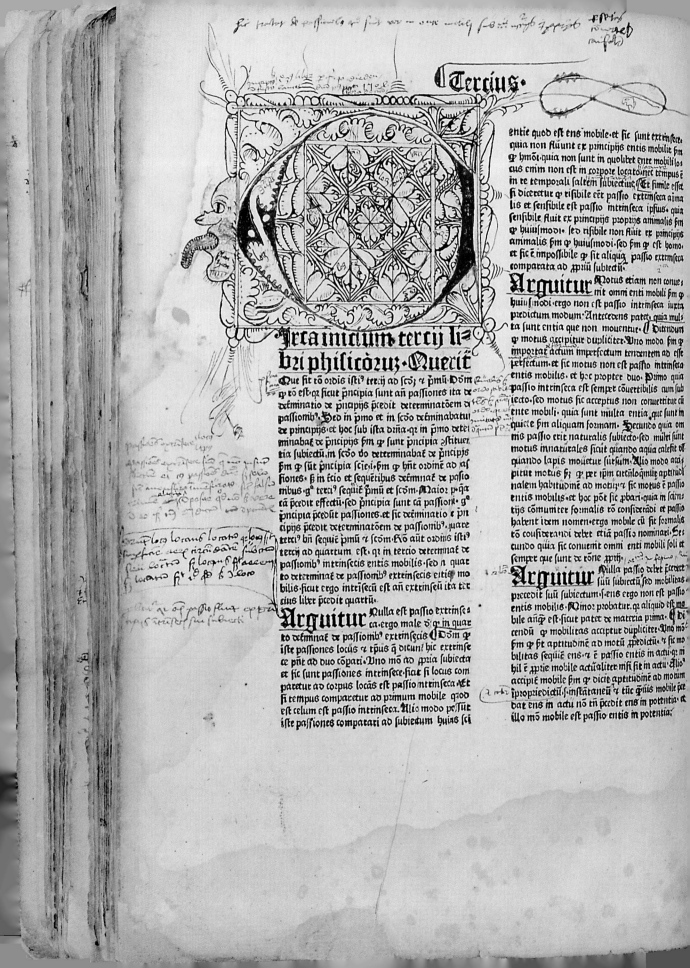

¶Irca inicium tercij li=
bri phisicorum · Querit

Que sit ro ordis isti⁹ tercij ad sc⁵m ⁊ pmū · Dōm
ꝗ ro est ꝗ sicut pncipia sunt an passiones ita ꝺe
ꝺeterminatio ꝺe pnapijs pcedit ꝺeterminatõem ꝺe
passiomb⁹· Sed in pmo et in scō ꝺeterminabatur
ꝺe principijs · et hoc sub ista ordia · qr in pmo ꝺeter
minabat ꝺe pncipijs ſm ꝗ sunt pncipia ⸗stituen
tia subiectū · in scō ꝿo ꝺeterminabat ꝺe pncipijs
ſm ꝗ sūt pncipia scie·i · ſm ꝗ hūt ordine ad pas
siones · ſȝ in tcio et sequētibus ꝺeterminat ꝺe passio
mib⁹ · ꝗ tercij⁹ seqꝰi· pmū et scōm · Maior ꝗꝗ
cã pcedit effectū · sed pncipia sunt cã passioⁿ · ꝗ
pncipia pcedit passiones · et sic ꝺeterminatio ꝺe pn
cipijs pcedit ꝺeterminatõem ꝺe passiomb⁹· quare
tcij⁹ bn sequꝰ pmū ⁊ scōm· Ro aut ordis isti⁹
tercij ad quartū est· qr in tercio ꝺeterminat ꝺe
passiomb⁹ intrinsecis entis mobilis· sed ñ quare
to ꝺeterminat ꝺe passiomb⁹ extrinsecis entis mo
bilis· sicut ergo intriseū est an extriseū ita ter
cius liber pcedit quartū·

Arguitur
Nulla est passio extrinse=
ca · ergo male ꝺr ꝗ in quar
to ꝺeterminat ꝺe passiomb⁹ extrinsecis · ꝰDōm ꝗ
iste passiones locus ⁊ tpus ꝗ ꝺicunt hic extrinse=
ce pñt ad ꝺuo cōpari · Uno mo ad ꝓpria subiecta
et sic sunt passiones intrinsece · sicut si locus com
paretur ad corpus locas est passio intrinseca · Et
si tempus comparetur ad primum mobile ꝗuod
est celum est passio intrinseca · Alio modo possūt
iste passiones comparari ad subiectum huius sci

entie ꝗuod est ens mobile · et sic sunt extrinsece
quia non fluunt ex principijs entis mobilis ſm
⁊ hmōi · quia non sunt in quolibet ente mobili lo
aus enim non est in corpore locato ·nec tempus ē
in re temporali saltem subiectiue· Et simile esset
si ꝺiceretur ꝗ visibile eēt passio extrinseca anima
lis et sensibile est passio intrinseca ipsius· quia
sensibile fluit ex principijs ꝓprijs animalis ſm
ꝗ huiusmodi· sed visibile non fluit ex principijs
animalis ſm ꝗ huiusmodi · sed ſm ꝗ est homo·
et sic ē impossibile ꝗ sit aliqua passio extrinseca
comparata ad ꝓpriū subiectū·

Arguitur
Motus etiam non conue
nit omni enti mobili ſm ꝗ
huiusmodi · ergo non est passio intrinseca iuxta
predictum modum · Antecedens patet quia mul=
ta sunt entia que non mouentur· ꝰDicendum
ꝗ motus accipitur dupliciter· Uno modo · ſm ꝗ
importat actum imperfectum tendentem ad esse
perfectum· et sic motus non est passio intrinseca
entis mobilis· et hoc propter ꝺuo · Primo quia
passio intrinseca est semper conuertibilis cum sub
iecto · sed motus sic acceptus non conuertitur cū
ente mobili · quia sunt multa entia · que sunt in
quiete ſm aliquam formam · Secundo quia om
nis passio est naturalis subiecto · sed multi sunt
motus innaturales sicut quando aqua calefit ꝿo
quando lapis mouetur sursum· Alio modo acci
pitur motus ſȝ · ꝗ ꝗ per ipm circiloꝗuiꝰ aptitu
dinalem habitudiñe ad motū·⁊ sic motus ē passio
entis mobilis · et hoc pōt sic pbari · quia in sciēn
tijs cōmuniter formalis rō consideradi ⁊ passio
habent idem nomen · ergo mobile cū sit formalis
rō cōsideradi ꝺebet etiam passio nominari· Se
cundo quia sic conuenit omni enti mobili soli ⁊
semper que sunt ꝺe rōne ꝓprij·

Arguitur
Nulla passio ꝺebet pcedere
suū subiectū· sed mobilitas
precedit suū subiectum · ens ergo non est passio
entis mobilis · Minor probatur · qr aliquid est mo
bile añ ꝗ est · sicut patet ꝺe materia prima· ꝰDi
cendū ꝗ mobilitas accipitur dupliciter· Uno mo
ſm ꝗ ſt aptitudiñe ad motū ꝓdictum · et sic mo
bilitas sequīt ens· ⁊ ē passio entis in actu· qr ni
hil ē ꝓprie mobile actualiter nisi sit in actu· Alio
accipīt mobile ſm ꝗ ꝺicit aptitudiñe ad motū
iꝓpriedictū· s·instātaneū ⁊ tūc qꝰuis mobile pce
bat ens in actu nō tñ pcedit ens in potentia· et
illo mō mobile est passio entis in potentia·

Arguitur

Ex hoc sequit q̄ tpus sit passio itrinseca entis mobilis qr tpus capiat p̄ tpali tūc couenit omni enti mobili quia ēē ens mobile est tpale. Dōm q̄ tpale accipit duplr. Uno mō put tpale capit p̄ illo q̄ est mensurabile tpe. et sic est verū q̄ tpale couenit omni enti mobili et sic nō ē passio qr passio debet inesse subiecto. sed q̄ mēsurat tpe nō est illud in quo est tpus. Alio mō accipit tpale p̄ illo in quo natū est esse tpus. sicut mobile in quo natus est ēē motus. et sic tpale qr̄ēt solų p̄mo mobili et nō oi enti mobili iō tpale nullo modo pōt esse passio itrinseca entis mobilis. Similiter dicendū est de locabili.

Qoniam autem natura est prin-

Postq̄ Aristo. determinauit de principijs rerum naturaliū iam determinat d passionib'. Et p̄mo ostēdit q̄ de istis passionib' est determinandū in isto libro. et hoc p̄mo de motu dein de alijs.s. infinito loco vacuo et tpe. Prima p̄bando pōt talem rōem. Phus naturalis habet determinare de natura sicut p̄batū est prius ergo h̄z determinare de motu qa tenz qr nō pt agnosci natura absq̄ cognitiōe motus qr ignorato motu necesse est natura ignorare. et hoc iō qr motus pōnit in diffinitiōe natre. s̄ ignorata diffinitiōe ignoraf z diffinitū

Determinantibus enim

Hic ostēdit q̄ naturalis phis h̄z determinare de alijs passionib'.s. infinito vacuo loco et tpe. et hoc probat duab' rōnibus. Prima est phus naturalis h̄z determinare de motu sicut p̄batū est. sed ista cōsequitur motū ergo ꝗ̄. q̄d sic p̄bat qr motus p̄ se est continuū. continuū aut multotiens diffinit p̄ infinitū ergo infinitū spectat ad rōem. motus ex tōne quia continuū. Locus aut habet ordinē ad motū qr principalis species mot' est motus localis. sed motus localis fit in loco. Et qr nō pt fieri motus localis sine vacuo q̄ etiam determinandū est a pho naturali de vacuo. Et tpus est mensura motus. sicut eni locus est mensura mobilis ita tpus est mēsura motus. qr ergo phs naturalis h̄z determinare de motu ergo etiam de omnibus alijs.

Arguitur

Motus nō est p̄ se continuus. qr continuitas est accis

Mot'

Mot' q̄ nō quērit sibi p̄ se. Dōm q̄ duplr aliq̄ couenit alicui p̄ se. Uno mō s̄m p̄mū modū p̄ se. et q̄ sic couenit alteri p̄ se est de sua diffinitiōe. et illo mō nō quērit motui ēē cōtinuū p̄ se. Alio mō quērit alicui aliq̄ p̄ se in scō mō p̄ se. z hoc p̄ tē accis q̄uit. et sic q̄uitur ēē p̄ se quērit motui qr est passio ei'. Circa q̄d advertendū q̄ dr in textu q̄ multotiēs ipsum pōnit in diffinitiōe q̄tinui ad denotandū q̄ continuū habet triplicē diffinitiōē. Una metaphisicale q̄ dat p̄ triscētēs sicut ista Cōtinuū est cui' mot' est un'. et in illa diffinitiōe nō pōnit infinitū. Alia est diffinitio data p̄ via cōpositiōis sicut in potcametis ubi dr. Cōtinuū est cui' ptes copulāt ad aliquē tminū cōem. et q̄ tal diffinitio daf s̄m via pstitutiōis q̄tinui iō dr dari s̄m via cōpositiōis. et in illa diffinitiōe iterū nō pōnit infinitū. Alia daf s̄m via resolutiōis siue diuisiōis. z in illa pōnit infinitū. sicut dicimus q̄ q̄tinuū est diuisibile in infinitum. et de illa loquitur textus.

Nam festum igitur ē

Hic pōnit scōa rō phīe q̄ de istis h̄z determinare naturalis phīs. et est de illis h̄z determinare phisicus que sūt cōia oib' reb' naturalib'. s̄ sic est de istis q̄ ꝗ̄. Maior ptz. qr in hoc libro phīcorū determinat de cōib' q̄ coitr quērunt enti mobili z in libris sequētib' fit ꝗ̄tractatio. Mnor p̄bat qr passiones sic assignate vr quērunt enti mobili quērtibiliter sicut mot' et infinitū. vel hūt ordinē ad ens mobile sicut tpus z loc' que q̄uis nō quērunt oib' entib' mobi libus p̄ inherentia tn hūt ordinē ad ēē ens mobile

Queritur

Utrū ignorato motu etiā ignoraf natura. Dōm q̄ sic. rōe qr ignorato eo q̄ ē de diffinitiōe alic' ncē ē etiam ipm diffinitū ignoraf. s̄ mot' est de diffinitiōe natre. qr ignorato motu ncē est natura ignorare. Maior ptz qr diffinitū agnoscif p̄ ptes diffinitēs sicut h̄ agnosci̇ē ex aial z rōnali Mnor patet qr nomē natre est nomē principij. q̄d est mot'. et si natura capiat absolute tūc etiam motus est de eius agnitione quo ad cognitiōem nrām qr nos agni oscim' natura ex motu

Queritur

Utrū cognito motu etiā cognoscaf natura. Dōm q̄ sic. cui' rō est qr effectus univoc' alicui' cāe ducit in cognitiōem cause quo ad quid est et quo ad quia est. sed motus est effectus univocus natre. ergo ducit in cognitionem natre s̄m propriam

The Epitome (1543)
Andreas Vesalius

Andreae Vesalii Bruxellensis . . . suorum de humani corporis fabrica librorum epitome. Basel, Switzerland.
Bound printed book, illustrated with woodcuts, 18 pp.; 13¾ x 20 in. (35 x 50.8 cm)

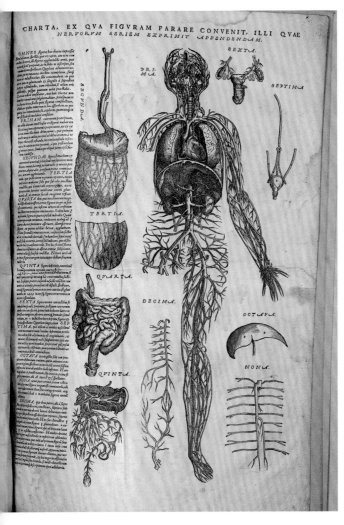

ABOVE: Before cutting out the figures on this page, Vesalius suggests that readers glue the page onto parchment and gives instructions on how to assemble the pieces and paste the resultant multilayered figure onto a base "muscle man" illustration. *Epitome*, fol. 14a

OPPOSITE: The woodcuts are arranged as if going through a dissection, from the outer parts to the inner muscles, bones, vessels, and organs. Naked "Adam" and "Eve" figures introduce the series. *Epitome*, fol. 10b and 11a

OVERLEAF: The fourth and fifth "figure of the muscles" conclude the illustrated/typographical dissection, showing more bone than muscle. They also present the anatomy of the head and brain. *Epitome*, fol. 7b and 8a

In autumn 1543, Andreas Vesalius (1514–64) arrived in Mainz, Germany, with a crate of freshly printed copies of his brand-new anatomical works. The offspring of a family of loyal medical employees at the Hapsburg court, Vesalius had traveled from Basel to meet the Holy Roman Emperor Charles V, and to present his credentials and *De humani corporis fabrica* (1543), the foundational text of modern anatomy. The anatomist offered the emperor a hand-colored copy (now in a private American collection), printed on vellum, illuminated in silver and gold. And he brought with him, also on vellum, a large, slim book, the *Epitome*, for Charles V's son Prince Philip (possibly, the copy now held at the Library of the Escorial in Spain).

Vesalius produced his "minor" anatomical book, dedicated to the young imperial heir, while working on *De fabrica* and while meticulously planning his future career. Perhaps on the advice of his publisher, Johannes Herbst (Oporinus), Vesalius realized that *De fabrica* was too long even for learned physicians, and too expensive for the general public he hoped to reach. But he had qualms about reducing his masterpiece: "Everybody knows the damages" that summaries and compendia "provoke in all sciences." So instead he conceived the *Epitome* as "a pathway or appendix" to *De fabrica*, "a more succinct and effective way" to present the richness and complexity of his anatomical studies.

The *Epitome* compresses every single part of the human body, according to Vesalius, "without any omission," into only a few pages of text and pictures. After the title page, twelve large in-folio leaves, printed on both sides, contain six pages of discussion (divided into six chapters, displayed on two columns) and six pages occupied by large anatomical woodcuts. Two unnumbered leaves, printed on only one side, follow. They present illustrations of organs, vessels, and bits and pieces of human anatomy as well as instructions on how to cut them out and paste them together. The reader, or rather the user, of the book is told to build with his own hands a multilayered anatomical paper doll and then glue it to one of the muscle figures represented in the lettered pages of the book.

Surprisingly, Vesalius—the ambitious and self-conscious founder of the new anatomy—found inspiration for this typographical artifice in the production of lowbrow, modest novelty prints that then circulated all over western Europe: anatomical "fugitive sheets" with superimposed flaps. His invitation to mutilate the *Epitome*, his pedagogical gimmick, was designed to aid the reader's memorization and understanding of the composition and spatial arrangement of the anatomical parts. It was a playful operation for his sixteenth-century readership, but unsettling for later bibliophiles, who venerated Vesalius and his monumental printed works.

There are three extant vellum copies of the *Epitome*. The National Library of Medicine's copy is not one of them. It is printed on paper and noteworthy because it is one of the few 1543 paper copies that have survived the spoiling effects of time—and the scissors of readers and owners.

—ANDREA CARLINO

HIC NON prolixior nominum ex-
ternarum hominis sedes locaue indican-
tium enumeratio instituitur, quàm
commodè imaginum uirilis muliebrisque
corporis superficie exprimentiū mar-
ginibus adhiberi potest. Quanquam
succinctam eorum descriptionem, ac
ueluti praesentium figurarum indicem duntaxat proponere
nihil obstet, quum eadem ferè nomina externis corporis sedibus ac ossibus, partibusque externae sedi subditis, accom-
modentur, quorum praecipua, ab iisque qui rectius dissecan-
di rationem aggressi fuerunt instituta, iam prius in oratio-
nis contextu, quantum proposita nobis Epitome requirit,
recensuimus. Solet itaque uniuersa corporis superficies ab
illius nominum institutoribus primùm in magnas sedes di-
uidi, ac dein illarum partes rursus nomenclaturis do-
nari. Atque ita Aegyptij medici corpus in Caput, Thoracem, Manus, & Crura diuidebant: Thoracem, perinde ac Aristoteles, nominantes, uniuersum corporis trun-
cum, à iugulo aut collo clauiculisue ad inguina & pubem,
aut magis ad femorum usque superiora pertinentem: non
autem tantùm, ut Galenus, nonnullis Anatomicorum pri-
mari, corporis sedem costis septam. Alij facultatum corpus
uniuersum dispensantium, animarumque sedibus mentem
adhibentes, quadrifariam quidem similiter ac Aegyptij corporis superficiem discernunt, ue-
rùm secus quàm illi corporis trun-
cum in duas sedes primùm distin-
guetis, manus & crura unius partis loco prima hac diuisione enu-
merat, illa quae Artus propriè uo-
catos constituunt, extremorū no-
mine complectetis. Ac in corporis trunco duas praecipuas locant
sedes, secundùm duas cauitates se-
cantibus inibi obuias: quarum inferior ab elatiori, interuentu septi
transuersi seiuncta, iecur naturalis
altricisue animae sedem sanguifi-
cationisque officinâ, ac insuper huic
subministrantia organa complectitur, partibus quoque generationi famulantibus parata. Superior cauitas cordi irascibilis animae fomiti uitalisque spiritus fonti,
illique subseruientibus organis af-
scribitur. Caeterum tertia corporis cauitas capi-
ti tribuitur, cerebroque potissimùm principis animae sedi, animalis usque spiritus promptuario sacra-
tur. Corpore in hunc modum obiter diuiso, singu-
larum partium superficies ita rursus distinguitur,
ut capitis totius pars anterior superciliis superpo-
sita, ac crinibus nuda, lineasque quasdam pro-
ponens, Frons nominetur. Hac superior & uersus capitis medium uergens, Sinciput, Vtrinque
ad sincipitis latus, supraque Aurem, cui Audi-
torius meatus inest, consistens, Tempus. Media
capitis sedes sinciput uersus posteriora superans,
Vertex, qui ueluti centrum est circuli crinium
originem circumscribentis. Post uerticem usque ad
musculorum qui utrinque in ceruicis summo prominentes, in medio foueam ostendunt, ac plerisque
Tendines dicuntur, elatissimam sedem Occiput
spectat. Prior autê capitis pars à frôte ad mentũ
spectat, Facies. Inferior enim frôtis pars, Superciliis ueluti eminêtibus, pilisque côstis terminis,
corundemque medio costis circunscribitur. His subsunt
Oculi, inferiùs & superiùs Palpebris intecti: quarum sedes ubi inuicem conniuent, & erectis ordi-
nataque in naribus remos spectamus, serie po-
sitis pilis, quos Cilia nuncupamus, ornatur, quo-
dammodoque cartilagineae sunt, Tarsi haben-
tur. Commissuras huius termini, Anguli sunt:
maior nasum, minor tempus spectat. In
quorum maiori angulo praeter Ca-
runculam palpebrarum medio praeter Album
candidumue oculorum apparet: in cuius medio
duo se offerunt circuli, quorum amplior Iris &
Corona est, minor Pupilla. Nasus oculos inter-
iacet, cuius foramina Nares uocantur: quarum
externa lateranasi Pinnulis seu Alis, interna uerô

Intersepto nasi constituuntur. Sedes ad nasi latera mali in modum pro-
minulæ

minulæ ac rubentes, Malæ, & quibusdam Genæ uocantur. Inter nasum ac malas mediæ nonnullis Concaua dicuntur, qui-
ne alij totam oculorum sedem à palpebris ad malas meitan-
runt. Faciei pars quam inflamus Bucca est, tota uerô ipsius pa-
perciliis ad elatiorem usque dentium seriem pertinens, Super-
xilla nominatur, reliqua autem quae in uiris Barba decoratur,
rior. cuius anterius extremum, Mentum nonnunquam foue-
tum educit, sub Labri inferioris rubore consistens. Elatiori-
sedes naso subdita, Sulculosque donata, Mustax censetur. Qua-
bris circunscribitur & continetur, Os, quo hiante Lingua, P-
Gargareon, Dentes, Gingiuæ, internaque Faucium sedes oce-
Quod caput ad clauiculas usque aut thoracem excipit, Collum &
uix est, & si posterius nomen magis posteriori parti accommo-
uti & anteriorem qua aspera arteria, & potissimùm Guttur
gentibus occurrit, Guttur dictam legimus. Humerus ueteribus
cabatur brachij ossis cum scapula articulus, unde & partem hu-
ad colli radicem thoracisque latera eminentem, Summum hum
dixerunt. Quod ab illo prorsum uersus Iugulum foucam ue ir
radice obuiam uergit, Clauicula est. Quod autem ab ipso ad ex
digitorum aciem protenditur, Manus: cuius prima pars ab
uitas Axilla aut Ala appellata, & musculis quos Tendines perr
illic uocant septa, consistit; ad proximum usque articulum Cub
flexum producta, Brachium, & Latinorum quibusdam Hum
dicitur. Posterior flexus illius sedes Gibberus est. Pars ab hoc ad
terminum articulum ducta, Cubitus, & Latinorum quibusdam
chium & Vlna. Ad cubiti extremum Summa manus incipit,
pars à cubito ad quatuor digitorum radices porrecta, in duas sedes
titur: ac cubito propinquior Brachiale est, alia Postbrachiale,
constructionis specie cum pectore etiam Pectus, à quibusdam Pa
nuncupatur. Huius interior sedes caua ac uarijs monticulis septa,
tisque lineis interstincta, Volam efformat, Reliqua sum
manus pars, Digiti sunt, singuli ternis partibus su
quam in acie locatis efformati, & exteriùs Vnguil
ornati. Horum maior alijsque actione oppositus P
lex est, illi proximus Index, dein Medius seu Impu
cus, cui proximus est Medicus & Anularis. Extima
uerô sedem occupat Paruus, Auricularis ue. Tho
cem hic nominamus corporis trunci partem Cost
septam, maximamque sedem Laterum efformanten
cuius anterior sedes Pectus est, quam Laterum
in illarum medio Papillæ cum obfusco ipsas ambien
circulo occupant. Abdomen constituit, cuius regio pectoris ossi carti-
lagini & costarū cartilaginibus illa humilioribus prox-
perinde Subcartilagina nuncupatur, ac uiscera
sum praecordia appellatur, sedes in quam id cartilaginibus illis complexa. Sic quibus septũ transuer
nomen obtinuit. quanquam rursus alij ita etiam thoracis anteriorem sedem nuncu
pent. Quod sub infimis costis & ilium ossis spina (que mulieribus multo magis quàm
uiris educitur) ossibus destituitur, tangentibusque cedit, Inania sunt & Ilia. in quor
ueluti medio Vmbilicus cernitur, sub quo mox Sumen, cuius infima sedes trunci
termino proxima, Aqualiculus nuncupatur. Pubes est & Pecten, ad cuius latera infima sedes trunci
Naturalia consistunt, Pubes est & Pecten, ad cuius latera infima sedes trunci
recensemus. Maris pudendi pars citra sectionem conspicua, Penis & Coles uocatur: cuius summitas magis quàm reliqua longitudo crasseces, Glandem esformat,
in cuius medio meatus urinae seminique communis conspicitur. Huius inuolucrum
Præputium est, licet alijs tota penis summitas ita nuncupetur. In inuolucro reliquaque
ad anum cute protuberante suturae modo lineam uocamus Suturam, & totam hã
exporrectam exuberantemque ad anum usque penis partem Taurum. Vti & sedem
inter testium inuolucrum (quod ex cute paratum Scortum dicitur) & anum conspi-
cuam, Interseminium nuncupamus. Muliebris pudendi rima, quæ uteri conspi-
est orificium. Sinus uocatur, quem Alæ & Colles utrinque prominentes, & cuti-
cularis in ipsius summo cervicis caro ornant. Recti intestini orificium per sedem
prodiens, à figura Anulus, & ab officio Strictor appellatur. Posterior trunci corporis pars, Dorsum aut Tergu ferè nuncupatur. Inter ipsas uerô mediũ & dorsi sedes hinc ad inf
thoracis sede Scapulis uocatur. Inter ipsas uerô mediũ & dorsi sedes hinc ad inf
mas usque costas, aut ubi id maximè in flexu protuberat, pertinens, thoraci dorsi
post septum transuersim consistit. Sedes uerô hanc ad latera ascribibit, ac
coplectitur. Sunt autê Nates carneæ & globosæ sedes, illū ossiũ occupates dorsum,
in quarum medio sacri ossis & coccygis posteriores processus ueluti excarnes dorsum
usque occurrunt. Vbi articulus femoris percipitur, magnusque Rotator exuberat, Co
xendix est, aut Coxa, quod nonnulli Femoriascribunt, ab inguinibus ad Genu
pertinenti: cuius posterior sedes & flexus Poples nuncupatur. Genu ad proximum
usque articulum pedis ue initiũ Tibia subsequitur, quæ nonnullis Crus nominatur, & si
plures id nomen simul tibiæ femorisque uelint esse commune. Anterior tibiæ sedes ossea
tangentibus occurrit, posterior autê ubi ipsius Venter seu Sura cernitur, & si
bera ad tibiæ imũ utrinque ueluti ossea tangentibus obuia, Malleoli, neutiquam uerô Ta
retrorsum prominens, Calx appellatur. Reliqua uerô pedis superficiariæ sedes pro
sus ossium nomenclatura assumunt, potissimùm autê Tarsi, Pedij seu Pectoris, quod
retrorsum prominens, Calx appellatur. Reliqua uerô pedis superficiariæ sedes pro
sus ossium nomenclatura assumunt, potissimùm autê Tarsi, Pedij seu Pectoris, quod
plerumque Planta, & Vestigium,

digiti hic nõ ex unguibus ornati sequuntur. Quanquã ubi de integro pede sermo instituitur, infima sedes qua calcamus
ipsiusque intersti nuus Concaui, superior uerô Tarsus nuncupatur.

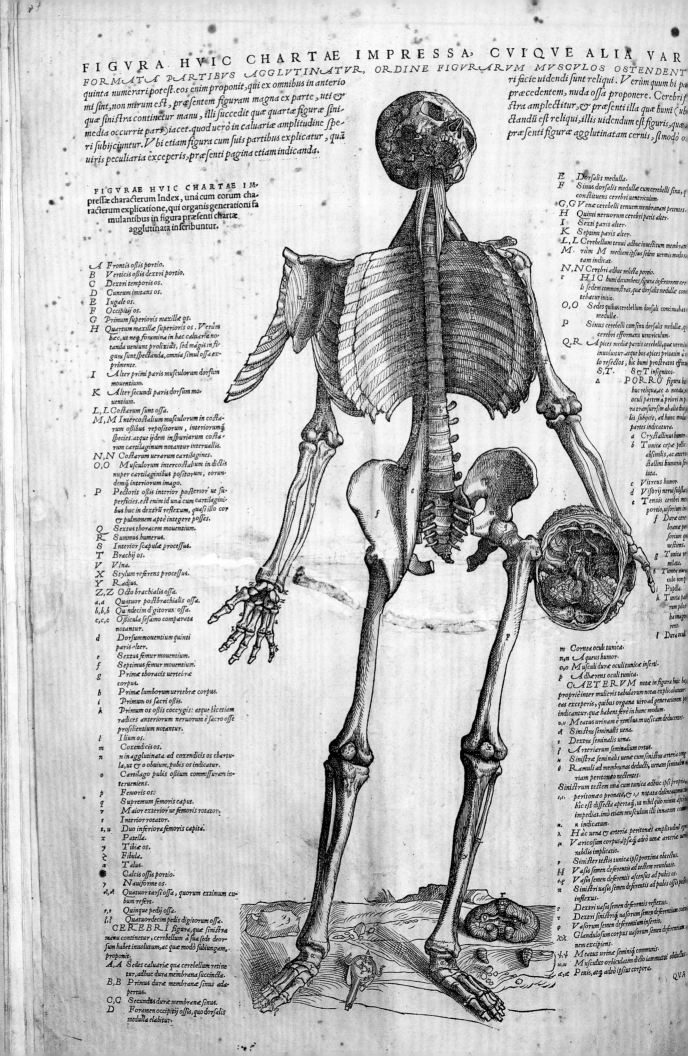

quinta numerari potest. eos enim proponit, qui ex omnibus in anterio
mi sint, non mirum est, præsentem figuram magna ex parte, uti &
quæ sinistra continetur manu, illi succedit quæ quartæ figuræ sini-
media occurrit pars) iacet. quod uerò in caluariæ amplitudine spe-
ri subijciuntur. Vbi etiam figura cum suis partibus explicatur, quã
uiris peculiaria exceperis, præsenti pagina etiam indicanda.

ri facie uidendi sunt reliqui. Verùm quum hi pa
præcedentem, nuda ossa proponere. Cerebri
stra amplectitur, & præsenti illa quæ humi ub
ctandũ est reliqui, illis uidendum est figuris, quæ
præsenti figuræ agglutinatam cernis, si modò o

FIGVRAE HVIC CHARTAE IM-
pressæ characterum Index, una cum eorum characterum explicatione, qui organis generationi fa
mulantibus in figura præsenti chartæ
agglutinata inscribuntur.

A   Frontis ossis portio.
B   Verticis ossis dextri portio.
C   Dextri temporis os.
D   Cuneum imitans os.
E   Iugale os.
F   Occipitij os.
G   Primum superioris maxillæ os.
H   Quartum maxillæ superioris os. Verùm
    hæc, ut neq; foramina in hac caluaria no-
    tanda ueniunt prolixius, sed magis in fi-
    gura sunt spectanda, omnia simul ossa ex-
    primente.
I   Alter primi paris musculorum dorsum
    mouentium.
K   Alter secundi paris dorsum mo-
    uentium.
L, L Costarum sunt ossa.
M, M Intercostalium musculorum in costa-
    rum ossibus repositorum, interiorumq;
    species: atque iidem in spuriarum costa-
    rum cartilaginum notantur interuallis.
N, N Costarum uerarum cartilagines.
O, O Musculorum intercostalium in dictis
    nuper cartilaginibus positorum, corun-
    demq; interiorum imago.
P   Pectoris ossis interior posterior ue su-
    perficies. est enim id una cum cartilagini-
    bus huc in dextrũ reflexum, quasi illo cor
    & pulmonem aptè integere posset.
Q   Sextus thoracem mouentium.
R   Summus humerus.
S   Interior scapulæ processus.
T   Brachij os.
V   Vlna.
X   Stylum referens processus.
Y   Radius.
Z, Z Octo brachialis ossa.
a, a Quatuor postbrachialis ossa.
b, b, b Quindecim digitorum ossa.
c, c, c Ossicula sesamo comparata
    notantur.
d   Dorsummouentium quinti
    paris alter.
e   Sextus femur mouentium.
f   Septimus femur mouentium.
g   Primæ thoracis uertebræ
    corpus.
h   Primæ lumborum uertebræ corpus.
i   Primum os sacri ossis.
k   Primum os ossis coccygis: atque hic etiam
    radices anteriorum neruorum è sacro osse
    prosilientium notantur.
l   Ilium os.
m   Coxendicis os.
n   n in agglutinata ad coxendicis os chartu-
    la, ut & o obuium, pubis os indicatur.
o   Cartilago pubis ossium commissuram in-
    terueniens.
p   Femoris os.
q   Supremum femoris caput.
r   Maior exterior ue femoris rotator.
s   Interior rotator.
t, u Duo inferiora femoris capita.
x   Patellæ.
y   Tibiæ os.
z   Fibula.
a   Talus.
β   Calcis ossis portio.
γ   Nauiforme os.
δ, ∆ Quatuor tarsi ossa, quorum extimum cu-
    bum refert.
ε, ε Quinque pedij ossa.
ζ, ζ Quatuordecim pedis digitorum ossa.

CEREBRI figuræ, quæ sinistra
manu continetur, cerebellum à sua sede deor-
sum habet inuolutum, ac quæ modò subiungam,
proponit.
A, A Sedes caluariæ qua cerebellum retine
    tur, adhuc dura membrana succincta.
B, B Primus duræ membranæ sinus ada-
    pertus.
C, C Secundus duræ membranæ sinus.
D   Foramen occipitij ossis, quo dorsalis
    medulla elabitur.

E   Dorsalis medulla.
F   Sinus dorsalis medullæ cum cerebelli sinu, q
    constituens cerebri uentriculum.
G, G Venæ cerebelli tenuem membranam petentes.
H   Quinti neruorum cerebri paris alter.
I   Sexti paris alter.
K   Septimi paris alter.
L, L Cerebellum tenui adhuc inuestitum membran
M   rũm M medium ipsius sedem uermis modo nu
    tam indicat.
N, N Cerebri adhuc relicta portio.
Γ   HIC humi decumbens figura inferiorem cer
    li sedem commonstret, quæ dorsalis medullæ com
    tebatur initio.
O, O Sedes quibus cerebellum dorsali continuabat
    medullæ.
P   Sinus cerebelli cum sinu dorsalis medullæ, q
    cerebri efforman's uentriculum.
Q, R Apices mediæ partis cerebelli, quæ uermis
    inuoluant: atque hos apices priuatim a
    lo resectos, hic humi prostratos effinxi
S, T   S & T insignitos.
∆   PORRO figura hu
    huc reliqua, & a notata,
    oculi partem a priori in,
    ra transuersim ab alia diuj,
    lis subijci, ad hunc modu
    partes indicatura.
a   Crystallinus humor.
b   Tunica cepæ pellic
    assimilis, ac anten
    stallini humoris se
    luta.
c   Vitreus humor.
d   Visorij nerui sub'sta
e   Tenuis cerebri mem
    portio, uisorium in
f   Duræ cere
    lineæ po
    sorium qu
    uestiens.
g   Tunica
    milata.
δ   Tunicæ sr
    culo comp
i   Pupilla.
k   Tunicæ pa
    rum pilos
    hæi magou
    rens.
l   Dura facu

m   Cornea oculi tunica.
n, n Aqueus humor.
o, o Musculi duræ oculi tunicæ inserti.
p   Adhærens oculi tunica.
CAETERVM notæ in figura huic b
proprie inter mulieris tabularum notas explicabuntu
teas exceperis, quibus organa uiro ad generationem p
indicantur, quæ habent ferè in hunc modum.
u, u Meatus urinam è renibus in uesicam deducentes.
α   Sinistræ seminalis uena.
ς   Dextra seminalis uena.
ζ   Arteriarum seminalium ortus.
η   Sinistræ seminalis uenæ cum sinistra arteria cong
θ   Ramuli ad membranas deducti, urnam seminalem
    riam peritonæo nectentes.
Sinistrum testem unà cum tunica adhuc ipsi propria
ι, ι peritonæo pronatæ, & ι, ι notata delineauimus
    hic est dissecta aperta, ut nihil quo minus obtu
    impediat. imò etiam musculum illi innatum co
κ   κ indicatum.
λ   Hæc uena & arteria peritonei amplitudini sp
μ   Varicosum corpus, ipsaq; adeò uenæ arteriæ co
    rabilis implicatio.
ν   Sinister testis tunica ipsi proxima obtectus.
ξ, ξ Vasis semen deferentis ad testem reuolutio.
ο, ο Vasis semen deferentis ascensus ad pubis os.
π   Sinistri uasis semen deferentis ad pubis ossis post
    inflexus.
ρ   Dextri uasis semen deferentis reflexus.
σ   Dextri sinistriq; uasorum semen deferentium inserto.
τ   Vasorum semen deferentium inserto.
υ   Glandulosum corpus uasorum semen deferentium
    nem excipiens.
φ, φ Meatus urinæ seminisq; communis.
ω, ω Musculus orbiculatim dicto iam meatui circum.
ꝗ, ꝗ Penis, atq; adeò ipsius corpora.

Q.V.A

ORPORIS SEDE SVB ILLIS, QVI SECVNDAE FIGVRAE SINISTRO LATERE EXPRIMVNTVR

itis proponit musculos, dextro quidē latere eos qui primū occur
caput humi collocata pariter iuuant. Tres uero in hac figura
tur, ac harum prima in integri hominis consistens capite, sinistro
at manibꝰhic cōtinetur : illa quae sinistra complectitur, ultimū locum

runt, sinistro autē quiꝰub ipsis adhuc cōduntur,quibus ostendendis
conspicuae cerebri partium imagines inuicē sectionis ordine sub
lateri secundae figurae capitis succedit, primam autem excipit quae
sibi uendicante.

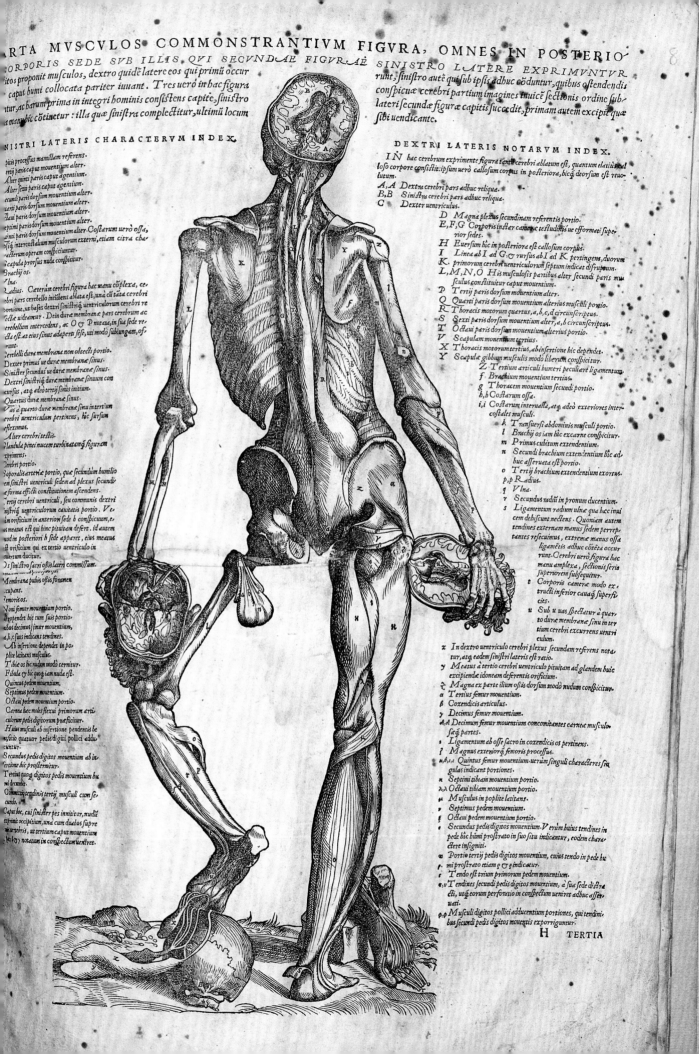

NISTRI LATERIS CHARACTERVM INDEX.

ꝑitis processus mamillam referens.
ertij ꝑaris caput mouentium alter
Alter quinti ꝑaris caput agentium
Aliter sexti ꝑaris caput agenium
eculi ꝑaris dorsum mouentium alter
uerti ꝑaris dorsum mouentium alter
seui ꝑaris dorsum mouentium alter
eptimi ꝑaris dorsum mouentium alter
inti ꝑaris dorsum mouentium alter. Costarum uero ossa,
isiꝗ, intercostalium musculorum externi, etiam citra cha
ecterum operam conspiciunt.
scapula prorsus nuda conspicitur.
Brachij os.
Vlna.
Radius. Caeterum cerebri figura hac manu cōplexa, ce
ebri pars cerebello incidens ablata est, una cū tota cerebri
ꝓrtione, ut bases dextri sinistriꝗ, uentriculorum cerebri re
ctae uideamur. Dein durae membranae pars cerebrum ac
erebellum intercedens, ac O & P notatae, in sua sede re
ctae est. at eius sinus adapertiꝰ sese, uti modo sublingam,ꝑ
runt.
erebelli durae membranae non obiecti portio.
Dexter primus ue durae membranae sinus.
Sinister secundus ue durae membranae sinus.
Dextri sinistriꝗ, durae membranae sinuum con
curfus, atꝗ, adeo tertij sinus initium.
Quartus durae membranae sinus.
Vas à quarto durae membranae sinu in tertium
erebri uentriculum pertinens, hic sursum
eflexum.
Alter cerebri testis.
Glandula pinei nucem turbinatamꝗ figuram
eximens.
Cerebri portio.
Soporaliꝰ arteriae portio, quae secundum humilio
en sinistri uentriculi sedem ad plexus secundi
eformae effici constitutionem ascendens.
tertij cerebri uentriculi, seu communis dextri
inistriꝗ, uentriculorum cauitatis portio. Ve
am oriscium in anteriori sede b conspicuum, e
us meatus est qui hinc pituitam defert . id autem
uod in posteriori b sede apparet, eius meatus
st quod ex tertio uentriculo in
auterium ducitur.
Os sinistro sacri ossis lateri commissum.
Membrana pubis ossis foramen
occupens.
emoris os.
Noni femur mouentium portio.
Dependet hic cum suis portio
ibus decimus, ꝗuer mouentium,
a, b, c suos indices tendines.
Ab insertione dependet in po
plite latitans musculus.
Tibiae os hic nudum modo cernitur.
Fibulae ꝗ hic quoꝗ iam nuda est.
Quintus pedem mouentium.
Septimus pedem mouentium.
Octaui pedem mouentium portio.
Carnea haec moles flexui primorum arti
culorum pedis digitorum praeficitur.
Huius musculi ab insertione pendentis be
issio quatuor pedis digiti pollici addu
cuntur.
Secundus pedis digitos mouentium ab in
sertione hic prosternitur.
Tertius quoꝗ digitos pedis mouentium hu
mi deiectus.
Coniuncti tendinis tertij musculi cum se
cundo.
Caput hoc, cui sinister pes innititur, nucli
etijni occipitium, una cum duabus supre
me uertebris, ut tertium caput mouentium
uerte (κ &) notatum in conspectum ueniret.

The Isagoge and Five Other Texts of the Articella (1210–30?)
Iohannitius (Hunayn ibn Ishaq al-Ibadi) and others

Paris. Bound vellum manuscript; 114 leaves; 6 x 8⅜ in. (15.3 x 21.3 cm)

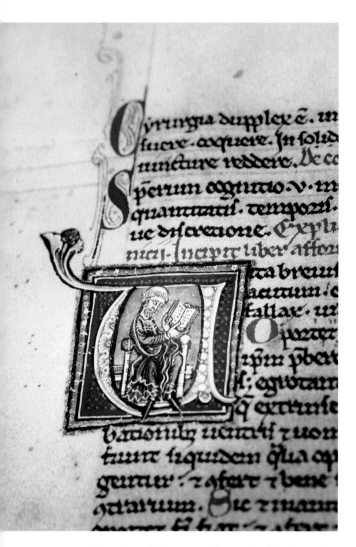

ABOVE: Master in cathedra expounding on the *Aphorisms* of Hippocrates. Initial *V* (rendered as a *U*) of "Vita brevis, ars vero longa," "Life is short, but the Art is long." *Isagoge*, fol. 15b

OPPOSITE: Left-hand folio: Master on bench pointing at a raised flask while lecturing on the *Book on Urines* of Theophilus. Initial *D* of "De urinarum differencia negocium" (The matter of the differences of urines). *Isagoge*, fol. 42b. Right-hand folio: Bearded master holding up a flask while explaining the diagnostic significance of urine to a student (or patient). Initial *U* of "Urina ergo est colamentum sanguinis" (Urine is the filtrate of the blood). *Isagoge*, fol. 43a

In the deluge of digital data and ephemera, and amid changes that challenge the "book" as a concept, this unique volume may appear as a quaint relic from thirteenth-century Paris. It is much more: a testament to the vital role of the written page; a product of the confluence of Greco-Latin and Judeo-Arabic legacies; and a witness to the emergence of the medical university and profession. The manuscript was created in a secular workshop rather than in a monastic scriptorium, but with an intense devotion that is evident in the fine vellum, steady hand, and exquisitely illuminated initials. Books are featured prominently in most of the illuminations, with a reverence normally reserved for the Bible. Reverence did not preclude use, however: the margins contain numerous though discreet annotations.

We do not know the original owner, but the volume was more likely intended for the classroom lectern than for the collection of an aristocrat or prosperous practitioner. The only subject outshining books in the illuminations is the *magister* (teacher), who is often depicted in the *cathedra*, or seat of authority—and who was on his way to appropriating the title of *doctor* originally held by the teacher of theology. The physicians and his students, like the teacher, belonged to the literate class, or clergy, marked by the tonsure, or shaven crown. As members of the faculty of medicine, on the other hand, they were dedicated to health rather than salvation, and to their Art rather than to the Church.

"The Healing Art," or (*technē iatrikē*), as celebrated in the Hippocratic tradition, followed the age-old conviction that writing gave medicine the foundation and constancy that were lacking in the cultivation of individual talent and transmission by apprenticeship. Recording allowed knowledge to accumulate and be passed on with relative uniformity in lectures and elucidating commentaries, although these were far less homogeneous than is commonly assumed.

This volume contains the "Little Art," or *Articella*, the writings that formed the core of the medical curriculum. The *Isagoge*, or introduction, to the basic definitions and parts of medicine is followed by the seminal *Aphorisms* and *Prognostics* of Hippocrates and two influential, though less historic, treatises on diagnosis by urines and pulses. The capstone of the collection is the *Tegni*, as Galen's key work on the Art was known.

These texts, and the methods of teaching them, aimed chiefly at replacing vague and deceptive impressions with precise and orderly reasoning. The preoccupation with distinctions and divisions led one master to schematize the treatises in elaborate diagrams that occupy almost one-eighth of the manuscript. Learned practitioners stood out by their ability to define and understand diseases, to recognize the symptoms, and to foresee the outcome, even when the cure was elusive. The illuminations do not show the physician as treating the sick but as identifying dropsy, explaining the diagnostic significance of urine, and pronouncing the prognosis of a bedridden patient's illness.

—LUKE DEMAITRE

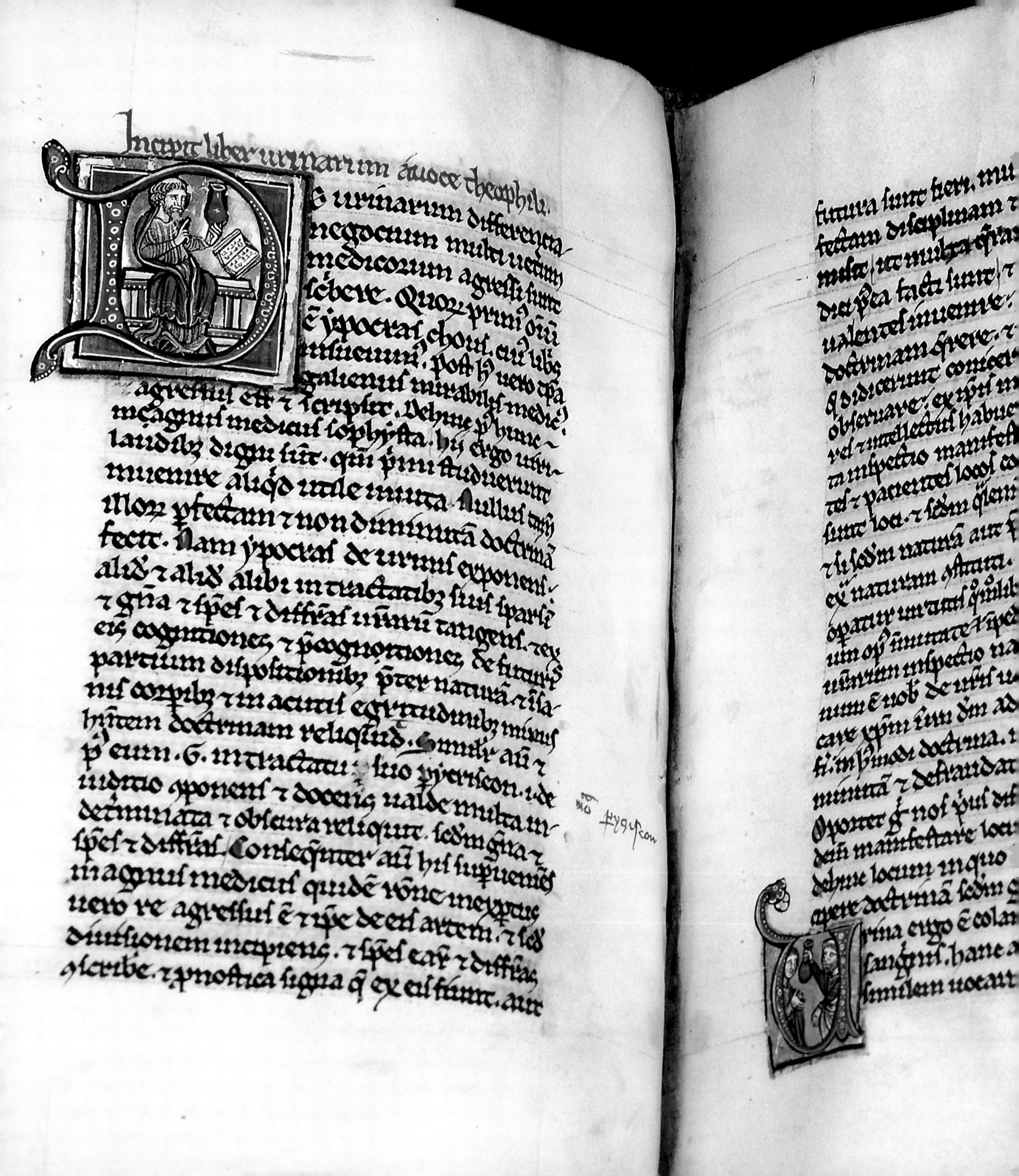

Incipit liber urinarum ẽ uoce theophili.

De urinarum differencia
negocium multi uetusti
medicorum agressi sunt
scribere. Quorum primi diu
ẽ ypocras, chorus, eius ube
ruerunt. Post hec uero tha
galienus mirabiles medici
agressus ẽ et scripsere. deinde phitrec~
magnus medicus sophista. hiis ergo uniu
laudibz digni sunt. qui primi audierunt
inuenire aliquid utile inuenta. Nullus ah
illorum perfectam et non diminutam doctrinam
fecit. Nam ypocras de urinis exponens
aliud et aliud alibi in tractatibz suis sparsim
et gra et spes et differencias uirium tangens. et ex
eius cognitiones, et pognitiones, de urinis
partium dispositionibz, propter naturam et sla
nis corpilz et in acutis egritudinibz minus
historiam doctrinam reliquid. Similiter aut et
p eum. G. in tractatu suo p risicon. ide
iudicio exponens et docens ualde multa in
determinata et obscura reliquit. secundum gena
spes et differencias. Consequenter aut hiis superuenies
magnus medicus quidem rone inexpertu
uero re agressus ẽ et ipse de eis artem. et sec
diuisionem incipiens. et ipes eas et differencias
pscribe. et pnostica signa que ex eis sunt. aut

[columna secunda]
futura sunt fieri. mul
testam disciplinam n
dicta facta sunt. et
ualentes inuenire.
doctrinam spere. et
q didicerunt conuen
obseruare. ex ipsis in
uel et intellectuis habui
ta inspectio manifest
tes et patientes locos
sunt loca. et secundum gena
ri secundum naturam aut
ex naturam statuta.
operatur in uirtutibz similib
uim oportet in unitate et speci
uirium inspectio na
nuim est nob de urinis u
care ipsum secundum diem
ti. in speciei doctrina.
minutam et destruenda
Oportet ergo nos prius di
dam manifestare loci
deinde locum in quo
apere doctrinam secundum
rina ergo ẽ colat
et sanguinis. hanc a
similem uocant

Coctura pōt— {qñdo fluxū / pinguedine tbulādo / euaporare faciendo / debilia gfortando} gña poſt ypo— {malum dñ... / peſſim... / hōīle corti...}

Suſpirium— {ex exnictione caloris / ex incendio cordis / ex ſollicitudine}

Syncopis cauentia ſpē— {pacciua aīe / p paſſione cors / ãt opilatione poroſi ſpitualium / ãt opilatione uene gtaue / ãt eucunōie ſang. inflōnia / ãt defectum ſpirituū / ãt egōnes nimias / ãt depdaōne ſubitā h̄ videtur v tipitaſ / ip dolore aliqꝯ utib ſpū ñue ruptꝯ}

Eff. paciens— {non reple. h̄. bal. pōt gſerre / reple. h̄. peccā— {qſi. bal. nocer / ſ?n. pōt gſerre}}

Incipiunt diſtinctiones ſuper libru pronoſticor ypocras

Morbor iīi. a— {alienatur r non curatur / alienatur r curatur / nec alienat nec curat}

Mors a— {naturalis— anticipat ſ̄ tñ ſubocciꝑari / caſualis— ab maꝑfectū uſū vel ñ ſhil... / fatalis— a rcbꝯ ñ uicecciſt. v nīueaus / ex na dei. non ualet medicꝯ}

Sunt bona ſigna— {
i. fortitudo cꝯ maꝗ ſit... vot. pꝯ — debilitas
ij. facilitas motionis eoꝝ̄ rpiū — granitaſ
iij. effugies cꝯ ſibi ſano ſilio — eſt difficiliſ
iiij. ſanū iſ̃. ꝗ̃ bo. appe. ad obt — agentū uſiam
v. ſomū cꝯ ſtī unione tārdie — ſōpni meꝯ
vi. facilitas inſpirōdi reſpir — diffi. iñpr. reſpir
vij. equalitas pulſuū — ineſt pul...
viij. fortitudo eat ega loc dꝯoꝯ — debilitas eat rō
ix. quenteſ exꝑt. iñ ꝓpe. re — ingue. exꝑt.
}

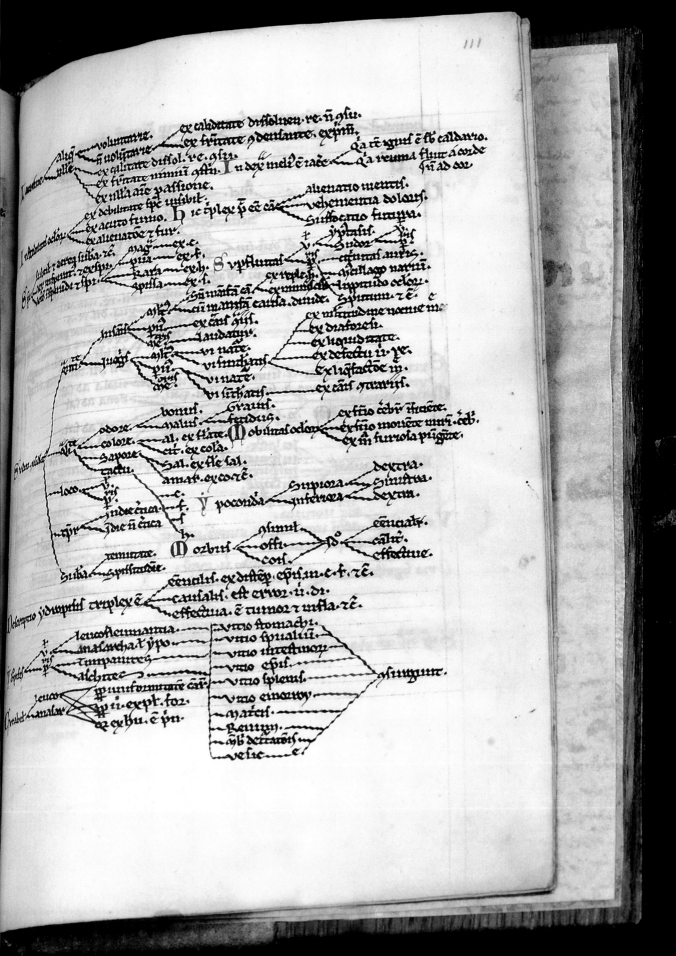

The Artificial Teledioptric Eye, or Telescope (1685–86)
Johann Zahn

Oculus artificialis teledioptricus sive Telescopium. Würzburg, Germany.
Printed book, 3 vols. in 1; 770 pp.; 8 x 12½ in. (20.5 x 31.5 cm)

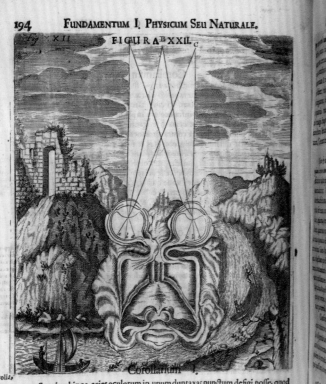

ABOVE: The eyes and optical nerves, removed from the body, stand in splendid isolation in a stylized baroque landscape to emphasize their singular importance. *Oculus artificialis teledioptricus*, vol. 1, p. 194

OPPOSITE: Natural philosophers contemplate the divine light of the cosmos. *Oculus artificialis teledioptricus*, vol. 3, between pp. 190 and 191

Installments of this lavishly illustrated encyclopedia of the anatomy, physiology, physics, mathematics, and instruments of sight—770 dense folio pages—began appearing in the city of Würzburg in northern Bavaria in 1685. Influential in its own time, the *Artificial Teledioptric Eye* ("Derived through a New and Lasting Method from Hidden Principles of Natural and Artificial Things, and Explained and Summarized from a Physical Foundation of a Threefold Nature, whether Mathematical-Optical, Mechanical, or Established through Practice") continues to fascinate historians interested in the invention of the "magic lantern" and the uses of the camera obscura, in the era before the invention of photography and cinematography.

Its author, Johann Zahn (1631–1707), was a German canon in the austere Premonstratensian monastic order. He was also a disciple of the Jesuit Caspar Schott (1608–66) and, via Schott, the Jesuit polymath Athanasius Kircher (1602–80). When Schott returned to Würzburg in 1655 to teach mathematics and physics, he earned his reputation assisting Kircher, whose dazzling array of writings on virtually every aspect of human knowledge included the *Ars magna lucis et umbrae* (*Great Art of Light and Shadow*), published in 1646 but revised in 1671 to include an image of a magic lantern. This treatise, along with Schott's works on curious technologies, inspired Zahn to produce his *Artificial Eye*.

Zahn crafted his publication to compete with the most lavish baroque encyclopedias of science, advertising it as a "curious theoretico-practical work embellished with a great variety of things" and including every new and useful art that a philosopher or practitioner of mathematics would want to know. Well-informed readers would have surmised his indebtedness to Kircher and Schott when reading his announcement that his book contained "many new, secret, and curious technasms"—a phrase that captures the phantasmagoric quality of their vision of technology—and his promise to bring the mysteries of the telescope "from shadow into light."

In his preface Zahn celebrates the German tradition of optics and mechanical invention. He had a broad understanding of the history of instrument making in the previous century and was well informed about the most recent developments in astronomy, including the debates over the rings of Saturn, Isaac Newton's invention of the reflecting telescope, and Danzig astronomer Johannes Hevelius's workshop for grinding lenses for the telescopes perfected in his famous rooftop observatory. It is a state-of-the-art discussion of instruments of vision and their utility in the progress of scientific knowledge and, at the same time, a great example of baroque Hermeticism: Zahn coupled his technical account of vision and the enhancement of the senses with a joyous celebration of the metaphysical qualities of light as the origin of the cosmos and a reminder of God's continued presence in the world.

Arguing that one cannot understand the "artificial eye" without an explanation of the "natural eye," Zahn begins with a discussion of the anatomy and physiology of the eye. He draws on the work of theorists such as Johannes Kepler, anatomists such as Thomas Willis, and Kircher, who provided an explanation of light and color. Zahn then builds a "material eye"—an experimental model—as a prelude to his critical assessment of the different kinds of

VAS ADMIRABILE.   OPUS EXCELSI.

MAGNUS DOMINUS   QUI FECIT ILLUM.

SIC TE NON
VIDIMUS OLIM

P.G. Axis Globi Solaris.
D.E. Æquator Solaris.
B.F.C. Spacium Solaris.
H.G.I. spacium Solis Boreale.
B.C.H.I. spacium Solis Australe.
A.A.A. putei lucis.
L.M.N.O.P.Q. et cæt.
Evaporationis una et
Macularum Solarum
Origo.

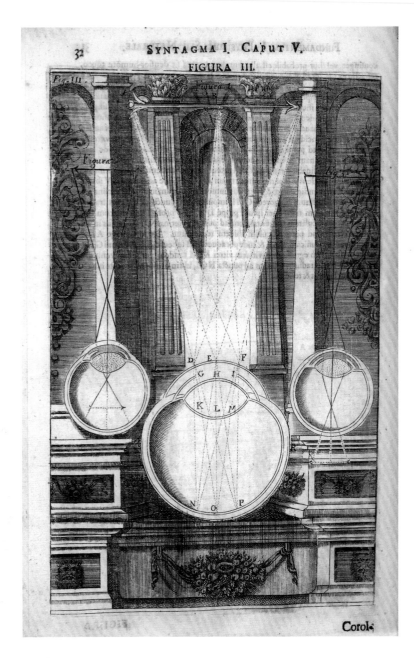

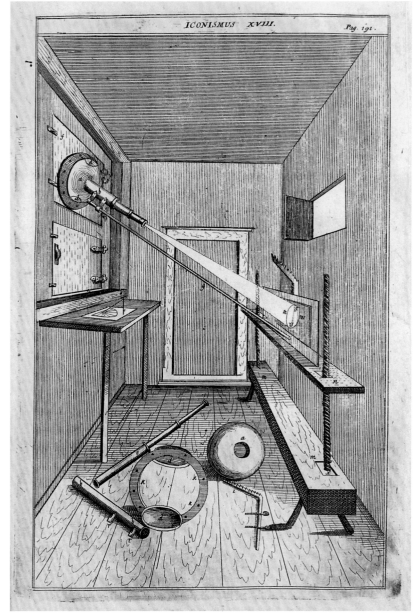

ABOVE AND OPPOSITE: Zahn's baroque diagram of the anatomy of vision (upper left) needs to be viewed in relation to his creation of a mechanical eye (upper right), the scioptric ball designed to project the image of the sun in a camera obscura. Zahn also provided different prototypes of the magic lantern (opposite) to delight readers with its curious possibilities, in this instance the projection of time on a wall. *Oculus artificialis teledioptricus*, vol. 1, p. 32; vol. 3, between pp. 190–91; vol. 3, between pp. 256–57

telescopes then available, and preliminary to his discussion of distorting (catoptrical) devices, binoculars, burning mirrors, and the camera obscura (which was used to view sunspots). He describes lens-grinding machines, the "English microscope" pioneered by Robert Hooke, and Newton's telescope. The book concludes with an account of the first device capable of projecting an image with artificial light—the magic lantern—whose basic principles Zahn credited to Kircher while offering concrete examples of how to build and use a projector. A virtuoso of the lens, Zahn experimented with combinations of lenses, built machines to focus and project images with light, and fostered the spread of the magic lantern.

We remember Zahn today as the man who almost invented the camera, but he did far more than that. Consider his telescope mounted in a scioptric ball with a steering rod to track the sun's movements and project its image into a darkened room. Zahn helps us to understand why the age of Kepler, Descartes, and Newton was also the era of the artificial eye. He allows us to envision this new age of instruments as an era of wonder, curiosities, and paradoxes animated in the shadows of his science.

—PAULA FINDLEN

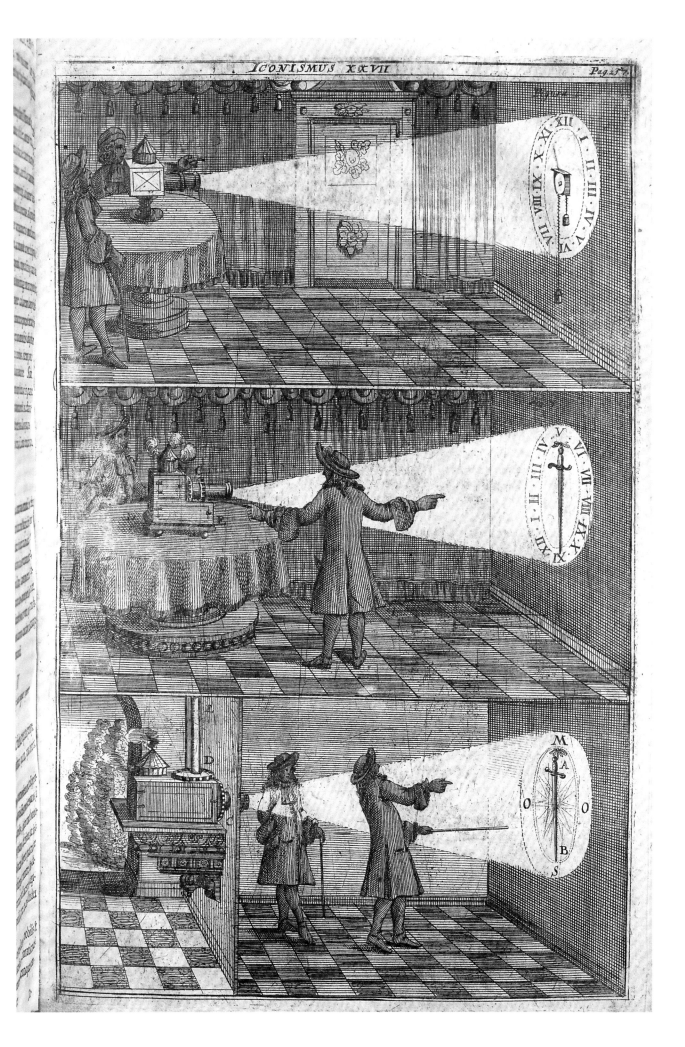

The Langenburg Manuscript (ca. 1580)
Walter von Nitzschwitz and others

Rossarzneibuch, Langenburger Handschrift. Southeastern Germany.
Bound manuscript on paper; 2 vols.; 358 folios + loose quire; 6⅛ x 7⅝ in. (15.5 x 19.5 cm)

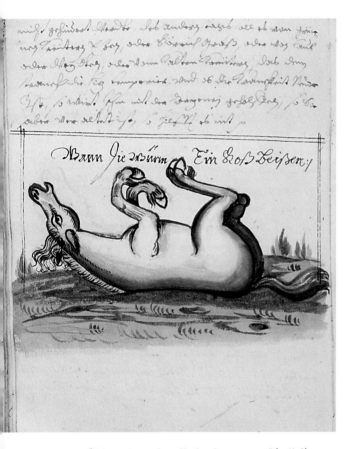

ABOVE: "When a horse is suffering from worms" (colic?).
Rossarzneibuch, vol. 1, p. 40b

OPPOSITE: "When a horse's body is pierced by arrows, blades, or thorns" (puncture wounds, lacerations). *Rossarzneibuch*, vol. 1, p. 56a

Just as there are many different kinds of people, so there are many different kinds of horses, each appropriate to an individual person's social standing and his way of life. God has ordained it to be thus." So wrote the Augsburg financier, humanist, and horseman Marx Fugger (d. 1597) in his 1584 treatise on horse breeding. Fugger's book is almost exactly contemporaneous with Walter von Nitzschwitz's treatise on the cure and treatment of equine ailments written in 1580 and revised in 1583. Several decades later Nitzschwitz's treatise, along with three other texts by different authors but dealing with similar subject matter, was copied and compiled into the two-volume Langenburg Manuscript now owned by the National Library of Medicine. The manuscript gets its name from the noble German family that originally owned the volumes in the seventeenth century.

As a compilation of texts focused on equines, the Langenburg Manuscript belongs to the pan-European culture of the horse that developed between 1400 and 1800. The horse, like the car in the twentieth and twenty-first centuries, proved essential to almost all members of society: for agricultural and commercial production, transport, warfare, entertainment, sport, and recreation. A person's very identity was bound up with the kind of horse he or she owned and the uses that the animal served. As Fugger's remark indicates, this linkage between horse and social status was not only recognized and appreciated but also regarded as part of the divine ordering of human society.

Because a horse was such a valuable asset, for labor or leisure, an owner would be concerned with keeping the animal in good health, no matter what illnesses or injuries might befall it. This was as true for humble farmers and tradesmen as it was for members of the nobility. Remedies and treatments for horses were passed down orally, written down in notebooks, diaries, and manuscripts, and eventually also printed in a variety of forms ranging from modest and easily affordable pamphlets to deluxe, densely illustrated tomes. The Langenburg Manuscript, written by and for members of the nobility, documents the concern of elites for the health and maintenance of their horses. By the select breeding of these animals, and by the artful manner of riding and performing on them, social and political preeminence was manifested and demonstrated. Fugger tells us that finely bred and well-trained horses fetched prices anywhere between 1,000 and 2,000 ducats. In comparison, Michelangelo was paid 3,000 ducats for painting the Sistine Chapel ceiling, a task that took him four years to complete.

The manuscript prescribes various methods of palliative and curative treatment. Some are unhelpfully vague. For example, for an animal experiencing "respiratory difficulties" it recommends that the reader "take some uncooked roots and give this to the horse mixed in with his feed." A favorite ingredient in many of the recipes is garlic.

Notable for its lively illustrations, the Langenburg Manuscript documents ways of knowing, visualizing, and interacting with animals that the Enlightenment and the Industrial Revolution would irrevocably change.

—PIA F. CUNEO

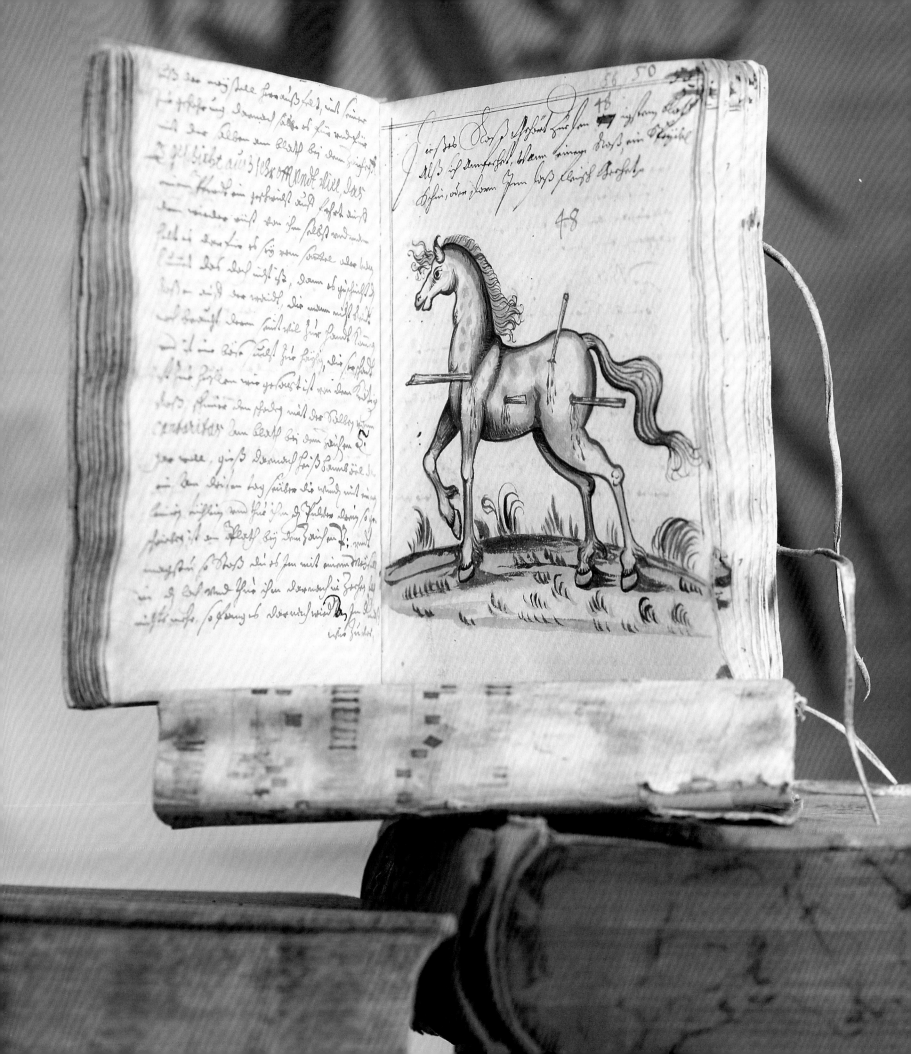

Wann ein Roß nicht dürsten mann.

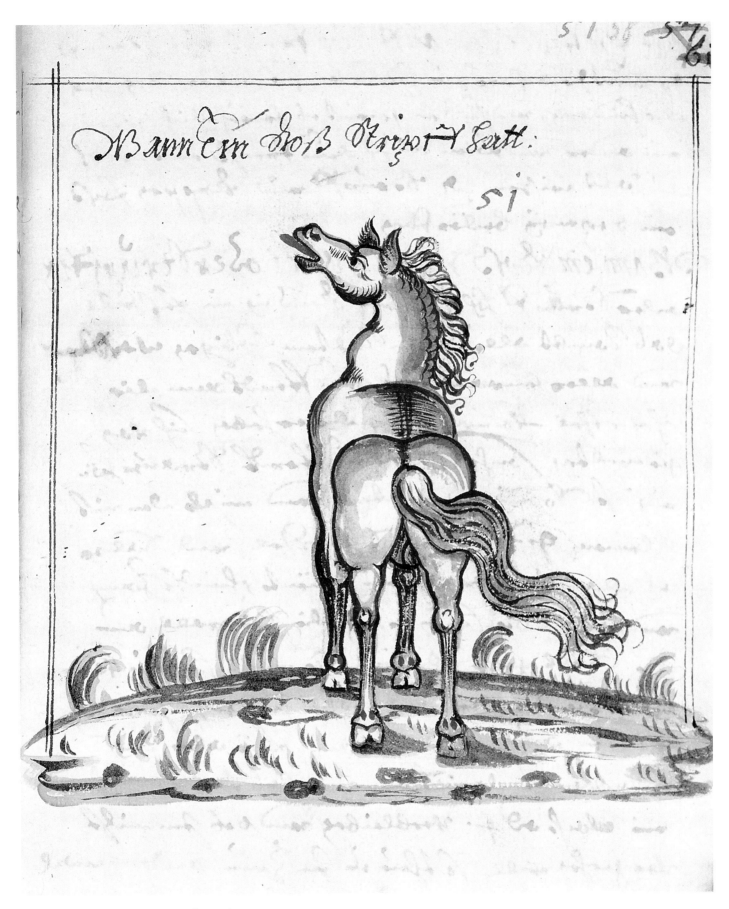

ABOVE: "When a horse has scratches" (fungal/bacterial dermatitis of the pasterns). *Rossarzneibuch*, vol. 1, p. 58a

OPPOSITE: "When a horse is unable to defecate" (constipation, intestinal blockage). *Rossarzneibuch*, vol. 1, p. 33a

Rare Plants of the Medical Garden of Amsterdam (1697–1701)

Jan Commelin and Caspar Commelin, with Frans Kiggelaer and Frederick Ruysch

Horti medici Amstelodamensis rariorum tam Orientalis, quam Occidentalis Indiae,
aliarumque peregrinarum plantarum magno studio ac labore, sumptibus civitatis Amstelodamensis…
Amsterdam. Printed book, 2 vols.; hand-colored copper-plate engravings; 9¾ x 15⅝ in. (25 x 40 cm)

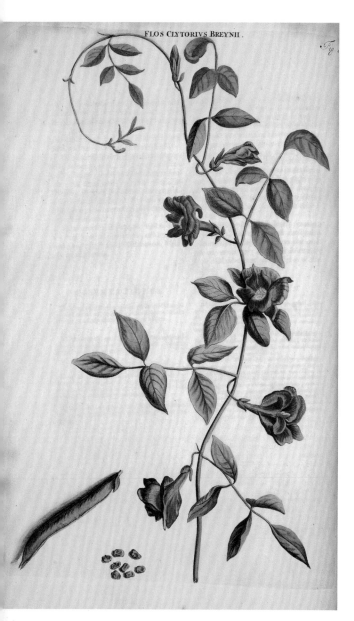

FLOS CLYTORIVS BREYNII.

ABOVE: "Flos Clytorius Breynii" (the clitoris-shaped flower described by Jacobus Breyn in his 1678 *Exoticarum Plantarum Centuria Prima*). *Horti medici Amstelodamensis*, vol. 1, facing p. 47

OPPOSITE: "Euphorbium Cerei," from the North African coast. The "euphorbium" of antiquity was reputed to be a powerful purgative; Commelin discusses whether this is that same plant. *Horti medici Amstelodamensis*, vol. 1, facing p. 21

*D*escription and Images… of the Rare Plants of the East and West Indies in the Medical Garden of Amsterdam, and of Other Exotic Plants Collected with Zeal and Effort in the Residences of Amsterdam, usually ascribed to Jan Commelin (1629–92) and Caspar Commelin (1667–1731), is one of several beautiful botanical atlases published in the Dutch Republic in the years prior to the work of taxonomist Carolus Linnaeus (1707–78). The atlas is based on the collections of the botanical garden in Amsterdam, a garden (or *hortus*) that had become one of the most important nodes in a network of collectors that stretched around the globe. Some collectors were academics (mostly professors who taught about the uses of plants in medicine), but most were enthusiasts, including some leading citizens of Amsterdam, who took a keen interest in growing unusual specimens in their own gardens and keeping up-to-date with descriptions of the latest findings.

Gardens like Amsterdam's were simultaneously sites for study; centers for the collection, acclimatization, and distribution of living plants; civic institutions for people seeking both pleasure and edification about God's creation; and displays of the ingenuity, power, luxury, and world-embracing connections of the city's patricians. Dutch printers, in turn, were adept in catering to the market of enthusiasts and academics through publications that ranged from simple lists to gorgeous atlases with lengthy descriptions and copper-plate engravings that could be hand-colored (for an extra fee). Possessing such an atlas allowed plant collectors elsewhere to experience vicariously the exotic riches cultivated in one of Europe's major entrepôts. The publication of a grand display piece required coordination among botanical experts, artists, engravers, and printers. Jan Commelin thus might be considered more the initiator of the enterprise than simply its "author"—indeed, he died in 1692, five years before publication of the first volume. Having become wealthy in the pharmaceutical trade, and having published a book in 1672 about his methods of raising citrus fruits in heated greenhouses at his private gardens near Haarlem, he was chosen to be a governor of the city's *hortus* in 1682 when it was reestablished outside the city walls. He and Joan Huydecoper (1625–1704) used their connections to acquire exotic plants from both the East and West Indies. They also commissioned excellent artists to make accurate watercolors of rare plants (the *Moninckx Atlas*).

Commelin himself wrote careful descriptions in Dutch of each exotic's appearance and time of blossoming, provenance, and names given in other publications. After his death, the governors of the garden, Huydecoper and Commelin's successor, Franciscus de Vroede (1641–1706), saw the first volume through the press. Working chiefly with the printing firm of Blaeu, they commissioned the celebrated physician Frederick Ruysch (1638–1731) and Frans Kiggelaer (1648–1722), a pharmacist from The Hague, to edit and annotate Commelin's descriptions and translate them into Latin, had the accompanying watercolors turned into engravings, and added a dedication and preface. Jan's nephew Caspar Commelin, a physician and his successor as garden botanist, brought out the second volume in 1701. The resultant masterwork delighted botanical enthusiasts of the day.

—HAROLD J. COOK

(21)

CAP. XI

EUPHORBIUM CEREI EFFIGIE, CAULIBUS CRASSIORIBUS, SPINIS VALIDIORIBUS ARMATUM. *Breyn. Prod. 2.*

Hanc liberalissime nobis dono transmisit Nobilissimus & Stren. D. Simon à Beaumond, Nobilissimorum Præpotentium D. Holl. & Westvisiæ Ordinum Secretarius, qui eam ex Africa, prope Zalé nactus est.

Ex ejus radice, in varios ramos subterra brachiata, super terram autem globosâ, crassâ, cortice griseo amictâ, caules prodeunt, Opuntiæ instar, aphylli, numerosi, in orbem dispositi, supati, multanguli, atrovirescentes, sentibus brevibus, acutis, terram spectantibus, ex angulis emergentibus, præditi; Horum rami exteriores ad exortum brachium crassi, sensim attenuantur, & spithamarum duarum longitudinem adæquantes, arcuantur.

Flores ex angulis quoque emergentes pentapetali, ex luteo virescentes, quibus succedunt vascula seminalia triquetra.

Utrum hæc eadem sit quæ à Dodonæo exhibetur, dubitandi ansam dederunt mihi spinæ, quæ in Euphorbio Dod. longiores, numerosiores, surrectioresque visuntur, in nostro verò, quod hic repræsentatur pauciores, minacioresque sunt spinæ, proniæque spectantes & breviores.

Hanc admodum teneram plantam multiplicavi ramis ad radicem abscissis, illicô terræ siccæ impactis, vaporatisque seculorum subterraneorum impositi; Caventes autem in amputatione ramorum ne succus lacteus nimis effluat, quò facili brevi vi perit; itaque illicô terræ conamrendi rami, sic sistitur ejus effluxus.

CEREUS GELYKENDE EUPHORBIUM, MET DIKKE STELEN, EN KLOEKE DOORNEN.

Deze Plant heeft den Ed. Heer Simon van Beaumond, Secretaris van de Ed. Groot Mog. Heeren Staaten van Holland en Westvriesland, alsmede bekomen van de Africaansche Kust, ontrent Zalé, en aan den Amsterdamsche Medecyn Hof, mildelyk vereert.

Uit deszelfs Wortel, dewelke onder de aarde in verscheyde dikke tuid-waerds schietende ter deeld, en (om zoo veel dessselfs boven de aarde uit-steekt,) rondom dik tuymangen van een groote scherfte, bruyn verde, daer tyven staende, stecku voort, dat van de Opuntia gelykende; dessse tuyten de ronte verspreid, veeltuylig, dukke groen van coleur, geruppee met korte scherpspekende, en voorwaerds springe doornen, dewelke uit de hoeken koten uit-spruit nemen; De boytuselfs dessse takken aan haar grond een arm-dik tuydt, komen allenkskens te verdunnen, en buygen om te kromnen, wylaa tuee spannen lang.

De Bloemen uit de hoeken werde nyten komende vyf vyfbladerig, groen geel van coleur, waer na volcheyd tuydig zaadbus kens komen te volgen.

De doornen dezer Geum daer my ryf feten, of die 'tseve met te, 't geen Dodonæus beschryft, aangesien desen tuyt ende meerder, en viger offtaendt tuyt 't geen in eigen afbeeldt wert, als dat in deffe, niet alleen Euphorbium Dod., als dat in deffe, mid Plante, welcken doornen minder in getal syn, scherpspekend, forter en minder in getal syn.

Deze seer teedere Plante heb ik verouigvuldigt door de takken, dewelke aan de grond afgesneden synde, aanstonts in drooge aarde te syn gezet, en in gesneeden in een broei-bak gezet werden; In 't afsnyden desser takken, moeten sorg dragen dat het melksagtig sap niet te seer uit en lekke, waer door desselve haaft me te lekke, waer door afsnyding haaft den uytgaen; welcken noveraaldig tuydt ken aanstonts in 't aardt-ryk weer geren, vervort de uytvlueyinge des saps verhindert.

L

The Anatomy of the Human Body (1386; copied mid-1400s)
Manṣūr ibn Muḥammad ibn Aḥmad ibn Yūsuf ibn Ilyās

Tashrīḥ-i badan-i insān. Iran? Bound manuscript with illustrations on paper; 24 leaves; 7 x 10¼ in. (18 x 26 cm)

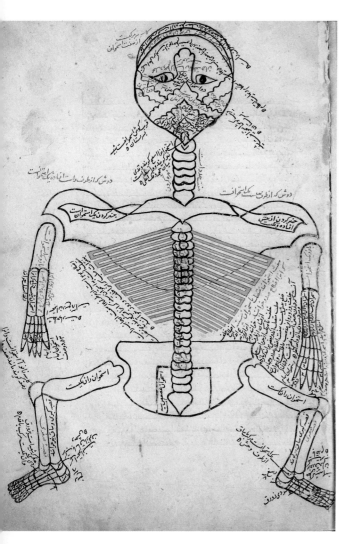

ABOVE AND OPPOSITE: A skeleton and the nerve figure, both viewed from the back, with the head hyperextended so that the mouth is at the top of the page—a posture suggestive of a dissection table. *Tashrīḥ-i badan-i insān*, fols. 17b and 14a

No anatomical illustrations of the entire human body are preserved from the Islamic world before the series of watercolor diagrams that usually accompany a Persian treatise composed in 1386 for the ruler of the Persian province of Fars and grandson of Tīmūr (the conqueror of Central Asia known to Europeans as Tamerlane). The author, Manṣūr ibn Muḥammad ibn Aḥmad ibn Yūsuf ibn Ilyās, was a physician from Shiraz. His treatise, *The Anatomy of the Human Body* (*Tashrīḥ-i badan-i insān*), was later referred to as *Manṣūr's Anatomy* (*Tashrīḥ-i Manṣūrī*).

The work consists of seven sections: an introduction; five chapters covering the skeletal, nervous, muscular, venous, and arterial systems; and an appendix on the fetus. Each chapter is illustrated with an annotated full-page diagram depicting the "system" under discussion. The skeleton is viewed from behind, with head hyperextended, so that the mouth is at the top of the page. On the head, jagged lines make a triangle and two bands, representing cranial sutures. The hands of the skeleton are drawn with the palms toward the viewer, again indicating that the figure is being viewed from the back. The nerve figure is also viewed from the back, head hyperextended, with the nerve pairs indicated by inks of contrasting color.

The placement of these figures, stomach down with the head drawn back, suggests a dissection table was used when the original was drawn. There is, however, no reference to dissection in the text. The only reference to an illustration comes in the chapter on the nervous system, where the different nerves discussed in the text are cross-referenced with those in a diagram, by the color in which they are drawn.

The muscle, venous, and arterial figures are shown frontally. Captions describe the muscles, while in the venous and arterial figures the internal organs are indicated in opaque watercolors with labels identifying the structures. The figures are all gender neutral and lack genitalia.

In the late nineteenth century similarities were noted between the five figures and twelfth-century European anatomical illustrations. The obvious element uniting the two sets is the curious squatting posture of the figures. The legs are spread apart and arms turned down, with elbows slightly bent. Three European diagrams present the skeleton viewed from behind with the head hyperextended and depict the bones and sutures of the skull in a manner identical to ibn Ilyās's skeletons. The origin of the European series remains a puzzle, but it clearly predates the Persian anatomy by at least 180 years.

Manṣūr's Anatomy concludes with the formation of the fetus, usually illustrated with a sixth diagram showing a pregnant figure—which, like the other figures, is gender neutral. The fetus, always in a breech or transverse position, is typically shown as a mature male. Unlike the treatise's other figures, the sixth has no labels. It is possibly the only contribution that ibn Ilyās himself made to anatomical illustration, all other elements deriving from earlier sources.

These squatting schematic figures remained the dominant model for anatomical illustration in the Islamic world until the introduction of European models in the genre of Vesalian anatomy.

—EMILIE SAVAGE-SMITH

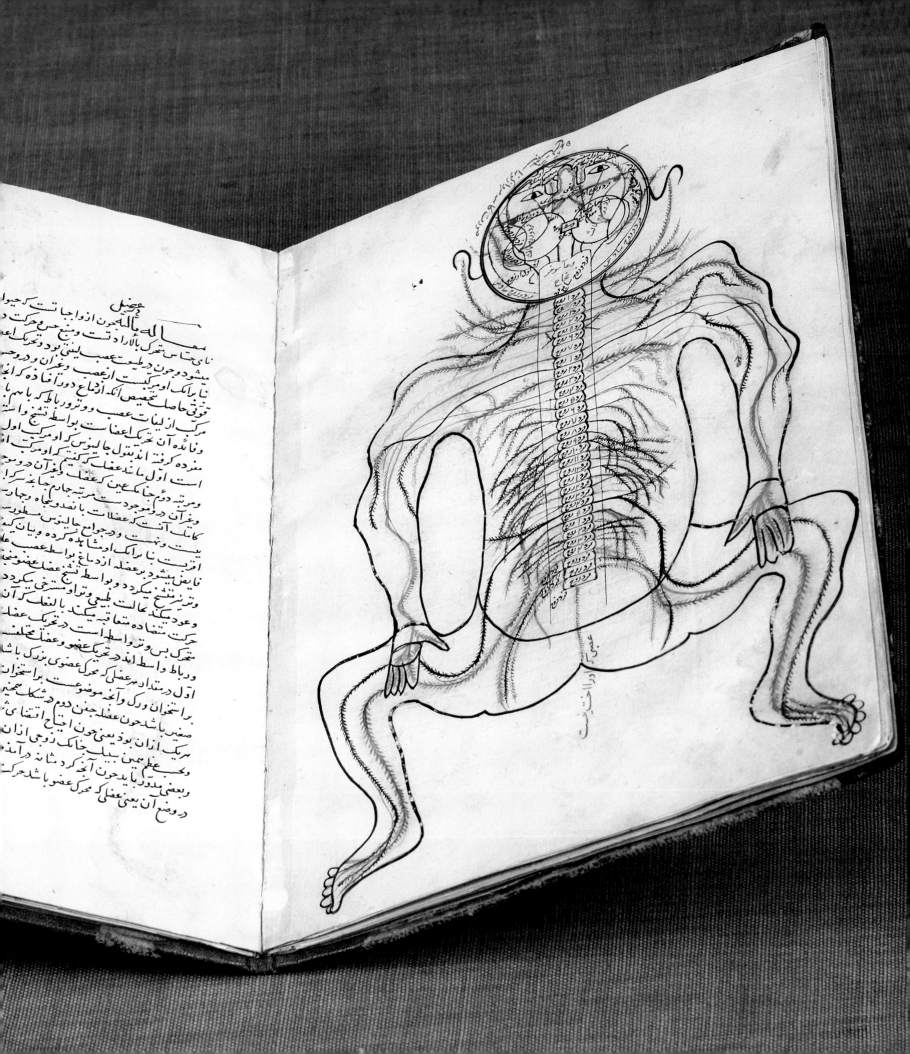

فصل

سمائه بالاجرون از واجبات است که جبو
نایجا س تحرک بالاراده است و منبع حس و حرکت د
میشود و چون در طبیعت عصب لینی بود و تحرک با
نا رابک او میل کند که در دفاع دون آفاده که اج
توتی حاصل تخصیص انکه عصب و و تزور ربا طکه با هم
مرکب از لینات عصب است و چون ربا ط بین تشح و اس
ونماده که فرتته اند قول جالینوس که او مرکب اول
است درجان که عقل باشنده عضله که فتیم و غیران دو موع
و غران دو موجود است که عقلات مرتبه نجات و جان
کامل وهشت و دو جوارح جالینوس سطور
بیت آنست که راک او مثا له فبرده و بیان که
اقربیت نا راک او عقل بردعقل از دماغ بردعضا عضو منی
نایض پیش در بک کرد و بواسط تشح بعض عقلا عضو منی
و تزر تشح کرد و بواسط تراو مسترخی یکرد
وتیرزیک میکنده جالت طبیعی و تراو مسترخی کند آن
و عود میکند شتا تبهریک کن ال بالغل عقلا
حرکت تراو واسط است که در حریک عقلا
متحرک بس و تراواسط عضو و عضلات مختلف
وربا ط واسط اند که تحریک عضوی بزرک باش
اول در تمدار مرعضلی که محرک عضوی است برای استخوان
برای استخوان و رک و آغه موضوع دشکل معین
صغین باشند جن عضله جن یعنی چون اختیاج انان
مریک از انان بود یعنی چون سبک خاک زوبی از ان
وحسب عظیم مین سبک خاک کرد شانه در آنده
وبعضی میتواند بایدجون آغه کرد شانه باش حرکت
دو وضع آن یعنی عضلی که محرک عضو باش حرکت

Examples of Chinese Medicine (1682)
Andreas Cleyer, editor

Specimen medicinae Sinicae, sive, Opuscula medica ad mentem Sinensium . . . Frankfurt-am-Main.
Printed book with woodcuts, copper-plate engravings, charts, and plates, 226 pp.; 6⅛ x 8 in. (15.6 x 20.3 cm)

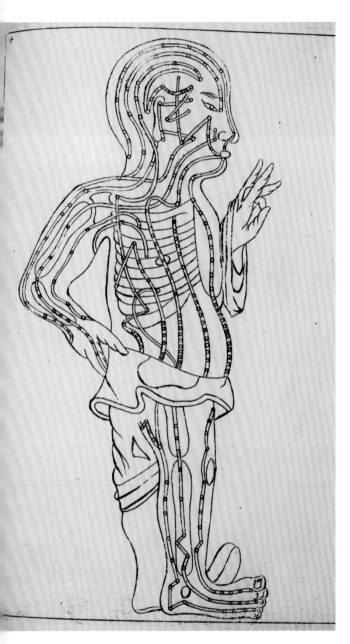

ABOVE AND OPPOSITE: Double lines indicating the channels of *qi/ki* flow in the body—sometimes called acupuncture meridians—were misinterpreted in the West as evidence of East Asian ignorance of anatomy. *Specimen medicinae Sinicae*, pls. 4, 1, and 2

In 1669 Andreas Cleyer (1634–98), a German physician working for the Dutch East India Company at Batavia (present-day Jakarta), wrote to Philippe Couplet (1623–93), a French Jesuit missionary in China, asking about Chinese medicine. Couplet was a confrère of Michael Boym (ca. 1612–59), another Jesuit who spent many years in China and translated several Chinese medical classics into Latin. Couplet sent Boym's manuscripts to Batavia, where Cleyer read them. Cleyer also consulted the famous Dutch physician and natural historian Willem Ten Rhijne (1647–1700), who had investigated Chinese and Japanese therapies while in Japan. Although Cleyer listed himself as editor rather than author when his book was published in 1682, Ten Rhijne complained to the Royal Society of London that his work had been plagiarized. In response the Society paid for the publication of Ten Rhijne's own introduction to acupuncture in 1683.

Cleyer's compendium, *Examples of Chinese Medicine, or Medical Essays According to Chinese Thinking*, contains an overview of Chinese medical theories, descriptions of *materia medica* and their uses, and translated excerpts from commentaries of Wang Shuhe's third-century *Mai Jing*, the *Pulse Classic*. Each pulse description combines diagrams from three different commentaries. Cleyer (or his sources) compared editions and diligently attempted to explain the tactile qualities of the pulse. Because the Chinese classics related pulse qualities to the conditions of internal organs as transmitted through channels (the "acupuncture channels" or "meridians"), Cleyer reproduced charts of the channels, shown here. He did not explain what the diagrams meant, however, leading many readers to conclude that they showed Chinese anatomical ignorance. Proper explication was provided in Ten Rhijne's book the following year.

Traditional Chinese diagrams of the major blood vessels are drawn with double lines. In their history of acupuncture Lu Gwei-Djen and Joseph Needham note that before the seventeenth century, diagrams of acupuncture channels had been drawn with single lines. It may be that in the seventeenth century Chinese and Japanese authors were starting to use double lines to represent the channels as physical vessels. Was this change provoked by Japanese interest in Western anatomy? A few Japanese doctors had been studying "Dutch learning" since the mid-1600s, some with Cleyer, who had been chief commissioner of the Dutch East India Company's trading post on Dejima Island in Nagasaki Bay in 1682–83 and 1685–86.

Cleyer's book blends his understanding of Galenic humoral medicine with Chinese ideas: *yin* and *yang* are rendered as *humidum radical* ("radical moisture") and *calor primigenius* ("original heat"). It also incorporates recent developments in Chinese medicine. The section on tongue diagnosis, for example, comes from a book written by a Christian convert and official physician. Tongue diagnosis was a mid-seventeenth-century innovation, which helps explain the Latin author's surprised note that his source disregarded other forms of diagnosis in favor of consulting only the tongue to indicate the cause of fevers. Cleyer's anthology of purloined translations is thus a snapshot of changing understandings of medicine, health, and disease in both Europe and East Asia.

—BRIDIE ANDREWS

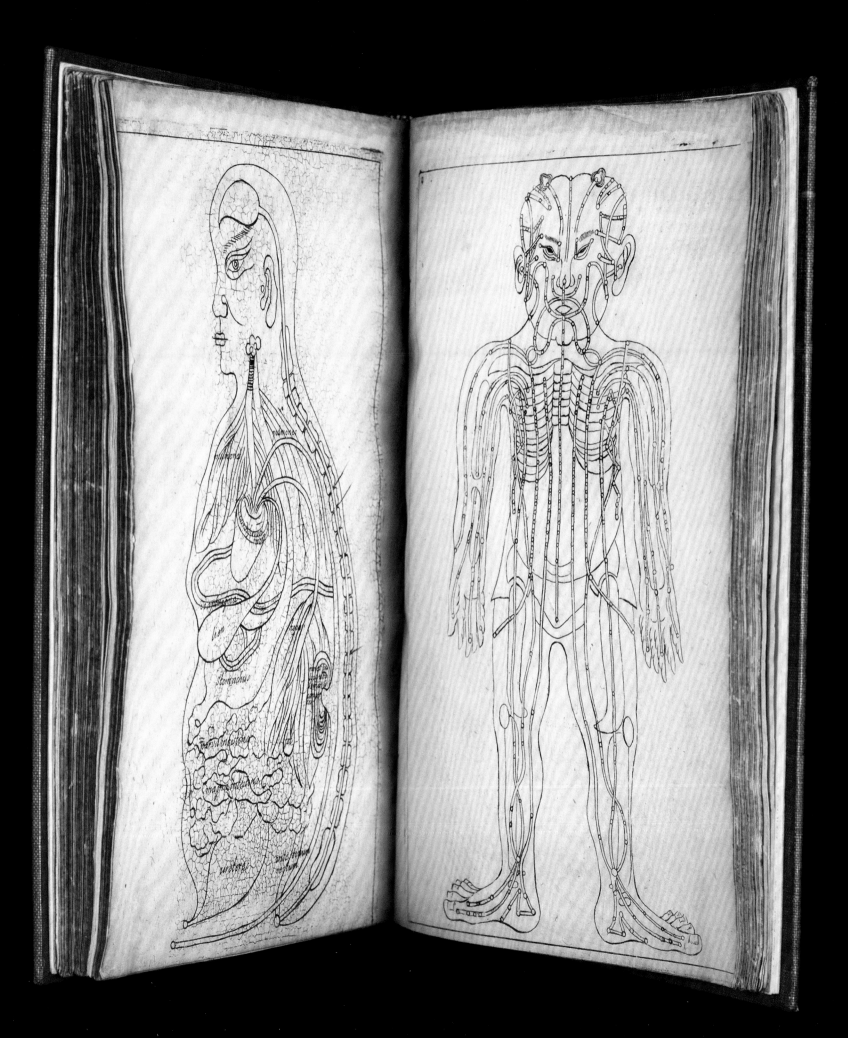

Anatomical Charts of Channel Acupoints for the New Acupuncture (1952)
Tang Xuezheng

Xin Zhenjiu Jingxue Jiepou Tu. Beijing. Printed accordion foldout book; 2⅞ x 7¾ in. (7.4 x 19.7 cm) folded, 77½ x 7½ in. (196.8 x 19.1 cm) unfolded

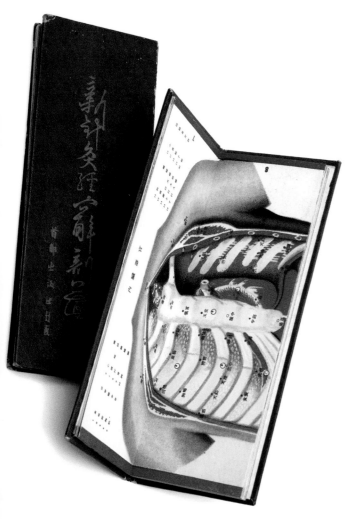

ABOVE AND OPPOSITE: Small circles locate acupuncture points in relation to anatomical structure, while the text suggests the imminent rehabilitation of acupuncture channels in "scientific" Chinese medicine. *Xin Zhenjiu Jingxue Jiepou Tu,* cover and foldout

This small accordion-style atlas documents a stage in the acceptance of acupuncture into the official medicine of the People's Republic of China. Literally a manifold, it is designed to display one of three different full-length views of the body and a cut-open view of the inner organs of the torso. In each view acupuncture points are located in relation to anatomy. The anatomical charts are not particularly detailed: rather the point is to map acupuncture and anatomy together, suggesting that acupuncture is scientific and modern.

This new role for acupuncture is signified by the title's use of the term "New Acupuncture," a phrase coined in the Communist revolutionary base areas during the civil war of 1945–49 by a woman doctor, Zhu Lian. Following Communist leader Mao Zedong's 1944 speech calling for a "United Front in Cultural Work," medical workers developed the policy of "scientizing Chinese medicine and popularizing Western medicine." Zhu Lian, who held several leadership posts within the wartime medical services, noticed that when acupuncturists accompanied mobile medical teams they needed far fewer drugs. She reasoned that a scientific acupuncture would discourage uneducated villagers from resorting to the superstitious or shamanic healing methods that the Communist Party was trying to eradicate. Zhu's New Acupuncture discarded the acupuncture channels and the concepts of *qi* (vital force) and *yin* and *yang*, as contrived and unscientific, instead organizing acupuncture points in military formations such as *bu* ("sections": head, upper limbs, etc.), *qu* ("divisions": eye, shoulder), and *xian* ("lines," as in battle lines or front lines).

The New Acupuncture was a response to the civil war period. The author of these *Anatomical Charts,* Tang Xuezheng (b. 1921), wrote during the Korean War (1950–53), when enthusiasm for Western models had cooled. This helps explain Tang's tentative rehabilitation of the idea that *qi* circulated along fixed pathways. The channels are not depicted, but the two pages of text visible near the bottom of the middle column describe the traditional fourteen channels and the order in which *qi* flows around them. The tables of acupoints on the back of the charts list points by channel *and* "line," and in relation to muscles, nerves, and blood vessels, and also describe how to use them. By the late 1950s nearly all acupuncture charts were once again depicting channels, and in the 1960s the government began sponsoring research to investigate their anatomical and physiological characteristics—a project that continues in China and in the West today.

Tang Xuezheng continued to explore the relationship between acupuncture and science. In 2000, aged seventy-nine, he was granted a patent for an ultra–high temperature electro-thermic needle for use in treating tumors.

—Bridie Andrews

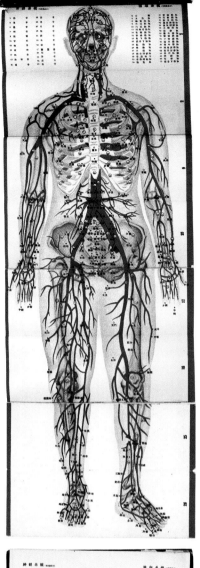

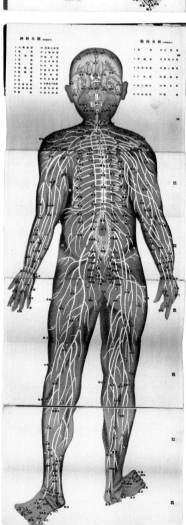

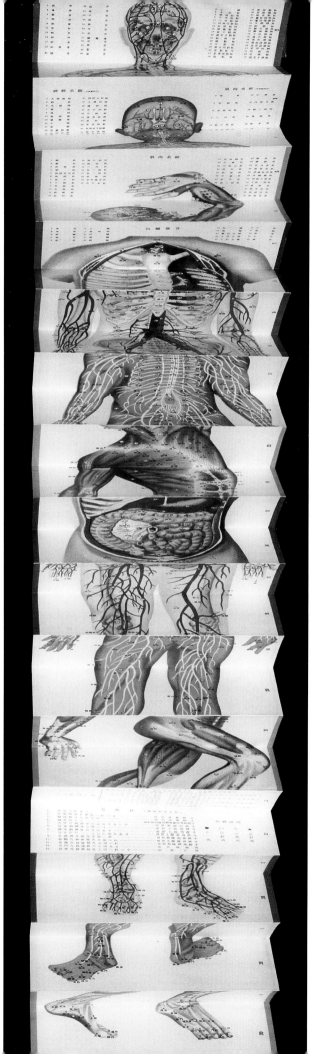

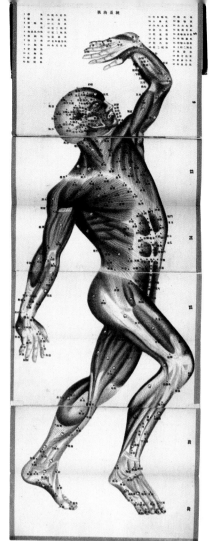

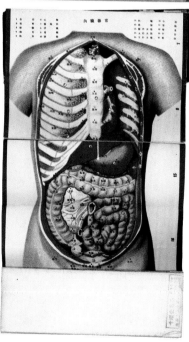

First: Science — Anatomy (1829–30)
"Clorion"

New Harmony, Indiana. Unbound manuscript; ink and pencil drawings with watercolor highlights; 28 leaves; 8⅝ x 11⅛ in. (22.5 x 28 cm)

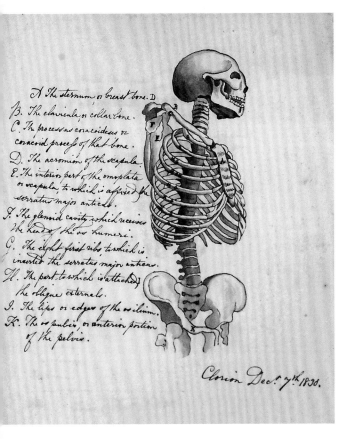

ABOVE: "The names of the bones forming the skeleton, viewed in front," copied from *The Medical Adviser*, n.s., 2 (1825), pl. 5, which in turn was copied from another unknown source. (The few originals printed in *The Medical Adviser* are all attributed.) Clorion's text is also copied from the weekly journal. Clorion, fol. 27a

OPPOSITE: The figure of the naked man tied to a dead tree, with fourteen numbered muscle groups, was designed to help artists develop mastery of the male form. Muscle men were traditionally featured in the art curriculum, where they potentially carried a (homo)erotic charge. Clorion, fol. 2a, copied from the frontispiece of *The Medical Adviser*, n.s., 1 (1825), from William Cheselden (1688–1752), *The Anatomy of the Human Body*, 5th ed. (London, 1740), pl. 19; artist Gerard Vandergucht (1696–1776).

Once upon a time, before originality was prized, copying was a very good thing. Pupils copied out passages from literature and long-division exercises. Art students copied masterworks or prints or casts (which were themselves copies). Medical students copied illustrations from anatomical atlases. And even when artists drew from human models in poses, and medical men drew from specimens and cadavers, such drawings were regarded as a kind of copy, an imitative representation of the observer's view. The act of drawing was a "heuristic device," a way to develop skill at rendering and powers of observation. There was a culture of copying, far removed from today's preoccupation with exclusive copyright and patent law.

In 1927 the Army Medical Library (now the National Library of Medicine) acquired a relic of that culture, some folded pages of drawings and notes from the hand of "Clorion," a resident of New Harmony, Indiana (the utopian community founded in 1824 by the socialist reformer Robert Owen).

Clorion's twenty-three faithfully rendered anatomical illustrations (in pencil, ink, and watercolor) were copied from a London weekly, *The Medical Adviser and Complete Guide to Health and Long Life* (1825), which claimed to offer "plain and easy directions for the treatment of every disorder incidental to the Human Frame," and was devoted to discussions of diseases ("Bilious Colic"), odd cases ("The Living Skeleton"), and healthy living ("Early Rising"). Every issue featured an anatomy lesson with captioned engravings. At the time, a knowledge of anatomy was a mark of refinement. Anatomical education enabled one to appreciate works of art, attain insight into God's design ("natural theology"), and contemplate human mortality (through images of skeletons and skulls). Anatomy was a subject where art, medicine, and philosophy converged.

Clorion's identity is unknown. Was he or she an aspiring medical student or artist or just studying anatomy and draftsmanship as an intellectual and moral exercise? The notebook consists entirely of copied material. Clorion offers no explanation but was almost certainly motivated by a desire for self-improvement. Acute observation improves drawing ability; drawing helps develop the ability to observe acutely. And both help the student to memorize information and reflect on its meaning. The Romantic pedagogical reformer Johann Heinrich Pestalozzi (1746–1827) preached that learning through doing, using the senses, was superior to methods that relied solely on the word. New Harmony had a Pestalozzian school.

Clorion's manuscript was a link in a chain of copies. *The Medical Adviser*'s engravings were themselves copied, without attribution, from illustrations that Gerard Vandergucht made for William Cheselden's *Anatomy of the Human Body* (1740) and from other sources. It's unlikely this was accounted as plagiarism. By 1825 Cheselden's engravings may have been so well known as not to require attribution. Or perhaps anatomy was a knowledge category that implicitly made a truth claim: here is the reality of humanity. If so, even derivatively, anatomical illustration could be taken as a report from nature, a transcription—and author and artist were irrelevant.

—MICHAEL SAPPOL AND EVA ÅHRÉN

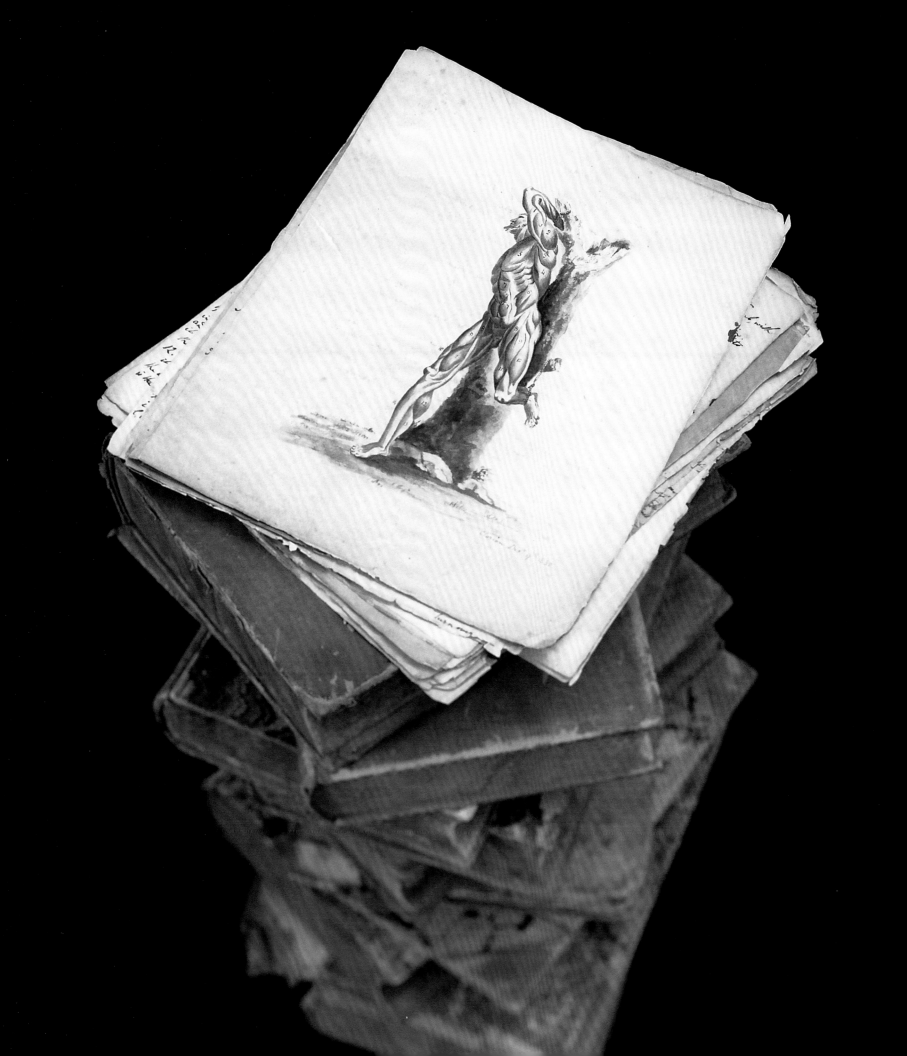

Complete Study of Human Anatomy (1831–54)
Jean-Baptiste Marc Bourgery, illustrations by Nicolas-Henri Jacob

Traité complet de l'anatomie de l'homme, comprenant la medicine operatoire, avec planches lithographiées d'après nature. Paris. 8 vols. with 8 atlases; hand-colored lithographs; 12⅜ x 16¾ in. (31.6 x 42.8 cm)

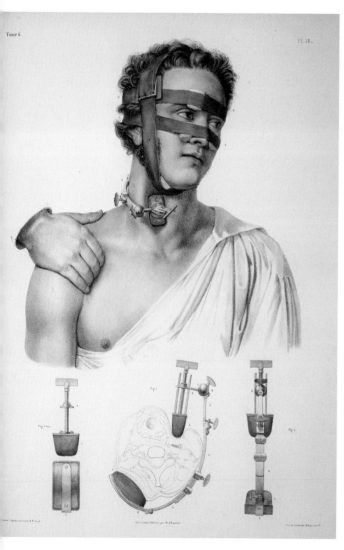

ABOVE: Top of page, a fastidious combination of straps and bandages compresses the patient's facial arteries. Bottom of page, three different angles of an instrument made to exert pressure on the carotid. *Traité*, vol. 6, pl. 18

OPPOSITE: At left, glass tubes and accompanying pumps (invented by V.-T. Junod) designed to constrict the circulation of the arms and legs—essentially a form of cupping—to cure rheumatism. At right, five methods for operating on crossed eyes and excessive squinting. *Traité*, vol. 6, pl. 28, vol. 7, pl. D

During the early decades of the nineteenth century the neoclassical ideal body—an aesthetic most forcefully delineated by Enlightenment antiquarian Johann Joachim Winckelmann (1717–68) and seized upon in canvas after canvas by history painter par excellence Jacques-Louis David (1748–1825)—was subject to an erosion as much literal as symbolic. This was especially true in France, where Romanticism's painters had knocked it from its pedestal: Antoine-Jean Gros laid it low in the *Battle of Eylau* (1808); Théodore Géricault had subjected it to cannibalization on the *Raft of the Medusa* (1818). Some, like aesthetic theorist Antoine Chrysostome Quatremère de Quincy, attempted to reinstate the ideal as the carrier of patriotic duty and cultural triumph. But in the early years of the century, as Xavier Bichat's teachings on pathology spread, Parisian medicine began to couple disease with expired organs. The balance of the four humors, to which the aesthetic ideal had been anchored, became history. And the result was irreversible. The ideal body's fragments were remnants of a lost world.

This wounded ideal appears throughout the *Traité complet de l'anatomie de l'homme* of anatomist J.-B.M. Bourgery (1797–1849). Initially a didactic set of pamphlets for the physician-in-training (volume 1 appeared in 1831), the *Traité* became a lavish, sixteen-volume masterwork, whose ideal bodies, Bourgery declared, would correct the physician's or surgeon's erroneous mental pictures of the body. But while the anatomist prided himself on the careful, cadaver-based empiricism he had learned at the École de Santé of Paris, the images in his atlas are bloodless and beautified. Over the twenty-three years of its publication, Bourgery and lithographer Nicolas-Henri Jacob (1782–1871), a student of J.-L. David, stressed the composition and reparation of ideally proportioned men and women. Picturing every inch of flesh in muscular, skeletal, and nervous anatomies with descriptions of surgeries of all stripes, they tamed their encyclopedic ambitions with soft chiaroscuro, pastel skin, and classical lines. Even Bourgery's depiction of a gruesome mastectomy (p. 48) was dictated by an insistence on upholding the ideal. In a variation on a theme found throughout the atlas, expert, disembodied hands extract a cancerous tumor from a stoic woman who remains as still as a statue, with perfectly coiffed hair, and who betrays no hint of pain, sweat, or fear.

The power of such images was recognized by Bourgery and Jacob's medical and artistic contemporaries, for whom visuality and surgery, spectacle and knowledge were closely bound. In 1845, after only five volumes had been published, the Académie des Sciences awarded the anatomist and artist a 5,000-franc prize for their contributions to the field of anatomy. A decade earlier, in a front-page review for the widely read *Journal des débats*, art critic Étienne-Jean Delécleuze had declared the *Traité* an "époque" in the history of anatomical atlases—a true collaboration between two men who felt a keen responsibility to each other's profession. But for Delécleuze, even Bourgery and Jacob's astonishing anatomical ideal had its limits. Made of stillness and silence, it could not cope with that most delicate principle of life, barely detectable by the senses—the inexplicable force separating the living from the dead.

—MELISSA LO

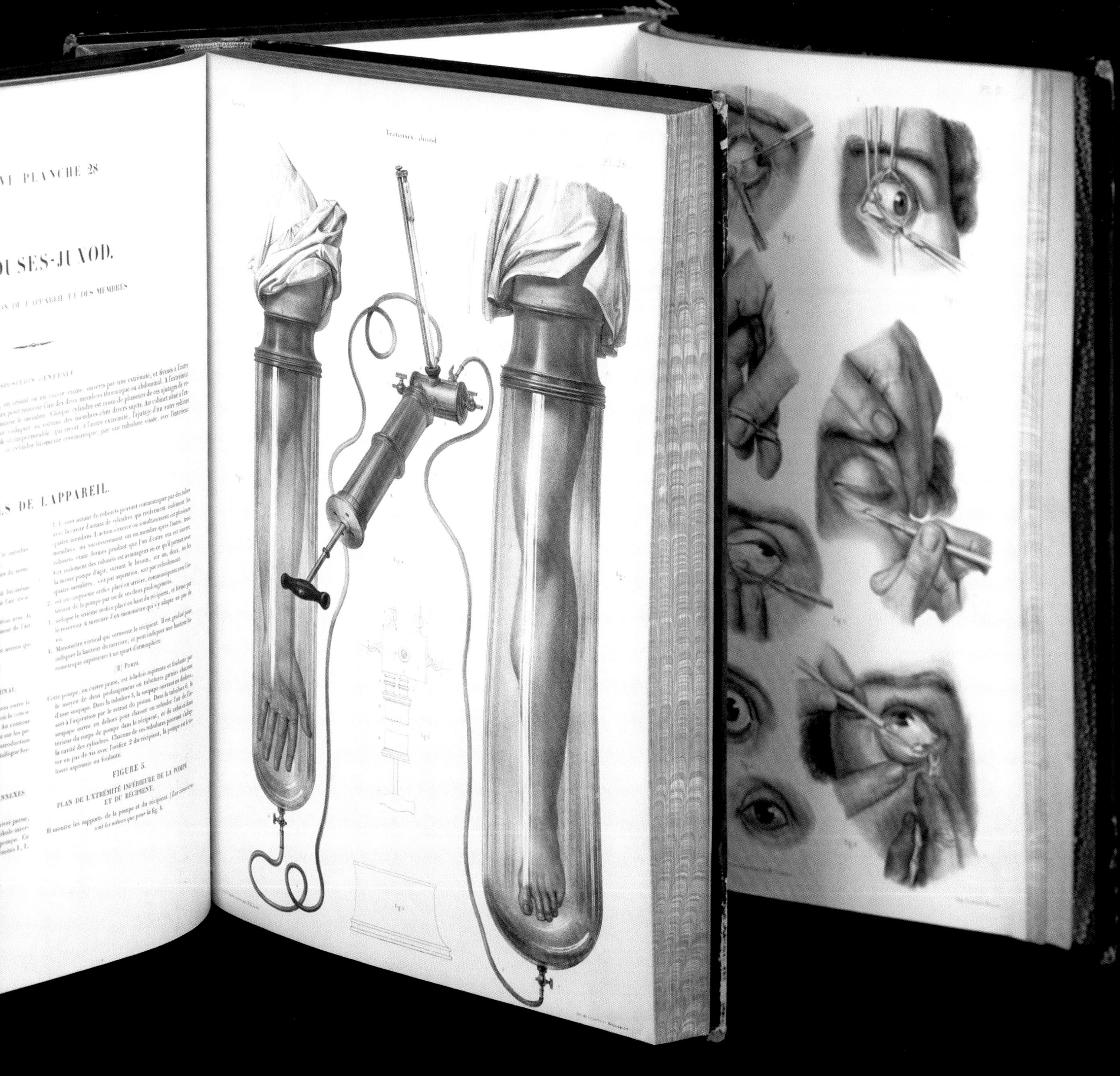

OUSES-JUXOD.

ON DE L'APPAREIL ET DES MEMBRES

S DE L'APPAREIL.

FIGURE 5.

PLAN DE L'EXTRÉMITÉ INFÉRIEURE DE LA POMPE
ET DU RÉCIPIENT.

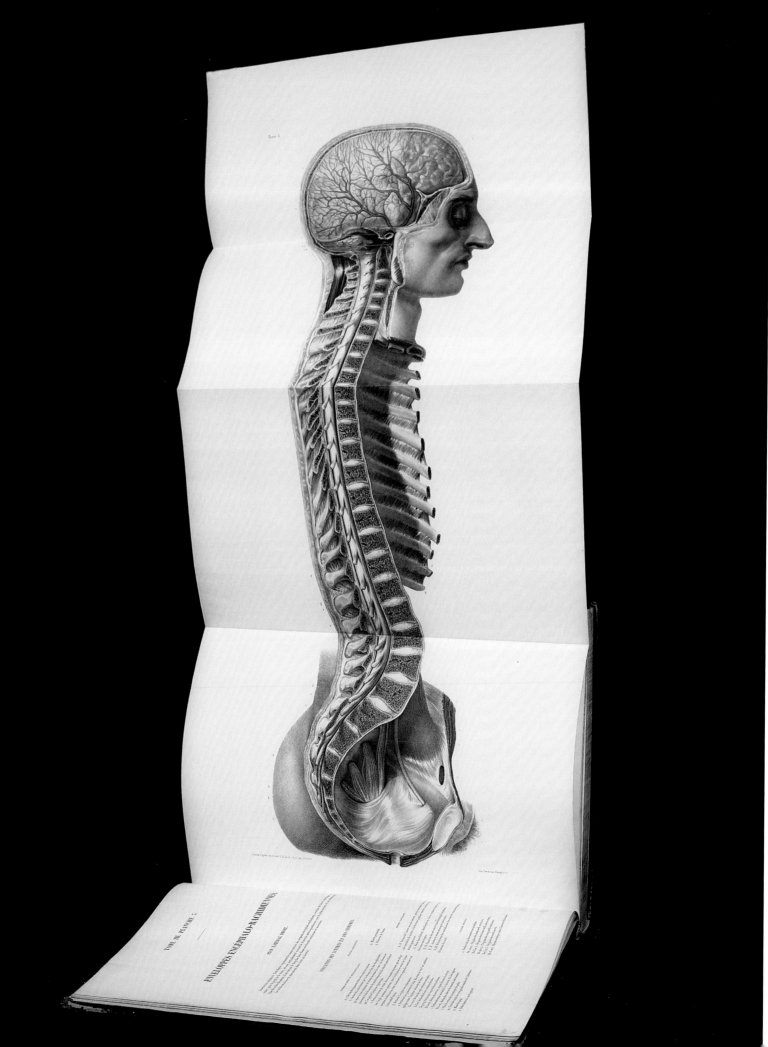

TOME II. PLANCHE 3.

ENVELOPPES ENCÉPHALO-RACHIDIENNES.

PLAN CÉRÉBRAL DROIT.

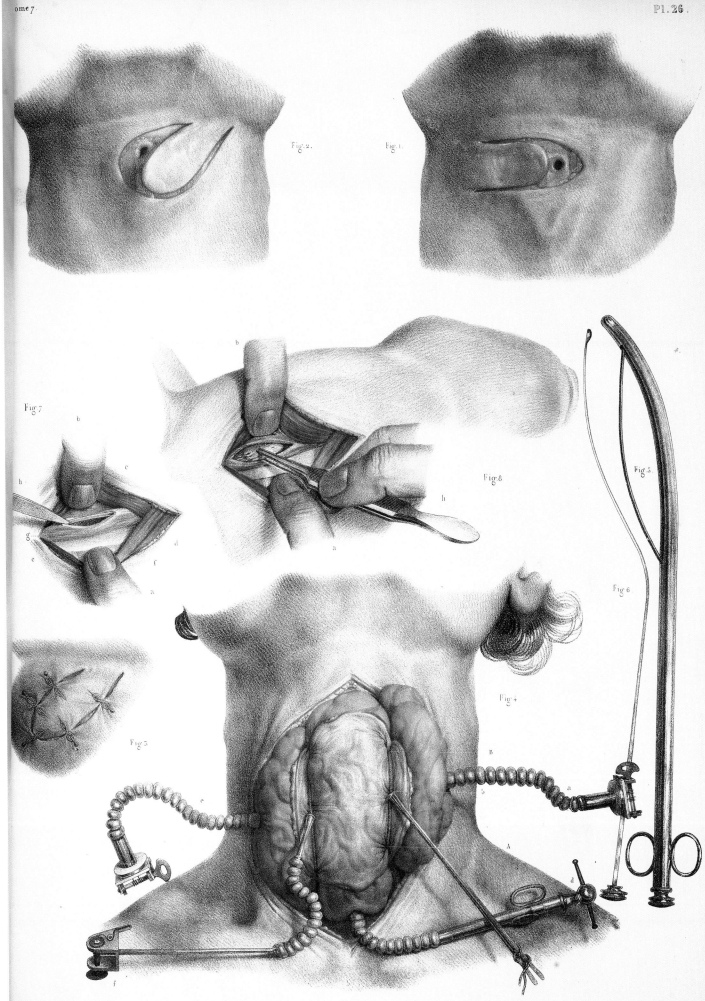

Fig. 2.

Fig. 1.

Fig. 7

Fig. 8

Fig. 5

Fig. 6

Fig. 4

Fig. 3

OPPOSITE: A transverse cut exposes an intricate view of the organs of the spinal column. *Traité*, vol. 3, pl. 3

RIGHT: The surgical repair of the bronchus (figs. 1–3); the Mayor technique for removing a cancerous goiter (fig. 4); and steps for cutting into the esophagus (figs. 7–8). *Traité*, vol. 7, pl. 26

Dessiné d'après nature par N. H. Jacob.

Imp de Lemercier Bénard et Cie

Fig. 1

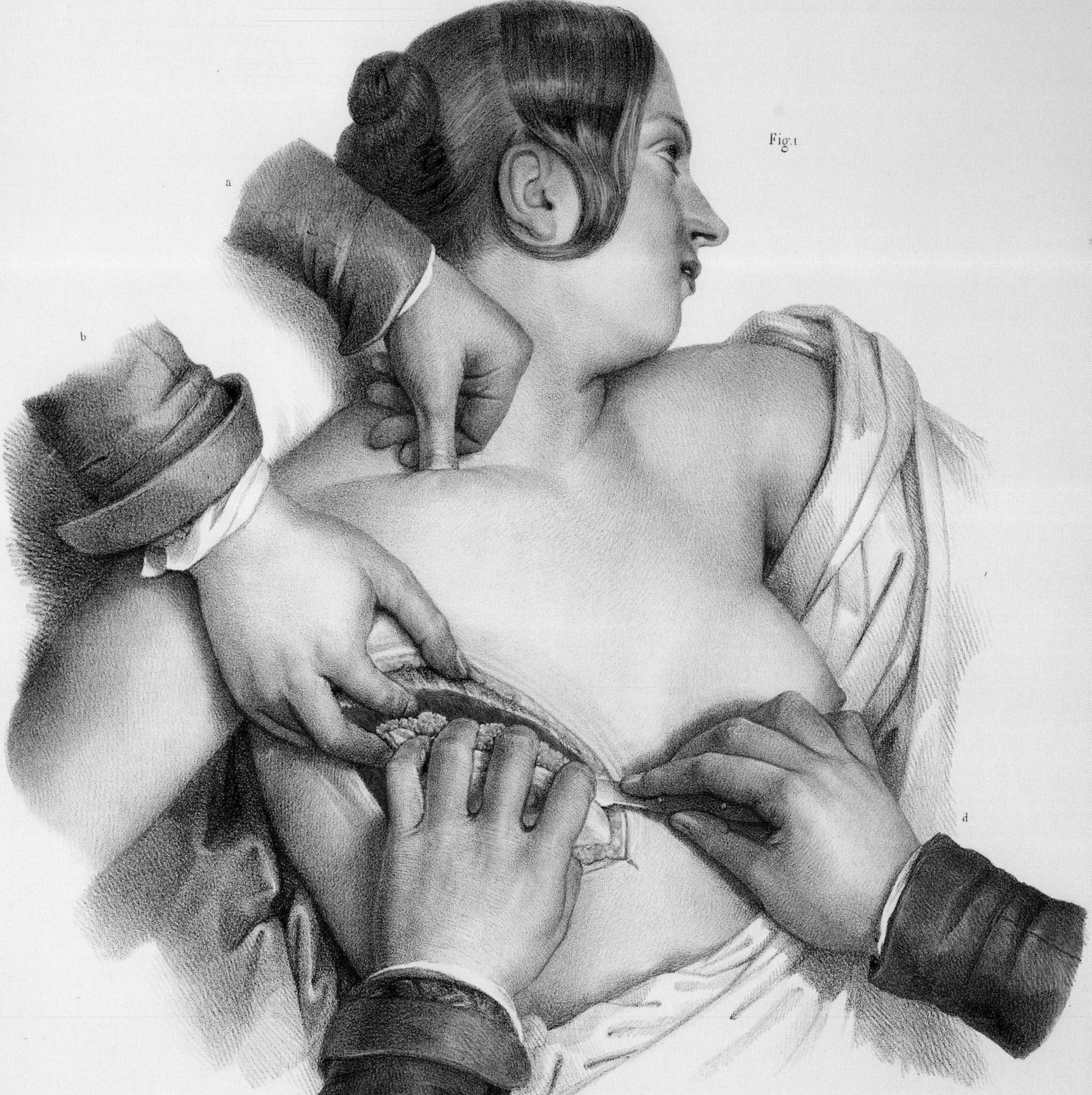

Fig. 2

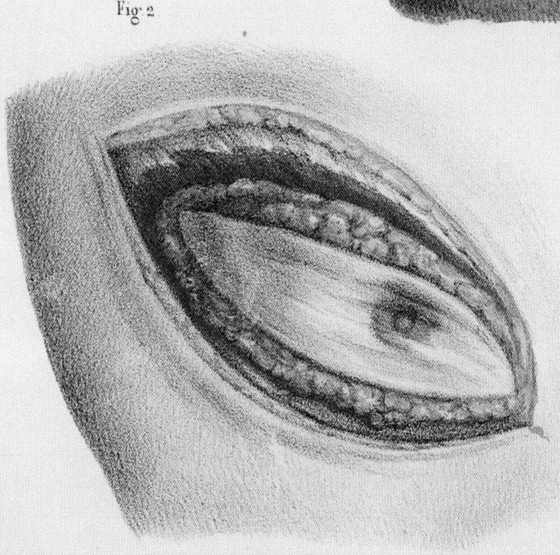

Fig. 3

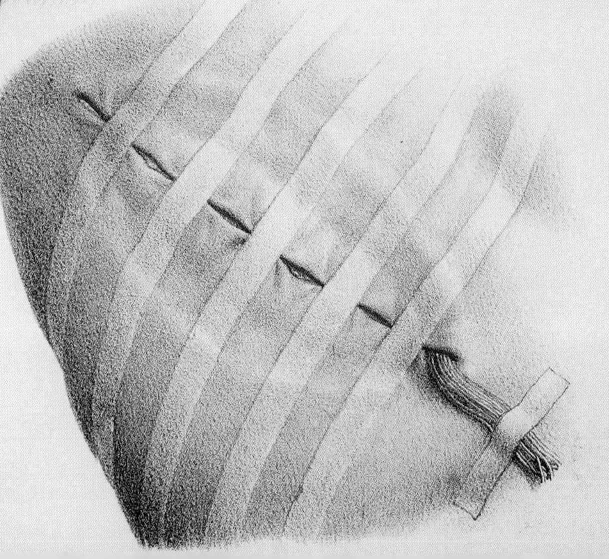

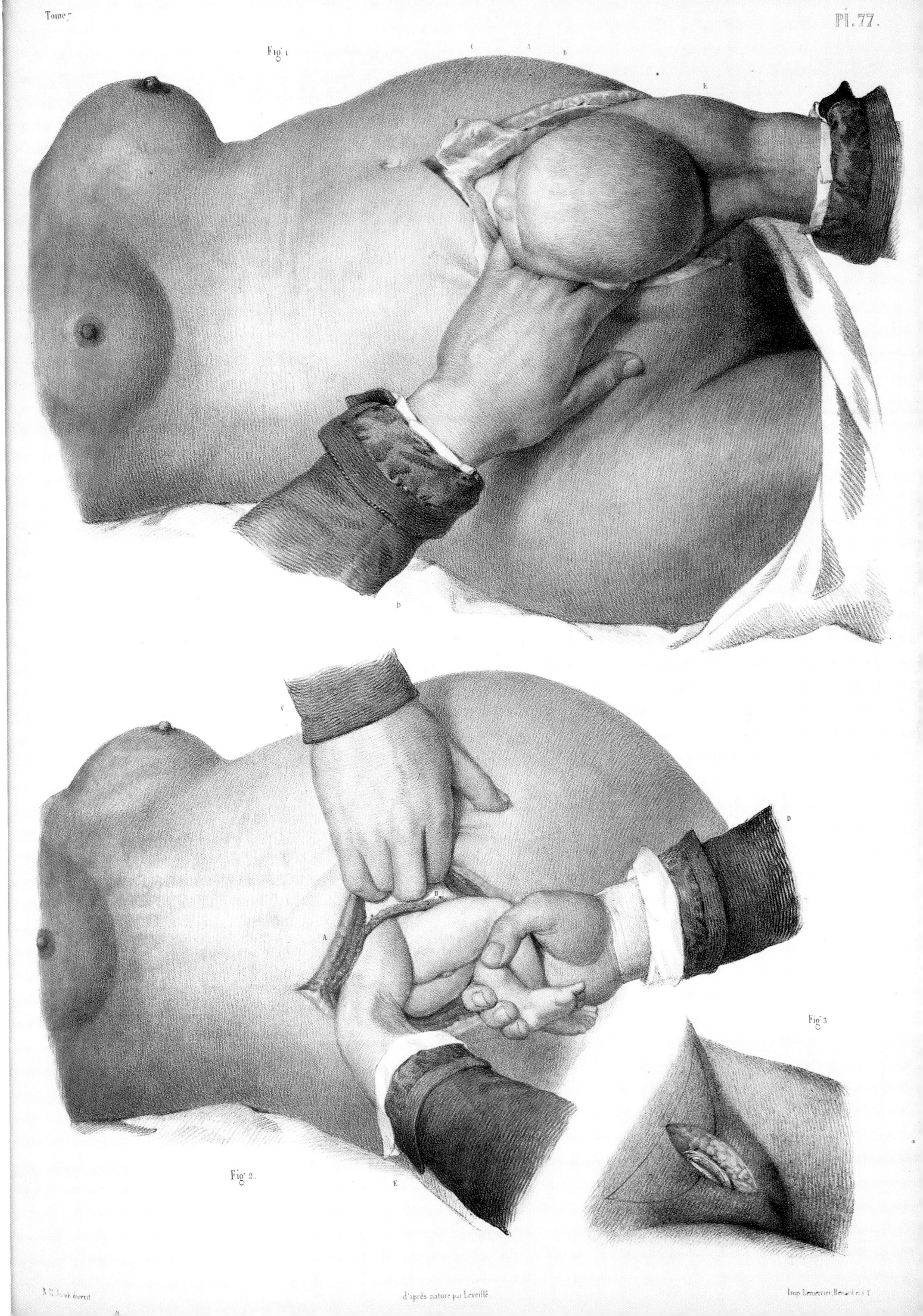

Fig 1

OPPOSITE: Mastectomy,
from deep incision to a
stratigraphic peek into the
breast (featuring layers
of skin, mammary glands,
lymphatic ganglia, and
portions of the pectoral
muscle) and finally the post-
operative bandaging of the
skin. *Traité*, vol. 7, pl. 27

RIGHT: Three different
caesarean methods: (1) a
vertical cut up and down the
belly and into the uterus;
(2) from the side; and (3)
an old technique called
symphysèotomie, in which the
surgeon creates an incision
closer to the pubis, carving
a flap that provides easier
access to the lower part of the
uterus. *Traité*, vol. 7, pl. 77

Fig 2.   Fig 3

Obstetric Tables; Comprising Graphic Illustrations (1835)
George Spratt

London, 2d ed. Printed book, with anatomical flaps; 2 parts; 8½ x 10½ in. (21.6 x 26.7 cm)

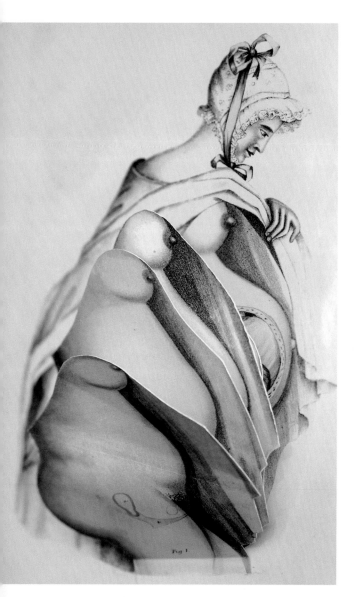

ABOVE: A temporal "dissection" showing progressive changes during pregnancy, including views of the "virgin" state and the end of each trimester of pregnancy. Lifting the final flap reveals a full-term fetus. *Obstetric Tables*, part 1, table 4

OPPOSITE: A combination of temporal and spatial dissection depicting a forceps delivery. The first two flaps show placement of the left and right forceps blades respectively; the third demonstrates the correct placement of the forceps prior to delivery. The final flap depicts the fetal head partially born. *Obstetric Tables*, part 2, table 8

This curious book, "intended to illustrate…midwifery, elucidating particularly the application of the forceps, and other important practical points in obstetric science," went through four editions in Britain and one in the United States. Its brilliantly colored lithographic plates consist largely of a series of flaps—small sections that can be lifted to "dissect" the figure. To construct the plates George Spratt (ca. 1784–1840) modified images he borrowed from other anatomical atlases and obstetric manuals. Most of the plates are spatial dissections, revealing ever deeper views into the body's interior. But Spratt also offers temporal "dissections" of the stages of pregnancy, difficult labors such as forceps delivery, and, in the American reprint, a caesarean section.

Flap books have a long history. They were first used in fifteenth-century astronomy and mathematics. In the sixteenth century, anatomical "fugitive sheets" depicted Adam and Eve with cutaway torsos, and Vesalius printed pieces to be cut out and assembled into flaps in his *Epitome* (1543) (see pp. 18–21). The flaps were intended to facilitate interactive learning in much the same way as virtual dissecting programs do today. (Readers had to open the plate overlays to see the sequence and, in a way, participate in the dissection or delivery.) The preface to Spratt's American edition raved, "The superiority of the present work over any other series of Obstetrical illustrations, is universally admitted. It is a happy combination of the *Picture* and the *Model*.… To the busy practitioner, who wants something to refresh his memory, it obviates the necessity for continual *post mortem* examination.… To the student it is equivalent to a whole series of practical demonstrations, with the advantage that it can be carried about with him and studied wherever he may desire." Reviews in contemporary medical journals were equally enthusiastic.

Spratt promoted his *Tables* as a way to help students who had insufficient opportunities for clinical training in obstetrics and anatomical dissection. Clinical training was expensive and time-consuming: obstetrical courses charged extra fees for clinical training, and physical contact with patients occurred only when students took the course a second time. The need to supplement dissection stemmed from a shortage of cadavers. Notwithstanding the passage in Britain and Massachusetts of "anatomy acts" designed to provide the bodies of "unclaimed" indigents to medical colleges and private anatomy schools, many anatomists faced chronic shortages and disruptions and struggled to obtain a legal supply of bodies. Spratt's work claimed to fill this need cheaply and efficiently.

Little is known about the author. Credited on the title page as "Surgeon-Accoucheur," Spratt worked as an illustrator as well as a medical practitioner. He published several lavishly illustrated botanical books, including *Flora Medica* (1829–30), along with wall charts and pocket books on poisonous plants, and collaborated with George Madeley, one of the lithographers of the *Tables*, on a popular series of composite caricature prints.

—MARCIA D. NICHOLS

TABLE VIII.

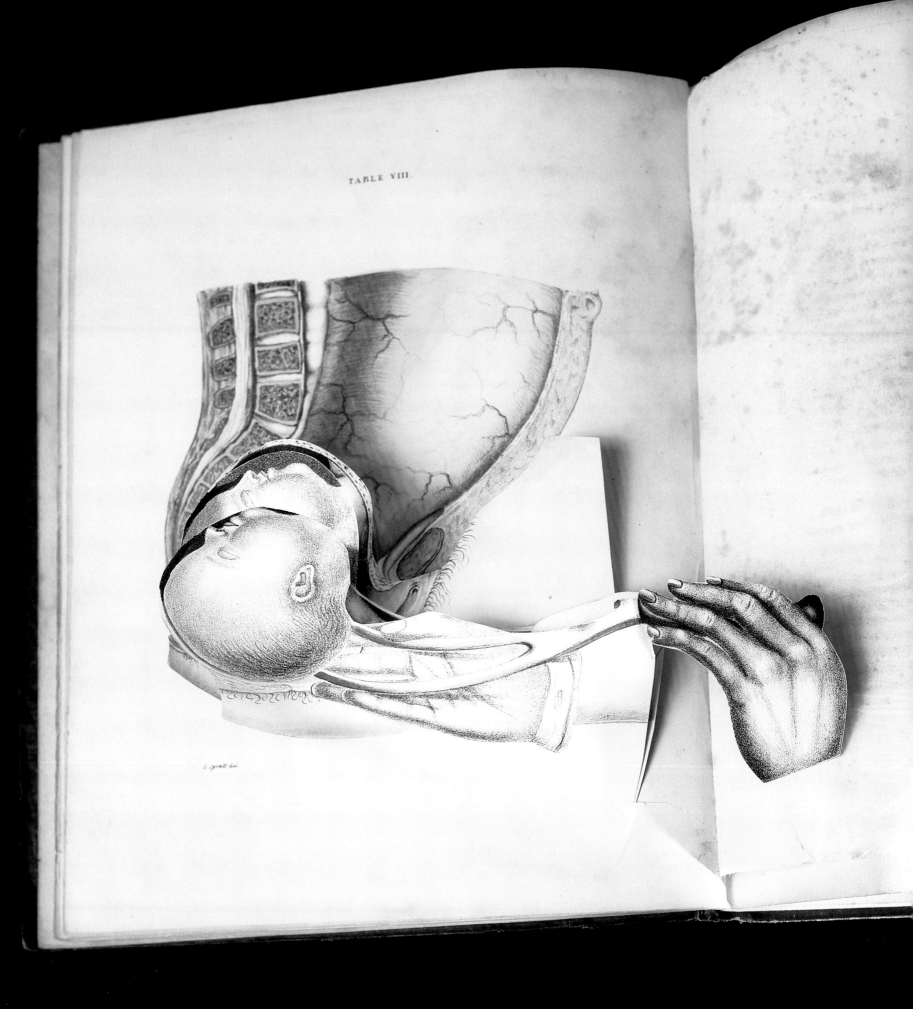

J. Spratt del.

Nurse Postcards Collection (late 1800s – mid-1900s)
Various manufacturers

Printed postcards, with handwritten messages and canceled postage stamps

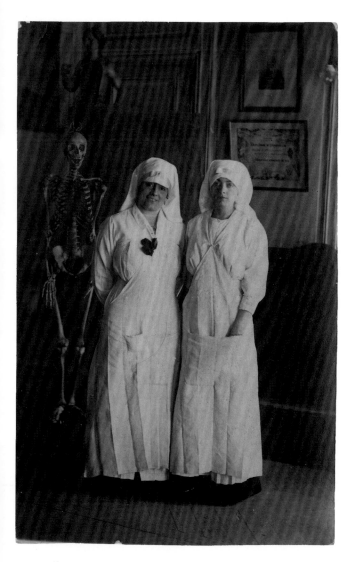

ABOVE: Two nurses pose before a skeleton and female anatomical manikin. Paris, early twentieth century.

OPPOSITE, LEFT TO RIGHT, TOP TO BOTTOM: Nurses giving women mud baths, Russia, early twentieth century. Nurses in gas masks at the trenches, France, ca. 1917 (U.S. postcard). White nurse with native nurses at the Red Cross School-Hospital, Pawa, Belgian Congo, 1939. Nurses with babies, U.S., twentieth century. Nurse giving woman an X-ray, La Cigogne, France, early twentieth century. Female nurses holding diplomas, behind two men on a dais, Albuquerque, New Mexico, early twentieth century.

I collect nursing postcards. My latest postcard, which some friends sent as a birthday present, shows a nurse advertising a girdle: "Brodies' tight fit corset"—"tight as can be."

The production of postcards on an industrial scale around the turn of the nineteenth century brought the figure of the nurse into millions of households across the globe. This was a time when nursing was expanding from the hospital into the home, school, and workplace. Postcards bearing images of nurses were used to mark hospital visits, celebrate graduation from nursing school, raise funds for philanthropic, medical, and religious activities that employed nurses, propagandize for war efforts and health campaigns, or just entertain. The rise of the postcard came with the expansion of working-class literacy. The postcard made only modest demands on the reading skills of sender and recipient and was cheap to buy and mail. It provided a speedy way for people to connect: a striking image that went with a brief handwritten message. Postcards and nursing were made for each other.

The more than one thousand postcards at the National Library of Medicine feature photographs, cartoons, chromolithographs, and paintings, populated by a prolific pantheon of nurses. The nurse is associated with the idealization of womanhood and motherhood (male nurses are rarely represented). She embodies heroic virtues, a valorous glamour that arises out of religious or quasi-religious devotion, a healing vocation.

There are also postcards that portray the nurse as seductress or object of seduction: busty, sexy innocents who unwittingly arouse bedridden male patients or wittingly fend off their advances. In some postcards the nurses wantonly tease and flirt. Most of these smutty nurse postcards were drawn in cartoon styles familiar to readers of men's magazines, but some were staged as a photographic tableau.

Most nursing postcards, however, have a documentary purpose. They show nurses at work or posing in a clinic, classroom, or field hospital, in a particular place and time. They usually feature white women, but some show nurses of color in colonial settings. Such postcards fit into the larger genre of travel postcards; they served as a souvenir of a trip or posting that a tourist, colonial administrator, settler, or missionary might send back home.

The two world wars provided the subject matter for many postcards. Wartime postcards typically show the nurse as the embodiment of patriotic self-sacrifice. Some postcards cast nurse and wounded soldier as lovers, the uniform acting as a reference point for both, a little melodrama. Other postcards sought to boost morale, recruit nurses, and build public support for the war effort. The Red Cross national nursing societies were prolific postcard makers, often adapting posters by well-known artists. But there was no uniformity: different countries adopted different styles.

My personal collection is small; as I look over the much larger collection of postcards at the National Library of Medicine I'm struck by the rich and contradictory figure of the nurse, who embodied authority and deference, professionalism and personal sacrifice, regionalism and empire, purity and eros, religion and science.

—Anne Marie Rafferty

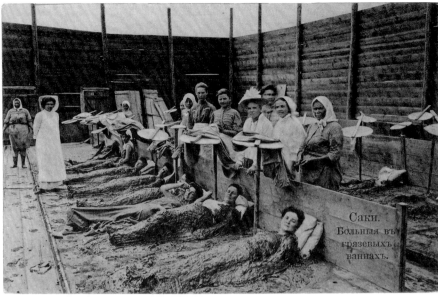

Саки.
Больныя въ грязевыхъ ваннахъ.

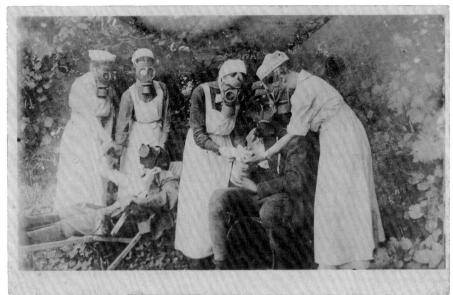

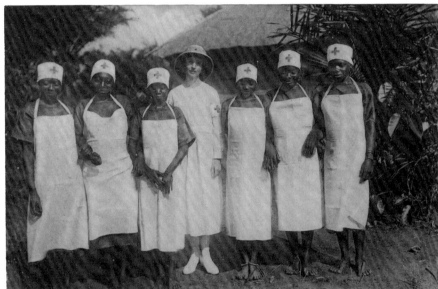

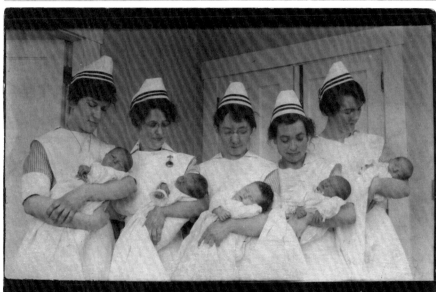

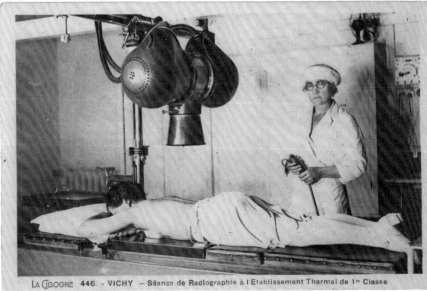

LA CIGOGNE 446. - VICHY - Séance de Radiographie à l'Etablissement Thermal de 1re Classe

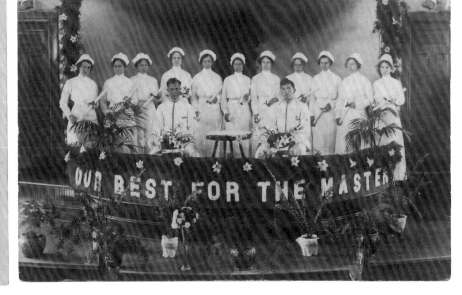

OUR BEST FOR THE MASTER

International Nurse Uniform Photograph Collection (ca. 1950)
Helene Fuld Health Foundation

Jersey City, New Jersey. 93 color photographs, glossy; 8 x 10 in. (20.3 x 25.4 cm)

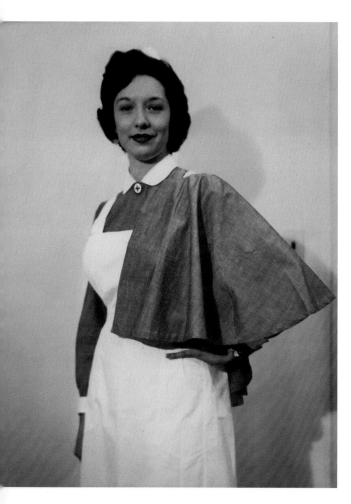

ABOVE: Nurse's uniform from Germany

OPPOSITE, LEFT TO RIGHT, TOP TO BOTTOM: Philippines, Denmark, British Honduras; Hong Kong, Madeira, Kenya; Nepal, Dominican Republic, Colombia

The nurse's uniform is a universal code for professionalism, decorum, efficiency, esprit de corps, and commitment to humanitarian values. Originally introduced to distinguish the untrained traditional nurse, who dressed in the everyday women's wear of her class, from the trained and licensed modern nurse, clad in a neat, clean, and well-fitting uniform, it was a synthesis of various influences—the parlor maid, the religious sister, and military apparel. It varied in time and place, but in every case it helped forge a common occupational and gender identity. Functioning as a sign of authority and institutional discipline for patients and lower-ranking employees, the nurse's uniform also signified service and subordination to doctors, who were usually men and not required to wear uniforms.

In the 1940s and '50s, the Helene Fuld Health Foundation, dedicated to the "relief of poverty, suffering, sickness and distress," focused many of its activities on nursing and produced this set of glossy photographs of nurse uniforms, each representing a nation or region, from Afghanistan to Zanzibar. The costumes differ in detail—the cuffs, capes, hats, aprons, and collars vary—yet all are recognizable as nurses' outfits. The starched whiteness signifies commitment to hygienic cleanliness, the apron a commitment to service, and so on. Noble traits, universal values. In 1950 the United Nations and World Health Organization were new and hopeful institutions; internationalism was rising. After the terrible war that had just been fought, a new global order seemed to be emerging. The Fuld Foundation surely intended these photographs to contribute to that order, to promote a utopian ideal of global harmony.

At the same time the photos have the look of advertisements. In the mid-twentieth century companies began manufacturing more smartly tailored uniforms, and they used women with modern hairdos and makeup who projected a sense of female independence and self-assurance to model them. Fussy styling and accessorizing was avoided; uniform design was meant only to echo the latest fashions while maintaining the modesty of the nurse.

Today the occupations of health care providers are not clearly signified by the informal clothing they wear, and some see the relaxation of dress codes as symptomatic of a decline in standards of care. But the transformation of the nurse's uniform came, in part, from a desire to democratize the medical workplace. Mental health nurses abandoned the uniform in the 1970s in an attempt to reduce the social barriers between nurses and patients. Around the same time, nurses began adopting a feminist view. The hierarchical distinction between doctor and nurse, and the requirement that nurses wear feminine (and sometimes hampering) uniforms, came under attack. The final blow to the formal uniform was the adoption of minimalism in dress in the interest of infection control. Today, in some settings, nurses and doctors are scarcely distinguishable: both don scrubs. But the nurse's uniform still represents authority over the patient and continues to be an iconic symbol.

—ANNE MARIE RAFFERTY

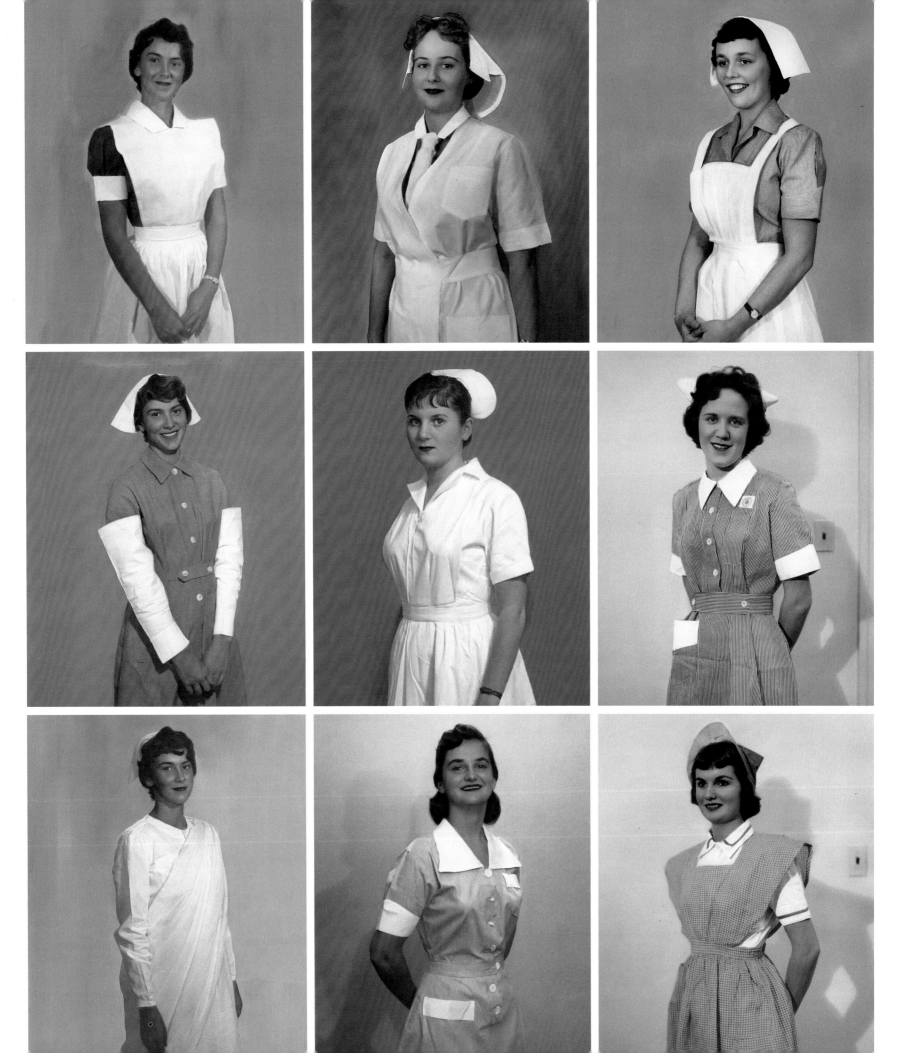

Midwife Dolls (mid-twentieth century)
American College of Nurse-Midwives Collection (1946–76)

Two dolls: handmade (fabric), height 12⅝ in. (32 cm); manufactured (plastic and fabric), 13⅛ in. (33.5 cm)

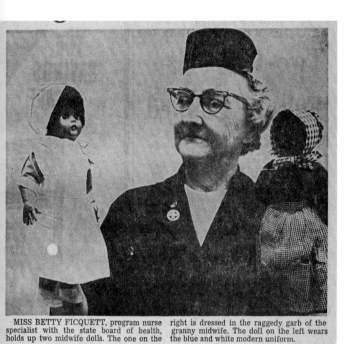

MISS BETTY FICQUETT, program nurse specialist with the state board of health, holds up two midwife dolls. The one on the right is dressed in the raggedy garb of the granny midwife. The doll on the left wears the blue and white modern uniform.

ABOVE: Photo accompanying a newspaper article that was part of a series on South Carolina midwives. *The State* (Columbia, SC), November 22, 1968

OPPOSITE: Laura Blackburn (1891–1955) made and used the doll on the right to depict the old granny-type midwife. Blackburn, midwife supervisor for the state of South Carolina, worked in counties that lacked an organized health department. The store-bought, factory-made doll (on the left) was dressed up in a clean, sterilized white uniform to epitomize the modern, formally educated midwife. Trainers at the Lee County Health Department, Bishopville, SC, used the dolls during summer midwife institutes.

There are forty-one cardboard boxes in the American College of Nurse-Midwives collection at the National Library of Medicine. In box number 10 I found the dolls.

The commercially manufactured plastic doll had become brittle and cracked and needed repair from a conservator. The handmade cloth doll, a bit worn, was perfectly intact. Together with the collection's letters, pamphlets, teaching manuals, and photographs, the dolls helped me piece together the story of "granny" midwives and the state and local programs that trained them as well as later generations of midwives.

For more than three centuries African American midwives, often referred to as "granny" midwives because of their advanced age and revered status in black communities, delivered babies and practiced folk medicine in the rural South. Without formal training, but much practical experience, the "granny" treated pregnant women, families, and other members of her community, in slavery and freedom and very often in dire poverty, under the most difficult sanitary conditions.

Before the 1920s, African American women became midwives through apprenticeship (usually a familial connection) or because they believed God had called on them to do so. After the 1920s, only women who had been recruited by a public health nurse to a state-sponsored midwifery training program could become midwives.

The sea change was fostered by the 1921 Sheppard-Towner Maternity and Infancy Protection Act. From 1921 to 1929 the act provided federal aid to state health departments for midwife training and regulatory programs. The programs were designed to be a temporary solution, to help fill the need for maternal and child health care services in rural areas, where hospitals and physician services were scarce, until trained physicians could take over obstetrical care. But in the rural South racial segregation and a weak regional economy made it difficult to attract enough doctors and build adequate new hospital facilities. Southern reformers compensated by seeking to expand and strengthen the role of midwives in maternal and infant care, even though elsewhere they sought to eliminate midwifery.

Instruction in the new midwife training programs was carried out through teacher demonstrations, role playing, and songs because most midwives had little formal education and many were illiterate. A nurse-midwife or public health nurse presented lessons and demonstrations using an anatomically correct life-size doll. The class curriculum covered pre- and postnatal care and potential complications. The dolls that I stumbled upon in the American College of Nurse-Midwives Collection were used in South Carolina training programs, not for birthing demonstrations, as one would expect, but to show the contrast between the traditional charming, but unsanitary, "self-made" granny-midwife and the modern hygienic, scientifically educated midwife.

—Sheena M. Morrison

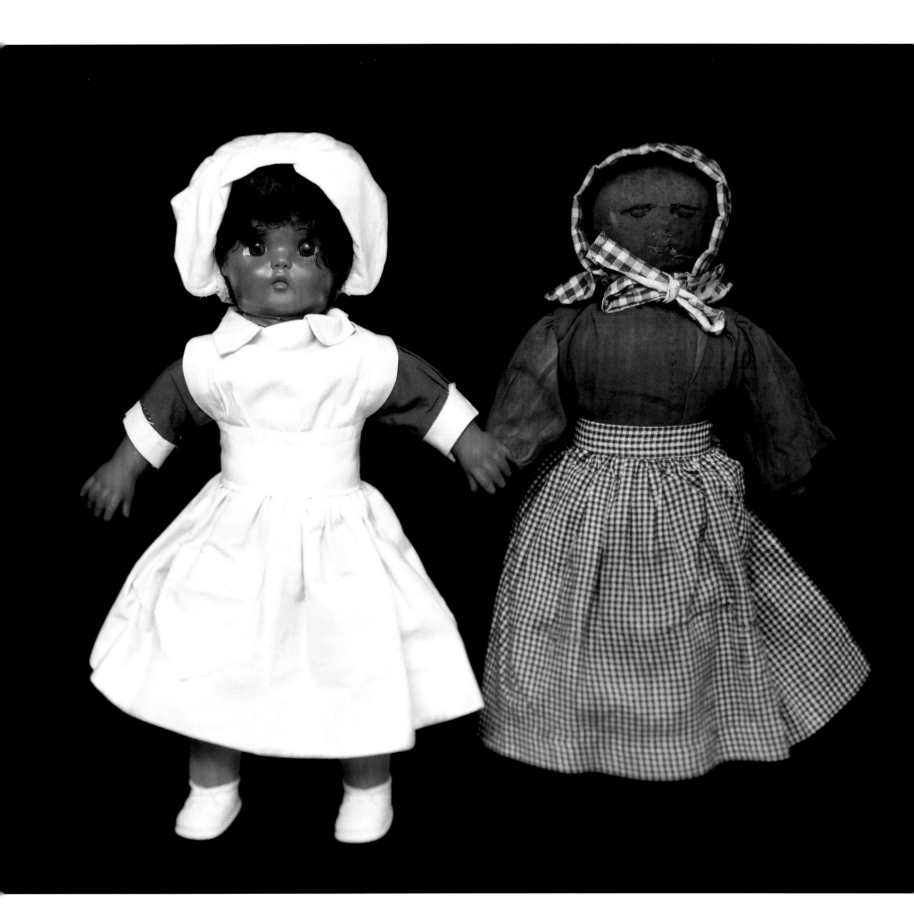

White's Physiological Manikin (1886)
James T. White & Co.

New York. Chromolithograph flaps sewn onto varnished cardboard; die-cut leaves; 23⅝ x 68½ in. (60 x 174 cm)

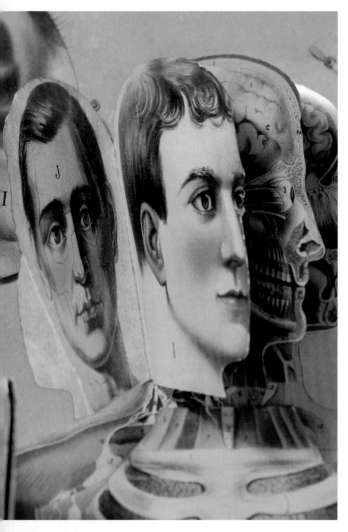

ABOVE: The head of *White's Physiological Manikin*

OPPOSITE: The manikin's flaps correspond to lecture topics such as the circulatory system, the brain and nervous system, the skeleton and muscles, venereal disease and the physiology of reproduction (male and female), first aid, and the dangers of corseting (visible in the far right). *Dr. Franke's Phantom* (1891), a deluxe edition of *White's Physiological Manikin*, also contains flaps showing the stages of gestation and possible positions of fetuses and twins—a pregnant hermaphrodite. The German "Dr. Franke" is probably a corruption of "Dr. Frank Hamilton," whose endorsement was featured in American versions and who wrote an accompanying booklet.

There he sits in retirement, still bearing the legend "Examined and Approved by Frank H. Hamilton, M.D." (a prominent surgeon and one of the four physicians who attended President Garfield). But during his career, the life-size manikin worked standing up, or, more precisely, hanging from a hook. Then he sustained a wound: the stress of suspending his 8.2 pounds wore out the cardboard and he fell. It might have happened front stage at a medicine show, where a pitchman of nostrums was getting the suckers worked up by enumerating the "thousand natural shocks that flesh is heir to." Or in a doctor's office, where the manikin served as a 100-in-1 quick reference wall chart. Or in a classroom, where he bore witness to lectures on the respiratory system, first aid, or nutrition.

He was stiff and sharply delineated, contained. Yet he came equipped with extravagant foliage—layers, sublayers, and openings—like some tropical plant that just can't stop growing. On the right half of his torso alone there sprouted seventeen flaps, printed on both sides. He was a gadget that does too much: a Swiss Army knife with a thousand blades.

A reviewer described him: "Besides exhibiting the form, position, color, and relation of the organs of a healthy body…the manikin is accompanied by a series of microscopical plates showing sections of lung, vein, valve, bone, hair, finger-end, skin, wall of stomach, cross-section of muscle, etc. The cranial, spinal, and sympathetic nerve systems, and their connections are also illustrated." Another writer raved about the many "surgical operations" presented in the manikin: "Ligations of Arteries, Amputations in the Seven Surgical Divisions of the Arm and Leg…, Lines of Exsections of Joints," etc.

Some openings were morally instructive. Colored plates demonstrated "the effects of alcohol and narcotics on the human stomach," deformations of the female rib cage caused by corsetry, and "microscopical sections representing pathological changes occurring in several maladies," including venereal diseases. The manikin—obviously masculine, but an effigy of the universal human—also contained both male and female organs of "generation."

At an 1887 educational exposition in Chicago it was showered with "special praise." At the time reformers claimed that every civilized person should have a basic knowledge of the human body and the laws of health. Twenty-five states required the teaching of physiology in public schools. But, for this task, books and lectures were insufficient. Visual and tactile aids were needed, argued Dr. Roger S. Tracy of the New York City Health Department. "Human dissection being out of the question," schools should buy three-dimensional "dissectable" manikins to "afford the pupil a vivid and exact conception" of the organs "in their situations, connections, and relative dimensions." But such papier-mâché manikins, imported from France, cost from $250 to $1,500—too expensive for financially pressed school systems. *White's Manikin*, in contrast, went for $35. The school superintendent of Woonsocket, Rhode Island, ordered four for his grammar school classrooms. It was marketed for at least twenty years. A deluxe edition was repackaged in Germany as *Dr. Franke's Phantom* (1891), clairvoyantly anticipating its current status: a ghostly relic of late-nineteenth-century anatomical pedagogy.

—MICHAEL SAPPOL

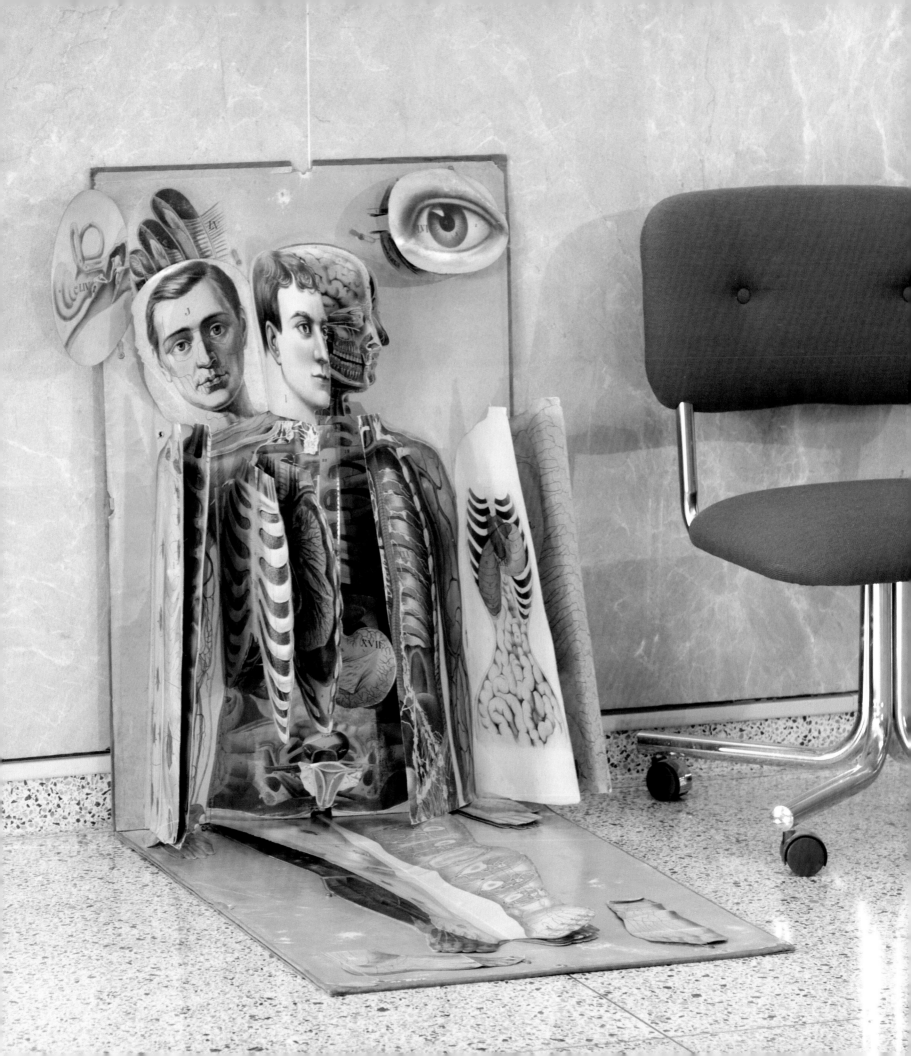

Sinhala Palm-Leaf Medical Manuscripts (1700s–1800s)
Author unknown

Sri Lanka. Untitled manuscripts, palm leaves with painted wooden covers; rope bound;
MS S6, 44 folios, 2 x 8 in. (5 x 20.3 cm); MS S1, 4 parts, each 1½ x 45¾ in. (3.8 x 114.6 cm)

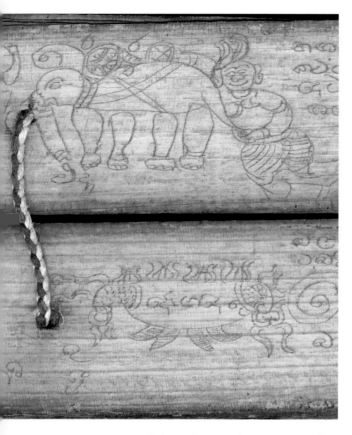

ABOVE AND OPPOSITE: Palm-leaf manuscripts are composed
entirely in prose, verse, lists, or some combination thereof.
Some also have illustrations and diagrams, as in this
manuscript.

RIGHT: Two decorated wooden covers and a single cord hold
together forty-four rectangular-cropped palm leaves—now
quite brittle—containing handwritten medical charms.

Throughout recorded history the island of Sri Lanka has been home to a variety of cultural and ethnic groups, with Buddhist Sinhala people the majority community in the south of the island and Hindu Tamils and Tamil-speaking Muslims prominent in the north and east of the island. At the same time, a variety of cultural, economic, and political networks connected Sri Lanka to other parts of the world, especially to South Asia. It is thus not surprising that the medical heritage of Sri Lanka is a composite, drawn from different medical traditions in India (*Ayurveda* and *Siddha*), Greek medicine (*Unani*) introduced by Arabs, and an indigenous medical heritage particular to the island. For many centuries medical practice in Sri Lanka was also a composite, with scholarly elements that looked to Ayurveda (which were transmitted in Sanskrit) bearing more prestige than the traditional local medical knowledge and practices.

The Sri Lankan medical manuscripts in the National Library of Medicine's collection originally belonged to Sinhalese physicians and are products of the lower-status Sinhalese local tradition. Even so, the physicians (called *veda mahattayas* in Sinhala) who owned these "books" deployed them as signs of their medical learning and prestige. Ownership of

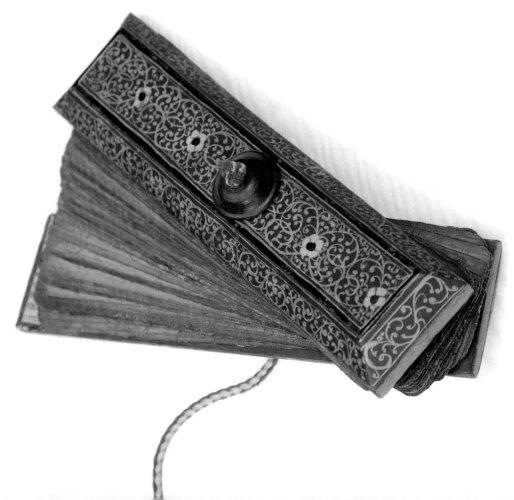

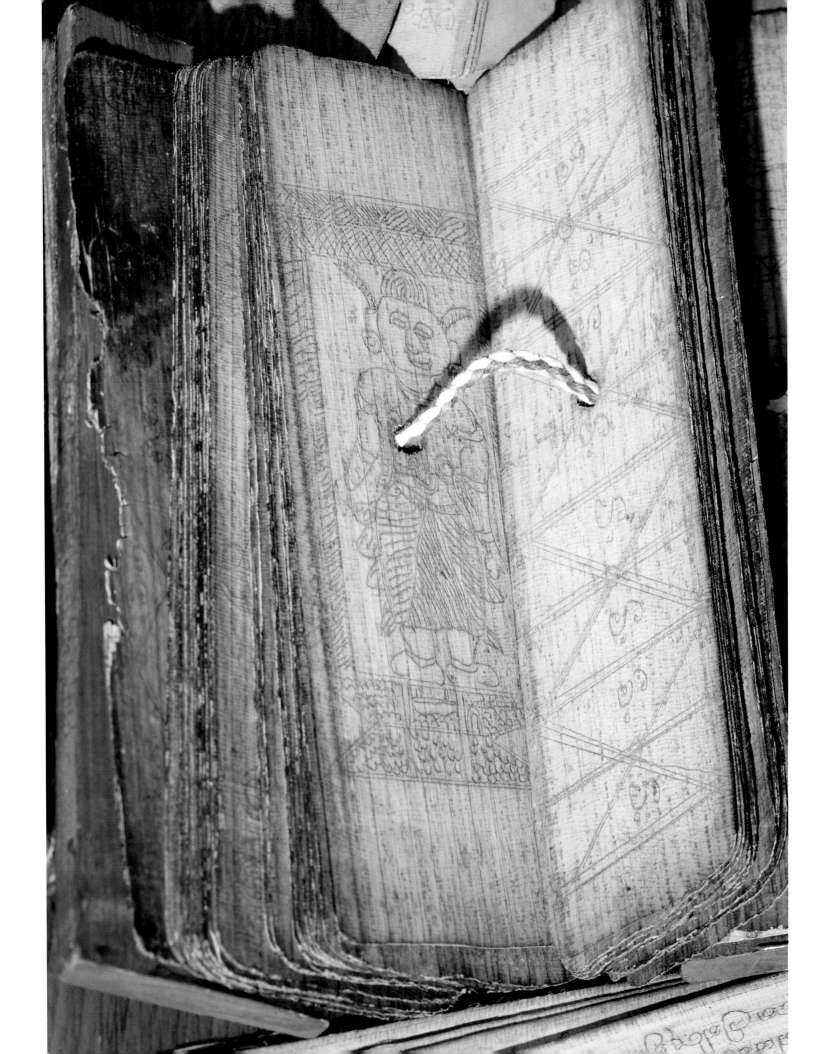

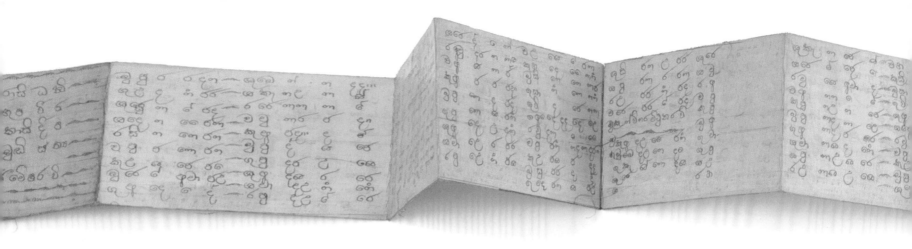

ABOVE: A rare folded Sinhalese palm-leaf manuscript astrological calendar (ca. 1800). The leaves have been shaped into small articulated panels, each about 1⅜ x 3½ in. (3.5 x 9 cm).

OPPOSITE, BELOW: The calendar resides in a small wooden box painted with flowers. Pasted on the inside of the box is a typewritten note describing the calendar and identifying its donor, Dr. Casey Wood (1856–1942) of Chicago, a prominent Canadian ophthalmologist and collector.

manuscripts signified and enhanced a healer's authority because of the painstaking effort it took to make a manuscript from the leaves of the *talipot* palm tree—the production of palm-leaf books largely stopped in the nineteenth century because it was so very labor intensive—and because of their aesthetic appeal, whether this took the form of a beautiful painted cover, artfully wrought text, or elegant handwriting. This is especially the case with the unusual folded manuscript pictured above. (Typically, manuscripts are held together by strings between wooden covers.) Its graceful and expressive handwriting, and the fact that some of its contents are in verse, connects it to the aesthetic contours of Sinhala literary culture, even though the verses were for ritual use. Beautiful books were among the accoutrements of a physician. The beauty of a manuscript suggested the kind of healing abilities its owner was possessed of—while the book's contents informed the actual medical practice. A Sinhala saying, "If you can't be a king, then practice medicine," reminds us that the lives of physicians, as well as kings, add something important and admirable to life in this world.

Traditionally, the practice of the healing arts in Sri Lanka went beyond medicine per se to include what we might consider to be religious practices, including exorcisms. The contents of the manuscripts are often brief; the books most likely served as an aide-mémoire for a healer. Some include recipes of remedies; others contain formulas for use in healing rituals.

The diagrams, text, and verses in these manuscripts were not part of a public system of medical knowledge: they were secret knowledge that belonged to individual healers. Much of the contents therefore were not meant to be intelligible to accidental readers.

—CHARLES HALLISEY

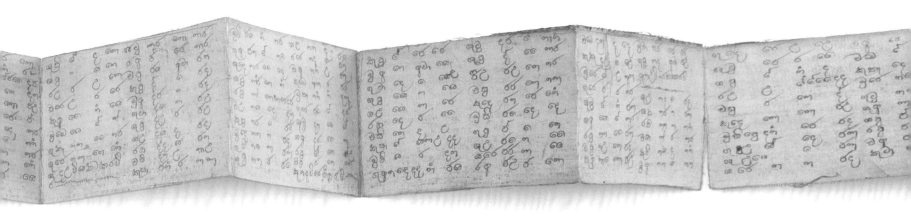

SINHALESE
ASTROLOGIC MONTHLY CALENDAR. A.D. 1800. (A)
****

This planetary scheme is available for
every day in the year, and affords information to the Native of the most favorable
hour at which to begin <u>any</u> enterprise, e.g.
when to ## commence a journey, to pick herbs
as a remedy for illness, when to get married,
etc. The decision to choose or to avoid a
particular hour is based on the individual's
horoscope — drawn and carefully preserved in
every true Sinhalese household. Calendars of
this sort are nowadays rarely written (on the
prepared leaf of the Talipot Palm) but printed in pamphlet form. They are often given to
Pilgrims to the temples. ** Presented by Dr.

China Illustrated (1670)
Athanasius Kircher, trans. François-Savinien d'Alquié

La Chine... illustrée de plusieurs monuments tant sacrés que profanes, et de quantité de recherchés de la nature & de l'art... Amsterdam.
Printed book, copper-plate engravings, 367 pp.; 9½ x 14½ in. (24 x 36.5 cm)

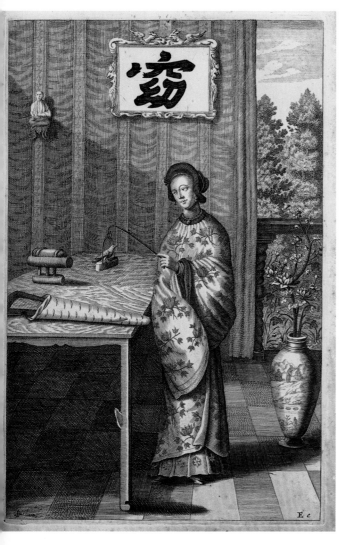

ABOVE: A Chinese beauty with tiny feet and European features. Half of a diptych reading "elegant and refined" (*yaotiao*), a learned allusion to the two-thousand-year-old *Shijing* (*Classic of Poetry*). The object wrapped in silk on the table is a *qin*, a zitherlike instrument sometimes called the Chinese lute. *La Chine*, between pp. 154 and 155

OPPOSITE: The frontispiece showing (clockwise from top left) Saints Francis Xavier and Ignatius Loyola, the co-founders of the Society of Jesuits; Matteo Ricci, leader of the China mission, with cartographic and astronomical tools; and Adam Schall, chief astronomer to the Qing court, wearing the Mandarin square of highest rank with a crane. *La Chine*, frontispiece

This lavishly illustrated French volume was originally written in Latin by the Jesuit polymath Athanasius Kircher (1602–80), who was famous throughout Europe for writing more than three dozen books on a staggering variety of topics: medicine, magnetism, optics, musicology, geology, astronomy, history, and linguistics. For his research into the eruption of Mount Vesuvius, Kircher had himself lowered into its smoking crater, but his book on China was composed without firsthand knowledge of any kind, relying instead on the published and unpublished writings of fellow Jesuit missionaries in the field, which he gathered together and embellished after his own fashion. That Kircher knew no Chinese at all, for example, did not prevent him from speculating at length that the "hieroglyphic" Chinese script was derived from the ancient Egyptians and must therefore contain Hermetic secrets and cosmic truths.

The best Dutch engravers were commissioned for the project, which took nearly five years to produce, at enormous expense. When the eagerly awaited volume was finally printed in 1667 by Johann Jansson van Waesberge, it was immediately pirated by a rival Amsterdam printer whose inferior copies found their way into many book collections. The authorized and widely read French translation that soon followed, however, was published with the original engraving plates and included a short Chinese-French "dictionary," the first of its kind ever circulated in Europe — even if it was only an eclectic word list.

Kircher's thinly veiled motives in writing the book were not only to illustrate the dazzling "spectacles" of China but also to showcase the work of Jesuit missionaries there and to plead for support of their mission. Thus the frontispiece (opposite) gives more prominence to the Jesuits illustrating China than to the China illustrated, and more than half the book is devoted to the progress of Christianity in China and to the indigenous religious beliefs that missionaries were trying to overcome.

Pride of place is given to the explication of a unique Tang Dynasty stone monument inscribed by Nestorian Christians a thousand years earlier in the city of Chang'an (modern-day Xi'an). Kircher provides a stunning double-page foldout of the 1,800-character inscription, including a few lines of Syriac, plus a verbatim translation, a pronunciation table for all the characters, and a second interpretive translation along with a detailed commentary. Modern readers are likely to skip over this section, which comprises almost the first quarter of the volume, in favor of the natural and cultural "spectacles" to follow — from dragon-shaped mountains to the Dalai Lama — but it contains the first bilingual critical edition of a Chinese text printed for European readers. Kircher argued that the discovery of the monument was a providential sign of favor for Catholicism in general and for the Jesuits in particular.

After describing the religions, government, and customs of China and adjoining regions, Kircher examines a number of Chinese spectacles from the standpoint of natural philosophy. He refutes reports of flying tortoises and wool-bearing hens as patently contrary

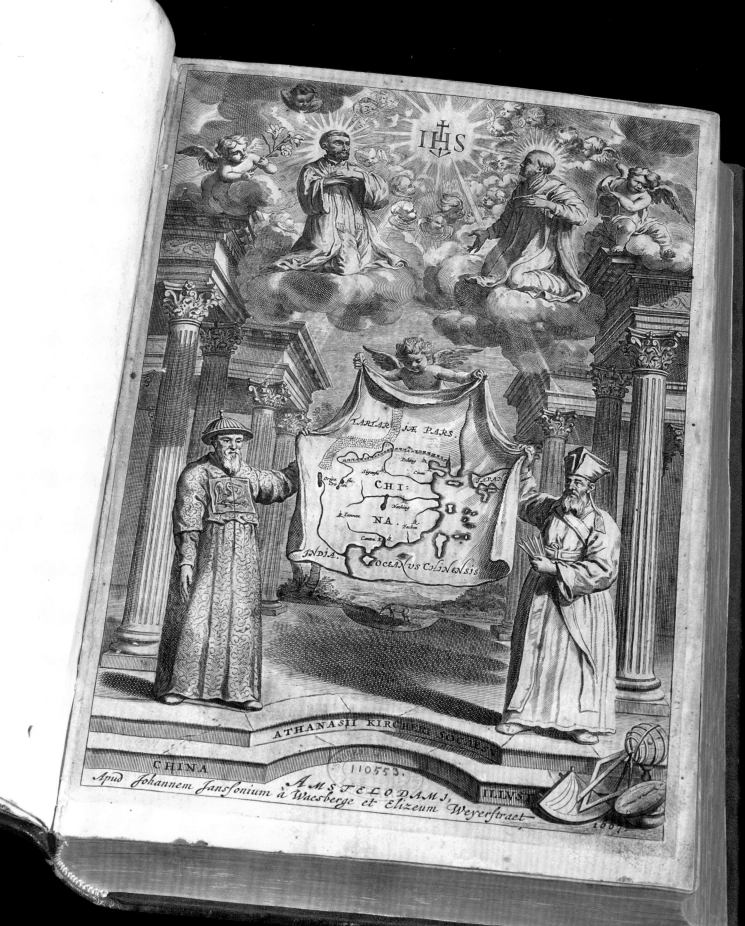

IHS

TARTARIÆ PARS.

CHI:
NA.

JAPAN

INDIA.

OCEANVS CHINENSIS.

ATHANASII KIRCHERI SOCIETS.

CHINA

110553.

ILLVST.

Apud Johannem Jansfonium AMSTELODAMI, à Waesberge et Elizeum Weyerstraet.

1667

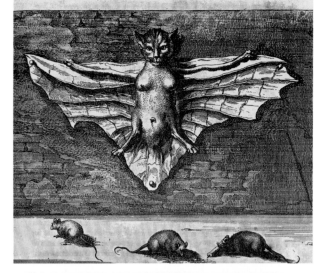

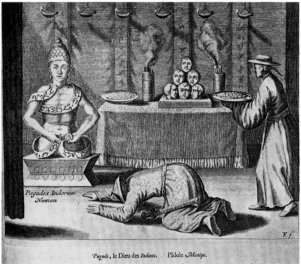

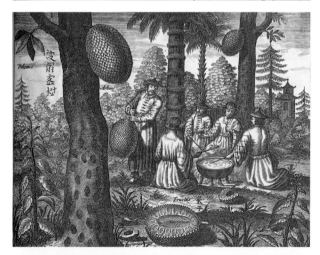

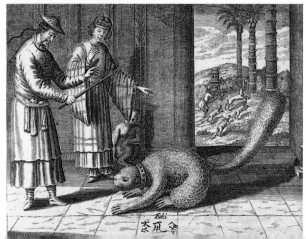

to nature (but well worth depicting anyway). Yet he credits reports of a stone found in the head of a serpent that can draw out poison on the basis of "sympathetic" virtue when applied to a bite wound, and he enthusiastically describes a yellow fish in the China Sea that metamorphoses into a feathered bird in the spring and then back again into a fish in the autumn, as a result of temperature changes and the "spermatic" influence of the birds' eggs it ingests.

As an authority on the plague Kircher was also interested in medicaments. He tells of a man-shaped root called *ginseng* that can warm the body, increase vital respiration, and even restore health to those near death, but he insists that it cannot bestow immortality as some believe. And he raves about a strong herb called *cha*, whose dried leaves are steeped in hot water to create a bitter broth that the Chinese drink at all times of the day. It is the reason they never suffer from gout or stones. It expels superfluous vapors and cures hangovers. It prevents drowsiness and wonderfully focuses the mind: it is Nature's noble gift to the Literati.

But the most precious substances were rhubarb and musk. Both had been memorably described by Marco Polo and were already in medical use in Europe, but the possibility of acquiring the purest and most potent varieties at their source was reason enough to support missionary work in China. Rhubarb, prescribed in both Europe and China as a purgative, could also be deadly in certain preparations. Kircher gives its Chinese name (*da huang*) and provides a half-page illustration of the "true" rhubarb plant—not particularly spectacular now but of undoubted interest to Kircher's readers. Musk from the wild Chinese musk deer was valued like gold, as a pharmaceutical and a perfume. It was prescribed against seizures and to improve circulation and was sometimes added to medicines as a catalyst. Kircher provides a full-page illustration of the strange creature, which nobody in Europe had ever seen before (including the illustrator). But it is also the one and only truly Chinese thing on the frontispiece (p. 65): that little animal grazing peacefully in the distance of an exotic landscape, just waiting for Europeans to come take him.

—TIMOTHY BILLINGS

LEFT, TOP TO BOTTOM: Spectacles of nature and art: a "flying cat," probably the giant flying squirrel; statues of a Tibetan Buddha and the many-headed Avalokiteshvara (confusingly called "Menipe," after the chant *Om mani padme hum*); the jackfruit (*puoluomi*), the largest tree-borne fruit in the world; and an exotic pet not recognized as a domesticated common squirrel (*song shu*). *La Chine*, pp. 113, 177, 251, 262

OPPOSITE: The proper brush grip for Chinese calligraphy, with an inkstone (enlarged) on the floor. The stylized characters on the wall, *shangfang* (Celestial Realm), along with the Ape of Nature, below, depict Kircher's belief that Chinese script is hieroglyphic in nature and thus contains secrets of creation. *La Chine*, p. 310

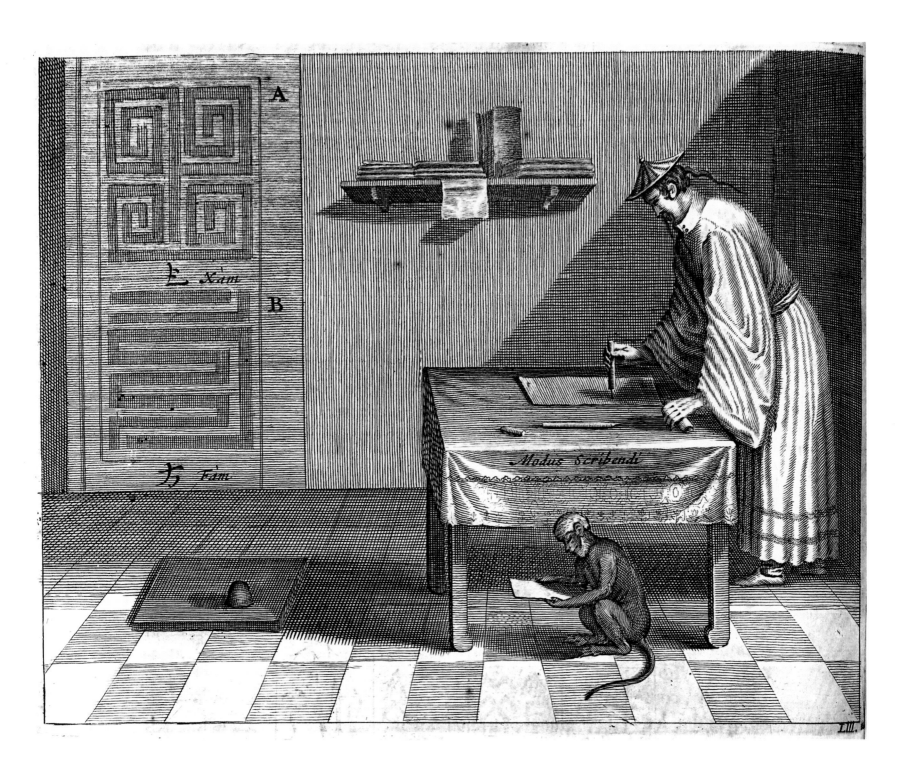

Darwin Collection (1859–1903)
Charles Darwin

London, New York, and other locations. Books, pamphlets, letters, photographs, engravings, lithographs

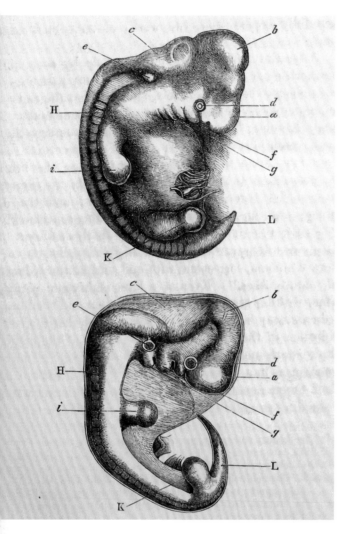

ABOVE: A comparison of a human and dog embryo at comparable stages of development. *Descent of Man* (1871), vol. 1, p. 15

OPPOSITE: *More Letters of Charles Darwin* (1903), vol. 2, frontispiece

An elderly gentleman with white beard and whiskers, swaddled in black cape and hat, leaning against a pillar entwined with a leafless vine. His eyes, bathed in shadow, convey an indeterminate expression. Is it tranquillity? Sorrow? Resignation?

This picture (opposite) may be the last formal photograph of Charles Darwin (1809–82). Although undated, it must have been taken in the final year or two of Darwin's life. His last book would appear in October 1881, just two months after the death of his beloved elder brother, Erasmus, and six months prior to his own death in April of 1882. He posed on the veranda of Down House, his home in the Kentish countryside about fifteen miles south of central London, probably for Clarence Fry, the senior photographic partner of the London firm Elliott & Fry.

Darwin had posed for photo portraits almost from the development of photographic processes in the late 1830s. A daguerreotype of him with his oldest boy, William, dates to 1842. Over the next four decades, Darwin had his portrait taken regularly—by his sons, who were keen amateur photographers, and by professionals. Initially, these were for family and friends. But Darwin's fame after the publication of *On the Origin of Species* in 1859 coincided with the explosive commercialization of the *carte de visite*. These 3½ by 2¼–inch photographs, printed on card stock, were less calling cards or even snapshots than the equivalent of trading cards. Photographers sold *cartes* of the rich and famous, politicians, actors, writers, scientists, and the like, to the general public, often in sets or albums. Darwin himself participated in this fashion, granting approval for the sale of his likeness and its inclusion in commercial albums, and he eagerly exchanged his photograph with other scientists. Such photographs, and the engravings made from them, contributed to the wide circulation of Darwin's image in Victorian culture.

Photography, and visual illustrations generally, also played an important role in Darwin's professional work. Because the *Origin* is, as Darwin famously described it, "one long argument," it uses words rather than pictures. Its single illustration, the famous "branching" diagram, was brilliant and important, but the lack of other illustrations in the book has tended to make us think of Darwin as a nonvisual thinker. Yet the *Origin* was unusual among Darwin's works, the rest of which were well illustrated—often copiously and sometimes innovatively. *The Zoology of the Voyage of the H.M.S. Beagle* (1838–43) featured colored lithographic plates of birds by John and Elizabeth Gould. *The Expression of the Emotions in Man and Animals* (1872) was among the first scientific books in English to be illustrated with photographs. Nearly two hundred zigzagging diagrams in *The Power of Movement in Plants* (1880) attempted to represent the movement of climbing plants. These images were never merely illustrative; rather, they worked with Darwin's words to advance the arguments of his books. In *The Expression of the Emotions*, for example, Darwin contended that human emotions, and our means for expressing them, are not unique to us but inherited from animals. The engravings of snarling dogs and affectionate cats in the book's earlier chapters thus prepared the way for the photographs of sneering, indignant, smiling humans in the later chapters.

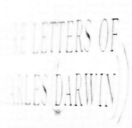

MORE LETTERS OF
CHARLES DARWIN

A RECORD OF HIS WORK
IN A SERIES OF HITHERTO
UNPUBLISHED LETTERS

EDITED BY FRANCIS DARWIN FELLOW OF
CHRIST'S COLLEGE AND A. C. SEWARD FELLOW
OF EMMANUEL COLLEGE CAMBRIDGE

IN TWO VOLUMES
ILLUSTRATED

VOL. I

Ch. Darwin

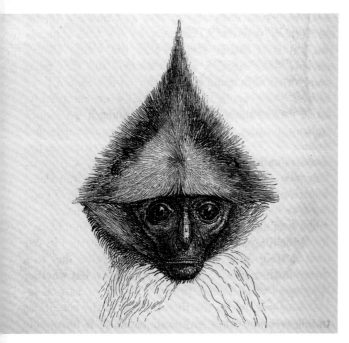

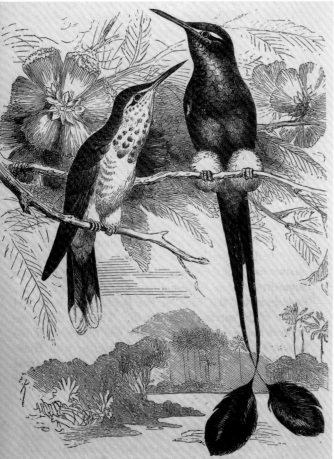

ABOVE, TOP: Monkey with a "curious crest" of hair to attract mates. *Descent of Man* (1871), vol. 2, p. 292

ABOVE: Tropical birds with brilliant plumage. *Descent of Man* (1871), vol. 2, p. 74

Photographs of the elderly Darwin helped to shape a benign and reverential image of him in the final decade of his life and in the years after his death. Here was not the wild-eyed, radical firebrand but the respectable paterfamilias, the learned philosopher, the wise lawgiver. He had begun his beard—an emblem of masculine authority for gentlemen of the period—to soothe his facial eczema but quickly recognized that it gave him a sage, even biblical, appearance. "Do I not look reverent?" he archly asked his relatives. His good friend the botanist Joseph Hooker joked that Darwin must have been the model for the fresco of *Moses' Descent from Mount Sinai* (1864) in the House of Lords. A well-known and widely respected naturalist when the *Origin* appeared, Darwin worried about his reputation, and his family, friends, and allies worked strenuously to protect it, a task made more difficult by Darwin's provocative arguments in *The Descent of Man* (1871) that not just the physical body of humans but our mental abilities, moral sense, and appreciation of beauty were part of our evolutionary inheritance from animals. And yet this giver of natural laws, the man whose views had raised such a stir among the orthodox in religion and science alike, would be buried in Westminster Abbey, the national church, in a public funeral.

This particular photograph, however, did not appear publicly until 1903, when Darwin's son Francis reproduced it as the frontispiece to the second volume of *More Letters of Charles Darwin*. An engraving made from one of the other photographs taken that day had been used by Francis as the frontispiece to the third volume of his *Life and Letters of Charles Darwin* in 1887. Francis's account of his father's life, and his presentation of his father's letters, played a major role in shaping the public's understanding of Darwin the man. So it is fitting that this photograph, like earlier ones of Darwin, contains no signs of his profession—no microscope or scientific tomes or animal bones. Except, ever so subtly, for that vine entwining the pillar.

Down House was covered with ivy and Virginia creeper, both of which had figured in Darwin's *Movements and Habits of Climbing Plants* (1875). This was a book in which Darwin, ever the boundary blurrer, had shown that plants were capable of movement and suggested that natural selection was responsible for preserving and developing it. Darwin had recounted observing the slow, sweeping motion of the Virginia creeper's tendrils, and he marveled at their adhesive power after attaching to a flat surface. "There are tendrils now adhering to my house," he wrote in *Climbing Plants*, "which are still strong, and have been exposed to the weather in a dead state for fourteen or fifteen years." Ill for much of his adult life, Darwin had doubted he would live very long. When, in 1844, he completed an essay laying out his theory of natural selection, the thirty-five-year-old Darwin left instructions for his wife, as his "most solemn & last request," to secure its publication in the event of his sudden death. Many years later the septuagenarian Darwin posed for one of his final photographic portraits with that tenacious plant, still strong many years after its death, a fitting companion.

—Jonathan Smith

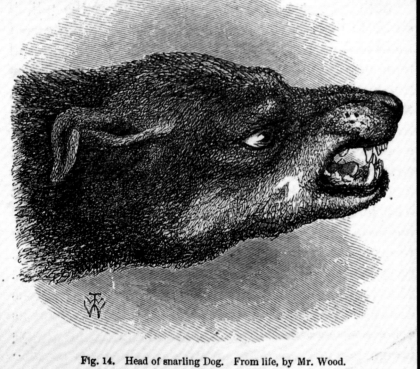

Fig. 14. Head of snarling Dog. From life, by Mr. Wood.

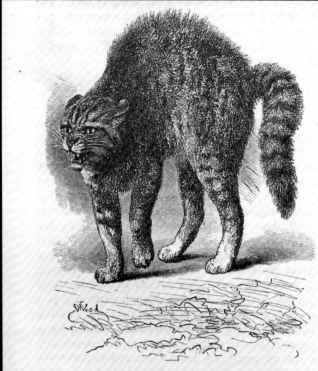

Fig. 15. Cat terrified at a dog. From life, by Mr. Wood.

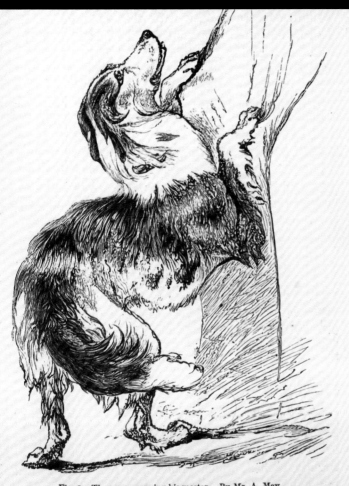

Fig. 8. The same caressing his master. By Mr. A. May.

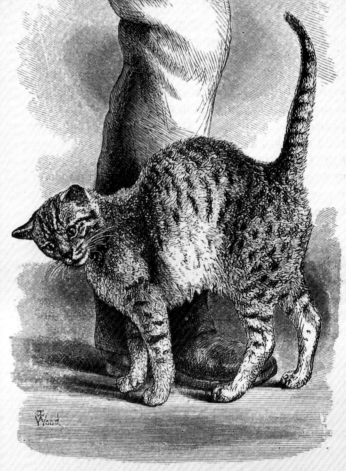

Fig. 10. Cat in an affectionate frame of mind, by Mr. Wood.

The expression of emotions in cats and dogs. *The Expression of the Emotions in Man and Animals* (London, 1872), clockwise from top left: pp. 118, 128, 59, 55

Manners, Customs and Dresses of the Hindoos (1799)
Balthazar Solvyns

Calcutta. Bound prints; 24 pp.; 251 plates, hand-colored etchings; 14⅝ x 20½ in. (37 x 52 cm)

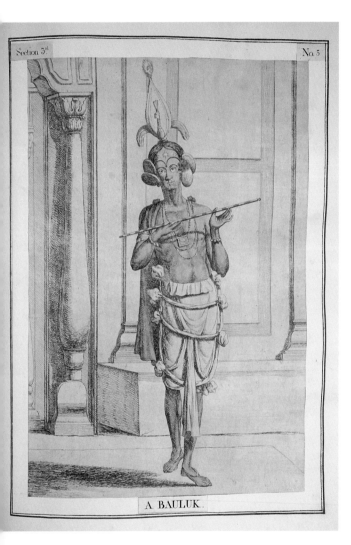

ABOVE: In *Les Hindous* (Paris, 1808) Solvyns describes three similar dancing boys dressed as *Krishna* (with painted faces, peacock feathers, metal breast plate inscribed with names of gods, feet adorned with little bells) and remarks that their "costume and danse take their origine from the remotest antiquity." *Manners*, sec. 3, pl. 5

OPPOSITE: According to Solvyns "an *Ooddoobahoo* is one who inflicts himself with pain and intolerable austerities, under the idea of its being acceptable to the Deity." Some keep an arm raised until it becomes "immoveable," others "sleep on a bed of pointed spikes and subject themselves to other incredible torments." The ocher shawl suggests that the figure shown is a Shivaite. *Manners*, sec. 7, pl. 10

By the late 1700s European printed images of India were beginning to shift from wonder-of-travel accounts by foreign artists, missionaries, and adventurers ("the picturesque") to more orderly "objective," "scientific" depictions by anthropological and colonial authorities ("the museological"). No single work better embodies this shift than Flemish artist Balthazar Solvyns's *Collection of Two Hundred and Fifty Coloured Etchings: Descriptive of the Manners, Customs and Dresses of the Hindoos.*

First published in Calcutta in 1796, this extraordinary volume features large, full-page etchings, based on original drawings, of the "residents of Hindoostan," divided into twelve sections including "Hindoo Casts [*sic*]," "Servants," "Faquirs," "Musical Instruments," "Festivals," and "Funerals." Together, they comprise a compelling social portrait of late-eighteenth-century Bengal. In the vein of other contemporary encyclopedic intellectual projects, Solvyns sought systematically to represent both the unfamiliar, such as costumes of foreign lands, and the familiar, such as typologies of peasants, craftsmen, and street vendors. Indeed, his collection of etchings was a prototype for the "Company School" paintings of occupational castes done by Indian artists for the British in the early nineteenth century. But, as the historian Richard Hardgrave suggests, it was also an ethnographic survey: the first European visual attempt to systematically portray the hierarchical ranking of Hindu castes. Other scholars have called it one of colonial India's first "para-ethnographies," predating by almost a century the photographic surveys of castes and tribes organized by British authorities.

The two plates shown here are typical of Solvyns's approach: portraits that present social types. *A Bauluk* represents the category of Bengali dancing boy but also portrays a specific dancer observed during the feast of *Jhulan Yatra*, where boys often performed along with dancing girls in *nautch* performances. The *Ooddoobahoo* print, based on observations of spectacular self-mortification practices at temples around Calcutta, is even more interesting. An *urdhbahu*, "one with upraised arm," is an ascetic who vows to keep an arm raised for twelve years or longer. Because fakirs had already become figures of fascination for Westerners, the *Ooddoobahoo* quickly became an iconic image of Indian asceticism.

Solvyns was not the first European artist to represent Calcutta life, but *Manners* far exceeds its predecessors in scope, scale, and ambition (by way of comparison, Thomas and William Daniells's *Views of Calcutta* offered only twenty aquatints). A marginal Flemish painter of ships and seascapes, Solvyns had fled turmoil in Europe to seek his fortune in India, where he produced *Manners* at tremendous personal expense. But the project failed. By contemporary European standards the etchings were adjudged crude and unfashionable. In 1803 Solvyns left India for France, where he redid the etchings for an exquisite folio of 288 plates, *Les Hindous* (Paris, 1808), which also failed owing to the Napoleonic Wars and the sheer cost of publication. But *Manners*, regarded then as a failure, succeeds brilliantly today as a tale of two cities: the colonial city, where British residents lived in their mansions, and Black Town, where migrants and Indian workers plied their trades.

—SITA REDDY

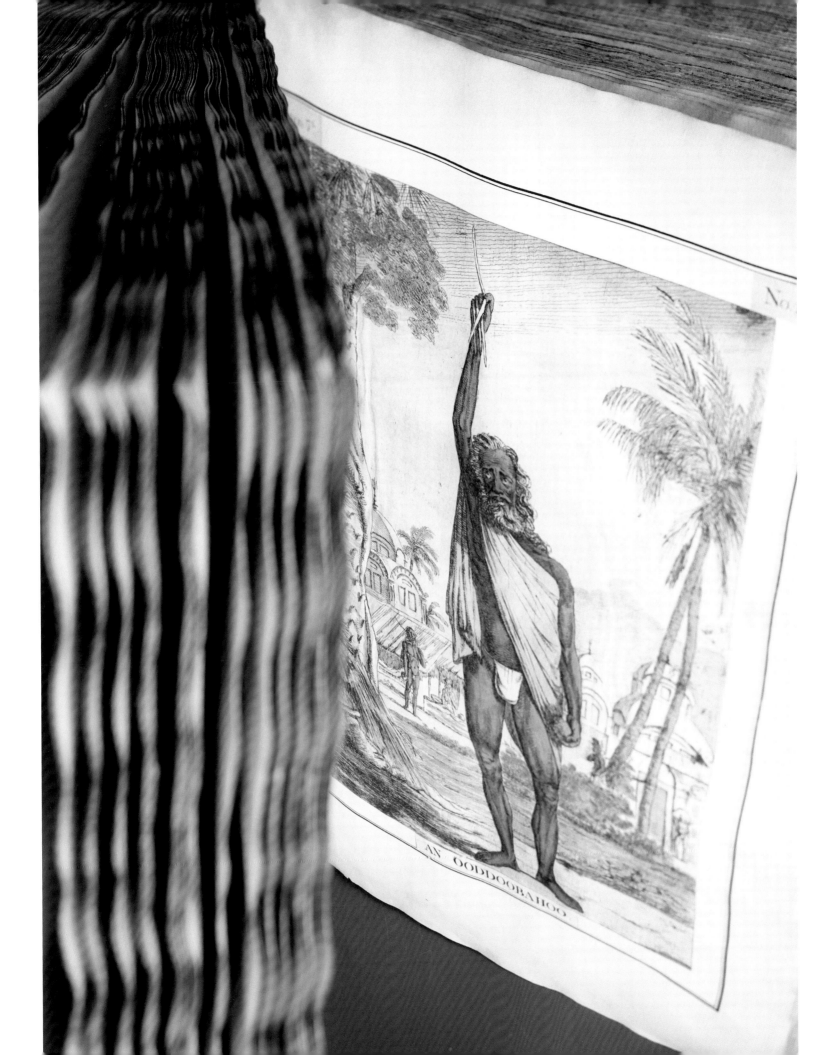

AN OODDOOBAHOO

Travels in the Interior Districts of Africa (1799)
Mungo Park

London, 2d ed. Printed book; copper-plate engravings, 377 pp. plus appendices; 8¼ x 10⅜ in. (20.5 x 26 cm)

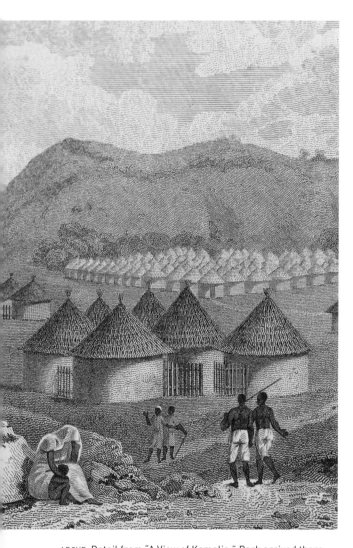

ABOVE: Detail from "A View of Kamalia." Park arrived there on September 16, 1796. In the foreground are the huts of the Kafirs, as Park termed them; in the distance are the huts of the Bushreen. *Travels*, facing p. 252; illustration by J. C. Barrow "from a sketch by Mr. Park."

OPPOSITE: "A View of a Bridge over the Ba-Fing or Black River." This river, which Park crossed in April 1797 on his return journey, is a principal tributary of the Senegal River. Park (shown seated and with sketchbook in the lower right-hand corner) reported that "the bridge is carried away every year by the swelling of the river in the rainy season." *Travels*, facing p. 338; illustration by J. C. Barrow "from a sketch by Mr. Park."

The Scotsman Mungo Park (1771–1806) was, by education and training, a physician and botanist. Prior to his voyage to Africa, he had worked in Sumatra as an assistant surgeon to the English East India Company. His account of his African travels "under the Direction and Patronage of the African Association in the Years 1795, 1796, and 1797" was sold through the London firm G. & W. Nicol. Sir Joseph Banks, the prominent English voyager and naturalist, and the broadly pro-slavery African Association were Park's patrons. They were motivated by geographical and commercial interests in West Africa (which included raw materials, minerals, and the medicinal properties of native plants) and by a concern with the then two-thousand-year-old, two-part "Niger problem": Which way did the river run (east-west or west-east) and where did it empty or reach the sea? Park solved the first part of the problem, establishing from direct observation that the "majestic Niger…[flows] slowly to the eastward." Effectively, he confirmed others' claims to this end but achieved fame by being the first European to see it and return safely.

Travels is a mixture of personal adventure (Park was beaten and stripped naked by bandits, his notes surviving only in his hatband), commentaries upon the trading networks of the interior, observations upon natural history, and ethnographic descriptions of indigenous peoples (Park described the Mandingo as "a very gentle race"). It has a sympathetic tone consistent with Scottish Enlightenment moral commentary. Park condemned Moorish slavers for their effect upon local peoples, but in the eyes of some later critics he was insufficiently critical of slavery itself.

Travels is not wholly Park's work. Upon his return to London he was assisted by Bryan Edwards of the African Association, who helped with the narrative, and eminent geographer James Rennell, who helped revise the maps and provided a lengthy "Geographical Appendix" on the Niger problem as well as a map of his own showing (erroneously) the course of the river.

Park presented his *Travels* as "a plain unvarnished tale, without pretensions of any kind, except that it claims to enlarge, in some degree, the circle of African geography." Generally, the book was well received and praised for its contributions to geographical knowledge. It provided significant new details on peoples, customs, and trade in a continent little known to Europeans. Given its success and later reception as a work of Enlightenment adventuresome travel, it is noteworthy that Park later admitted, in conversation with Sir Walter Scott, Dugald Stewart, and Adam Ferguson, that he had omitted "many real incidents and adventures" for fear that his public might think his narrative incredible.

That Park's 1799 *Travels* is still in print is testimony to its enduring importance as a work of late Enlightenment geographical exploration and to its sympathetic depiction of West African peoples and cultures. Park never solved the second part of the Niger problem: he drowned at Boussa Falls on the Niger, at age thirty-five, on a second expedition to determine where the river reached the sea.

—CHARLES W. J. WITHERS

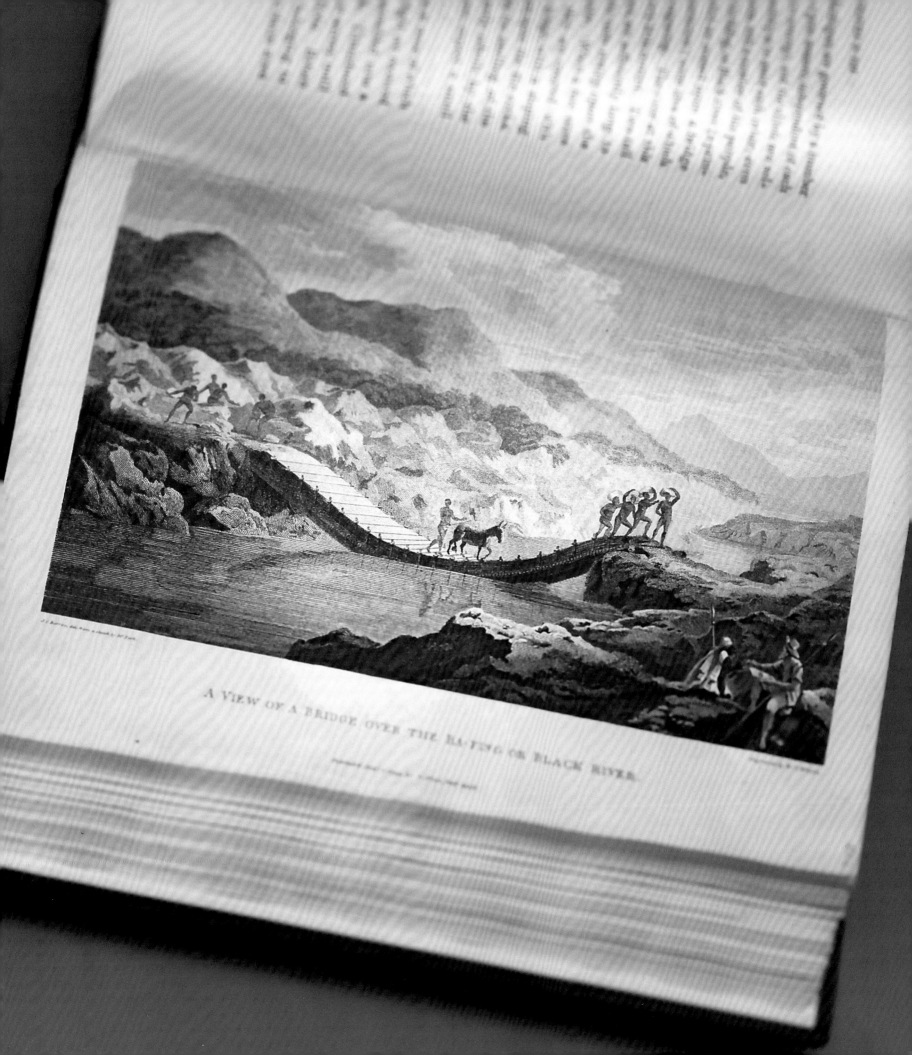

A VIEW OF A BRIDGE OVER THE RISING OR BLACK RIVER

The *Sūtra of Great Liberation* (ca. 1880–1920)

Thar pa chen po'i mdo ... Mongolia. Unbound manuscript on paper; 102 leaves, wrapped in silk with illuminated wooden boards; 3½ x 13¾ in. (9 x 35 cm)

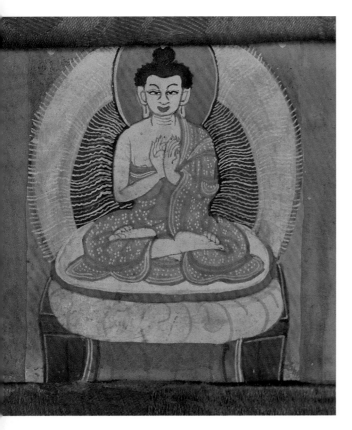

ABOVE AND OPPOSITE: The text of *Thar pa chen po'i mdo* is written on black paper with an ink that can contain gold, silver, copper, coral, lazurite, malachite, and mother-of-pearl. The unbound sheets are kept between two wooden boards covered with brocade, each with sunken compartments containing illuminations of the Eight Medicine Buddhas.

A *sūtra* is a text ascribed to the Buddha himself. This scripture bears the full title *Sūtra on Eliminating Misconduct by Means of Confession and Contrition Increasing toward Great Liberation, an Array to Attain Buddhahood*. It corresponds to a still extant apocryphal Chinese work and is one of a group of Buddhist texts translated from Chinese into Tibetan. It sets out a method of purifying bad karma and defilements through rituals of confession and repentance and by chanting the names of different Buddhas.

The earliest known Tibetan version is a fragment discovered in Dunhuang, which was a major stop on the ancient Silk Road. Tibetan catalogues of Buddhist collections prepared in the ninth century list this work, and it was included in several *Kanjur* editions of later centuries. (The *Kanjur* is a collection of mainly Buddhist works translated from Sanskrit, other Indian languages, and Chinese; the texts in the *Kanjur*, although predominantly of Indian origin, were compiled in Tibet.) In the late sixteenth century it was translated into Mongolian as the *Yekede tonilyayči sudur* (*Great Liberator Sūtra*) and, in revised form, was part of the Mongolian *Kanjur* edition prepared in the first half of the seventeenth century under the Mongol ruler Ligdan Khan (1588–1634).

The worship of *sūtra*s gained enormous popularity among the Mongols and also among the Tibetans of eastern Tibet. Soon a liturgy developed. Blo bzang nor bu shes rab (b. 1677 or 1737), a Mongolian native and Gelugpa monk, composed and propagated a meditation ritual based largely on the "Means of Accomplishment" of Buddha and the sixteen Arhats (saintly predecessors or disciples of Buddha) and on the recitation ceremony to uphold the eight Mahāyāna precepts of "abandoning" worldly pleasures and sins. This and other liturgical developments encountered vehement resistance from the monastic establishment. The eminent scholar Blo bzang chos kyi nyi ma (1737–1802) denounced these new practices in a brief work entitled *Removing Mistakes in the Recitation Method of the Great Liberation Sūtra, Sealing the Mouths of Fools*, but scholastic opposition could not stop its spread.

Read aloud, or copied by commission in Mongolian or Tibetan writing, the *sūtra* enabled believers to accumulate religious merit and extinguish sins, and it was especially featured in funeral ceremonies to purify negative karmic obstructions of the deceased. In this copy the text is written in seven lines on black paper with an ink made of precious substances known as the "Seven Jewels" that can contain gold, silver, copper, coral, lazurite, malachite, and mother-of-pearl. The long-leafed, unbound sheets are kept between two wooden boards covered with light blue brocade. Both boards possess sunken compartments with illuminations of the Eight Medicine Buddhas—Dharmakīrtisāgara, Abhijñarāja, Bhaisajyaguru, and Buddha Śākyamuni (on the upper book cover) and Sunāman, Svaraghosa, Suvarṇabhadravimala, and Aśokottama (on the lower). This beautifully embellished manuscript offers its reader the possibility of a long and healthy life and, freed from the consequences of moral wrongdoing, a good rebirth or even the "Great Liberation" from the cycle of rebirths: *nirvāna*.

—OLAF CZAJA

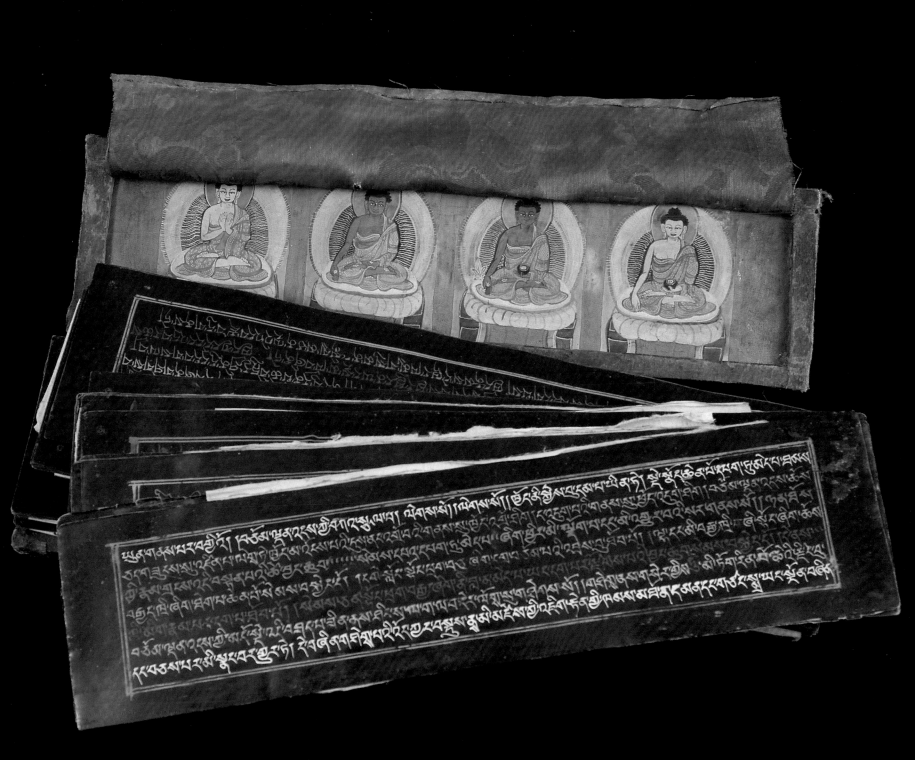

Marvels of Things Created and Miraculous Aspects of Existing Things (mid-1200s)
Al-Qazwini

Ajā'ib al-makhlūqāt wa gharā'ib al-mawjūdāt. Western India; Persian translation, nineteenth century.
Bound manuscript on paper; 210 leaves; 5¾ x 8½ in. (14.5 x 22 cm)

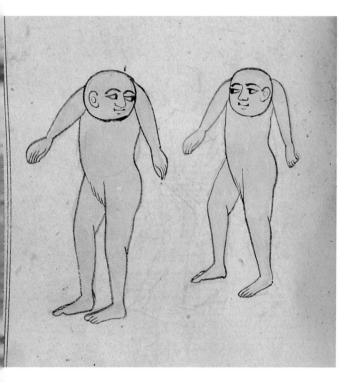

ABOVE AND OPPOSITE: Al-Qazwini's narrative of exotic places, peoples, and creatures—monkey men, mermaids, animal-headed demons, and dragons—drew on a tradition stretching back to antiquity. The neckless humans (above, fol. 59a) and centaur (opposite, fol. 24b) would have been familiar to Herodotus (fifth century BCE).

Al-Qazwini, an astronomer, geographer, geologist, mineralogist, botanist, zoologist, and ethnographer as well as cosmographer is best remembered as a compiler and synthesizer who raised cosmography to a literary genre. His *Marvels of Things Created and Miraculous Aspects of Existing Things*, often known as the *Wonders of Creation*, is the best-known Islamic cosmography. Abu Yahya Zakariya ibn Muhammad ibn Mahmud was born in 1203 in the city of Qazwin in northwest Iran, hence his sobriquet "al-Qazwini." He spent much of his life in Baghdad until his death in 1283.

Al-Qazwini's long text is divided into two discourses. In the first, on supraterrestrial things, he describes the heavenly bodies—the moon, sun, planets, and fixed stars—and the inhabitants of heaven, the angels. He ends with a consideration of the various calendars of the Arabs, Greeks, and Persians. The second discourse, four times as long as the first, treats terrestrial matters. It opens with a disquisition on the elements, the winds, and heavenly phenomena such as rainbows, thunder, and lightning. It then moves to the division of the earth into seven climes, describing all known seas, rivers, and islands, the causes of earthquakes, and the formation of mountains and wells. The author continues with a review of the three kingdoms of nature: mineral, vegetable (trees, plants, fruits, vegetables), and animal. The discussion of the animal kingdom, which forms half of the discourse, also considers man, his character and anatomy, and the characteristics of human tribes, and then moves to jinns and demons, animals, birds, and creeping things. A concluding section covers remarkable monsters and angels.

Al-Qazwini's impact can be seen in the many copies of this work, which enjoyed widespread popularity in several languages. There are not only four different Arabic versions, but also numerous Persian and Turkish translations and revisions. Its subject matter lent itself to illustration, and many manuscripts have hundreds of paintings of astronomical tables as well as plants, animals, and various beings.

The earliest copies in Arabic were produced in Iraq in the late thirteenth century during the author's lifetime. Many others were made in later centuries for a wide range of patrons. The Ottoman prince Şehzade Mustafa, son of Suleyman the Magnificent, transcribed one in Turkish, which was left unfinished at his execution in 1553. In the late sixteenth century, several fine Arabic copies were produced at the court of the 'Adilshah sultans in the Deccan plateau in India; they imitated those made several centuries earlier. Persian translations were particularly fashionable in Iran and India.

Manuscripts such as this Persian translation, copied in nineteenth-century India, were made for a popular audience, probably for sale on the open market. This copy, unsigned and undated, is illustrated with many full-page depictions of animals and other beings (opposite). The images were drawn in ink and then colored with wash to bring the text to life. It is no surprise, therefore, that al-Qazwini's text was one of the most widely read books in the Islamic lands.

—SHEILA S. BLAIR AND JONATHAN M. BLOOM

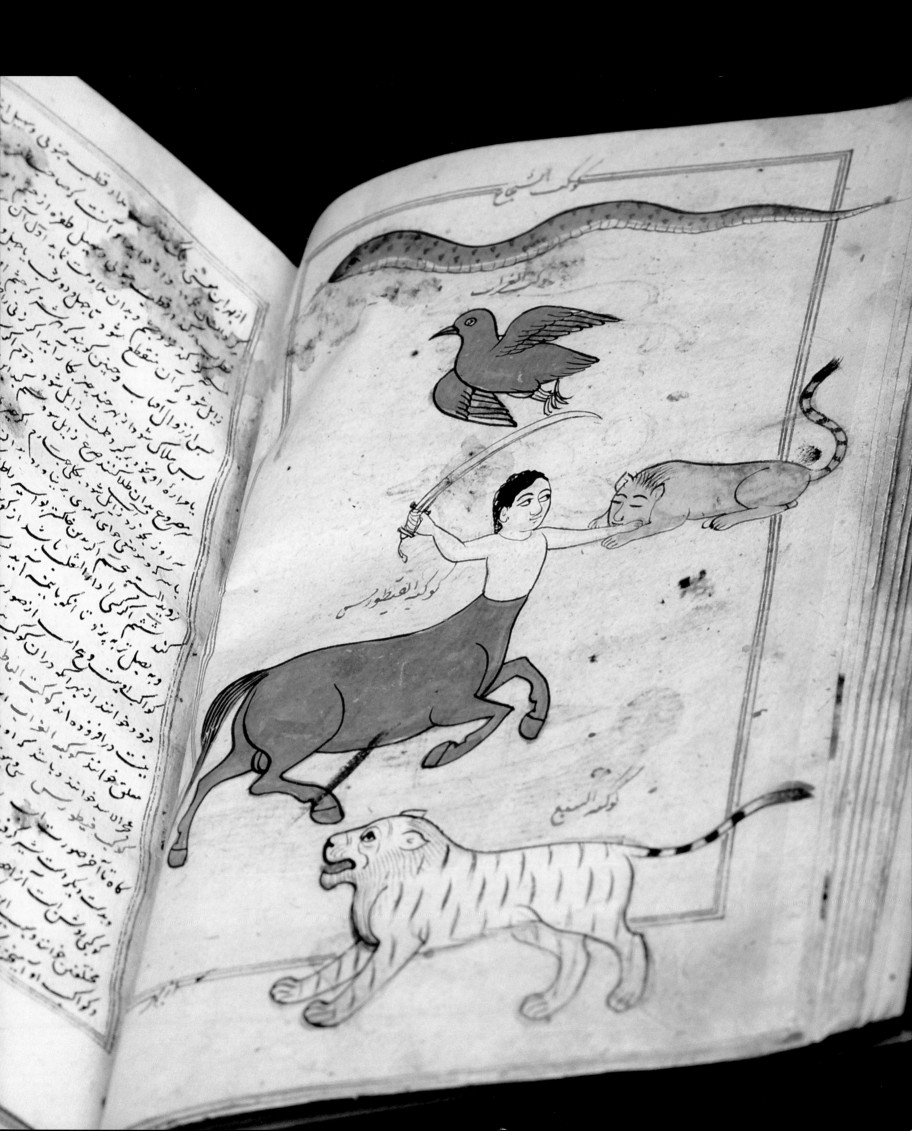

Complete Notes on the Dissection of Cadavers (1772)
Shinnin Kawaguchi

Kaishi Hen. Kyoto, Japan. Printed woodblock book, color illustrations; 28 leaves; 7⅜ x 10¾ in. (18.7 x 27.2 cm)

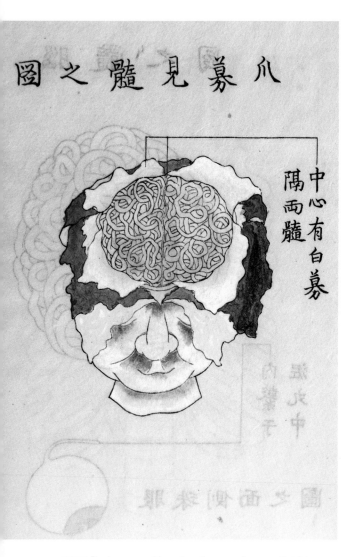

ABOVE: Brain exposed by retracting membranes. *Kaishi Hen,* 19a

OPPOSITE: Rib cage, heart, and lungs exposed by cutting open rib cage. *Kaishi Hen,* 10b

Japan's first book on human anatomy was published in 1759 by Toyo Yamawaki (1705–62), a court physician. In April 1754 Yamawaki dissected an executed criminal with permission from Tadamochi Sakai, the governor-general of the Kyoto region. Yamawaki's studies were published five years later as *Zoshi.* Despite deficiencies, such as not distinguishing between large and small intestine, and the absence of the head (unavailable owing to the execution procedure), *Zoshi* became one of the foundations of modern medicine in Japan.

The second anatomical text produced in Japan, *Kaishi Hen* (*Complete Notes on the Dissection of Cadavers*), was published in 1772 by Shinnin Kawaguchi (1736–1811). *Kaishi Hen* was a true anatomical atlas. Kawaguchi was the official physician of the Koga domain, based in what is now Koga, Ibaraki, in Japan. In 1770 Kawaguchi personally dissected a criminal executed at the Kyoto execution grounds, and the book is a record of what he found. The studies of the head, brain, and eye were the first such dissections recorded in Asia. Kawaguchi's dissection was also a key development in that it was personally performed by an actual physician (and not a surrogate or assistant). In little more than a decade, Japanese medical science had made great progress, and the beautiful colored prints in *Kaishi Hen* are much more precise than those of Yamawaki's *Zoshi.* The illustrations were produced by Shukuya Aoki (? –1789), a student of the renowned *nanga* painter Taiga Ike.

Kaishi Hen was followed in 1774 by the publication of *Kaitai Shinsho,* a translation of *Ontleedkundige Tafelen,* a Dutch version of Kulmus's anatomy (see p. 84). A group of Japanese physicians led by Genpaku Sugita and Ryôtaku Maeno had taken this work with them as a reference when they observed a dissection of an executed criminal in Edo three years earlier. Astounded at its accuracy, Sugita and Maeno decided to translate it into Japanese. *Kaitai Shinsho* became well known in Japan and is even referred to in elementary school textbooks. It surpassed *Kaishi Hen,* which is now mostly known only to specialists.

When these books were published, the Tokugawa Shogunate had isolated Japan, banning its subjects from interacting with foreigners and allowing only restricted diplomatic and trade contacts. The only information that Japanese physicians could get about Western medicine was what filtered into the country via a Dutch trading post at Dejima in Nagasaki.

There was another obstacle to the adoption of Western medicine: the cutting open of a body to examine what was inside was considered unethical and treated as taboo, requiring special permission from the authorities. Until these anatomies were published in the second half of the eighteenth century, people in Japan mainly used *kampo* herbal medicines derived from traditional Chinese medicine. The Western approach of using surgical instruments came as a great surprise to the Japanese. When physicians were suddenly confronted with representations of the structure of the human body—and the opportunity to dissect—they began to incorporate Western medical practices and ideas into their medicine. Because the new medicine had reached Japan via the Dutch, it was called *rampo* (Dutch-method) medicine, in contrast with *kampo* (Chinese-method) medicine.

—MAMI HIROSE

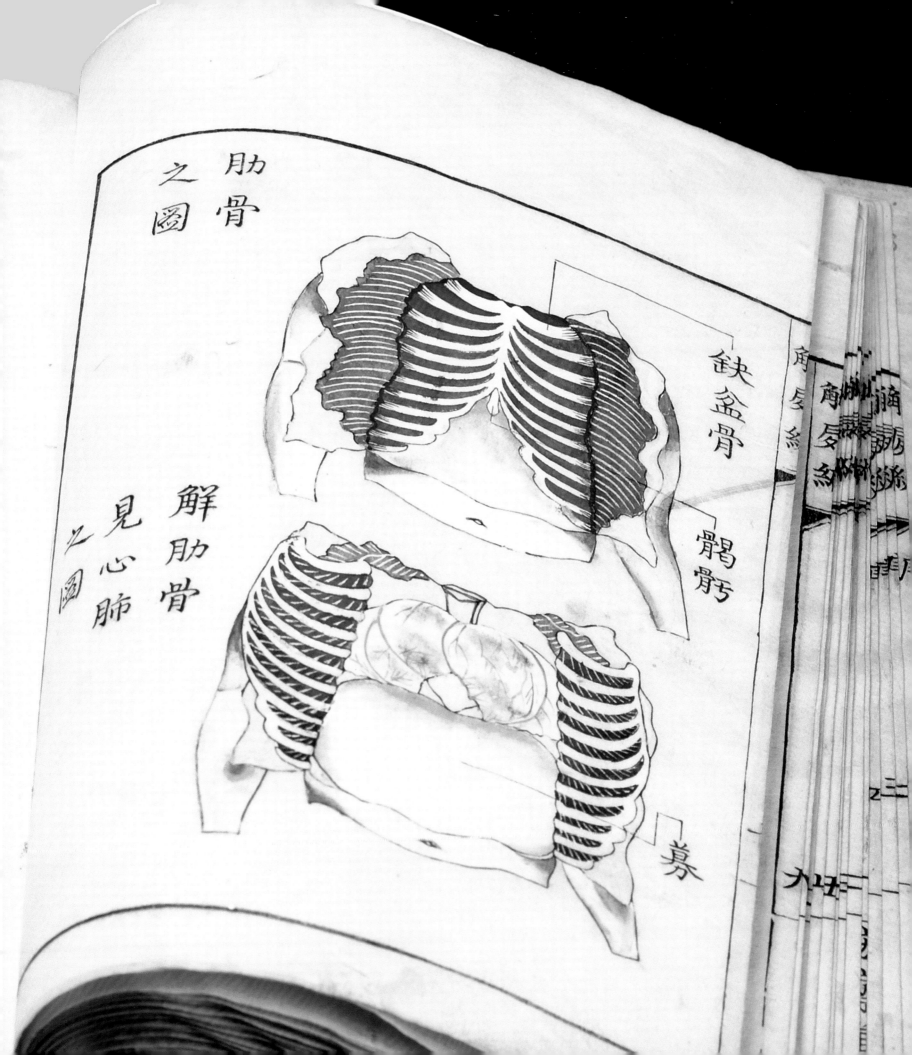

肋骨之圖

解肋骨見心肺之圖

鈌盆骨

骷骨

募

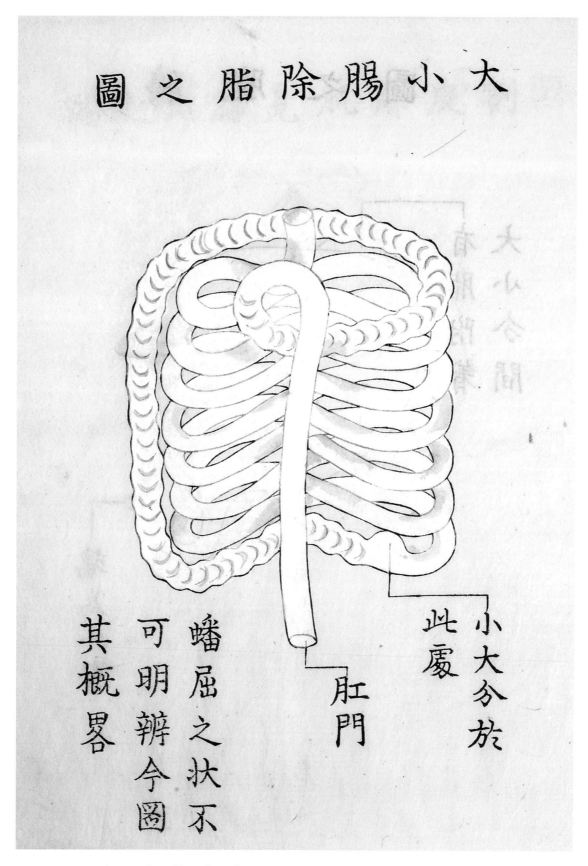

大小腸除脂之圖

蠕屈之狀不
可明辨今圖
其概畧

肛門

此處

小大分於

ABOVE AND OPPOSITE: Large and small intestines after removing fat, *Kaishi Hen*, 21a; muscles and attachments, 14a

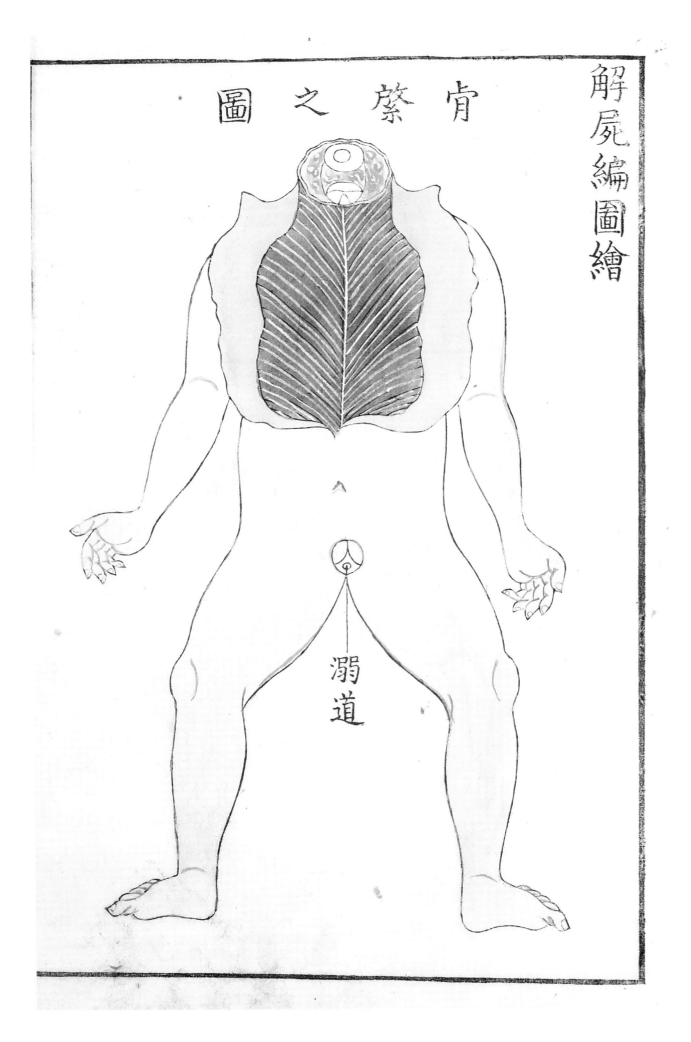

肓縶之圖

溺道

New Book on Anatomy (1774)
Johann Adam Kulmus and others; translated by Genpaku Sugita and Ryôtaku Maeno

Kaitai Shinsho. Tobu, Japan. Printed woodblock book, 5 vols.; 7 x 10½ in. (17.7 x 26.5 cm)

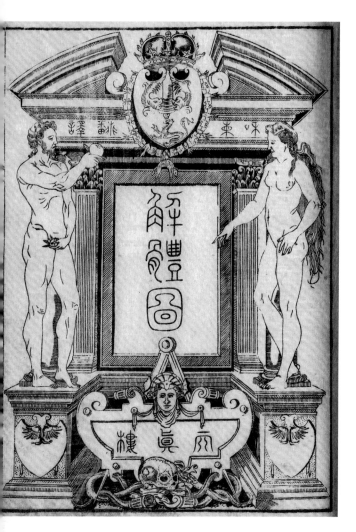

ABOVE: Some of *Kaitai Shinsho*'s illustrations were taken from sources other than Kulmus—a detail that reminds us that the translators consulted a variety of Western texts to help them understand their text. The frontispiece was drawn from Juan Valverde de Amusco's *Vivae imagines partium corporis humani* (1566). *Kaitai Shinsho,* prologue vol., frontispiece

OPPOSITE: For Genpaku Sugita, Western anatomy offered not only new ideas about the body but a new and more precise way of seeing. The figures of the floating abdomen and the hanging dissected cadaver derive from Andreas Vesalius, *De humani corporis fabrica* (1543), but are reversed (in Vesalius the cadaver is suspended by his right shoulder and the abdomen appears in the upper right corner of the plate). *Kaitai Shinsho,* prologue vol., 9b and 10a

single drop of oil that spreads to cover an entire pond." The influence of his book had been like that, Genpaku Sugita (1733–1817) mused near the end of his life. Reflecting on how its publication had changed the whole country, he felt, even in his eighties, like dancing with joy.

Kaitai Shinsho (1774), literally "Understanding Body New Text," initiated the modern transformation of Japan. As the first published Japanese translation of a Western anatomical text, it revealed many structures previously unknown to Japanese doctors and transplanted the idea of dissection as the foundation of medicine. Even more importantly it opened the door to the study of Western languages and science. Other translations on other subjects soon followed.

On the fourth day of the third month of 1771, Sugita, Ryôtaku Maeno (1723–1803), and Jun'an Nakagawa (1739–86) attended their first ever dissection of a human cadaver. It was a revelation: the three men were stunned by the close match between the organs exposed before them and the illustrations in the anatomical guide that they had brought along—a Dutch version of the German-language *Anatomische Tabellen* (1722) of Johann Adam Kulmus (1689–1745). True knowledge of the body, they concluded, was found here, in Western texts, rather than in the revered medical classics of ancient China. Japanese doctors had to completely relearn their science. As the three men walked home from the dissection, Sugita excitedly proposed the idea of translating Kulmus's manual. They began work the next morning.

It was an ambition of dizzying boldness. A translation? Sugita and Nakagawa were doctors but they scarcely knew even the Western alphabet; Kulmus's text was more than two hundred pages long. Maeno's Dutch vocabulary was limited to some seven hundred or eight hundred words; there were no dictionaries or grammars to consult. The three, along with other collaborators, would sometimes spend whole afternoons puzzling over the sense of a single phrase.

They inevitably mistook some meanings, and a few details ("talus bone," for example) stumped them to the end. The retranslation later published by Sugita's disciple Gentaku Ôtsuki (1757–1827), *Chôtei Kaitai Shinsho* (1826), would be more exact and complete. Still, their achievement was impressive: in just three years they crafted a translation that got most things mostly right. Many of their neologisms for alien concepts such as "nerve" and "artery" remain basic to modern Japanese.

Pictures are key to this tale. Beyond guiding the translators in their struggles to decipher words, anatomical plates inspired the very idea of translation: Sugita's immediate conviction in the truth of Western medicine was a response to the precise and detailed realism of the European copper-plate engravings. The enthusiastic reception of *Kaitai Shinsho*, in turn, owed much to Naotake Odano (1749–80), an artist recently trained in Western techniques, who made woodblock prints from Kulmus's illustrations. The opening of a new world of knowledge turned crucially on the transfer of a style of picturing that no one had seen before.

—SHIGEHISA KURIYAMA

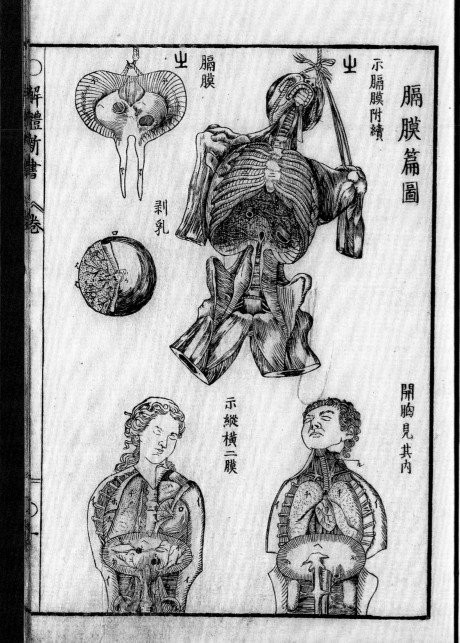

膈膜篇圖

示膈膜附續

膈膜

剥乳

開胸見其内

示縱横二膜

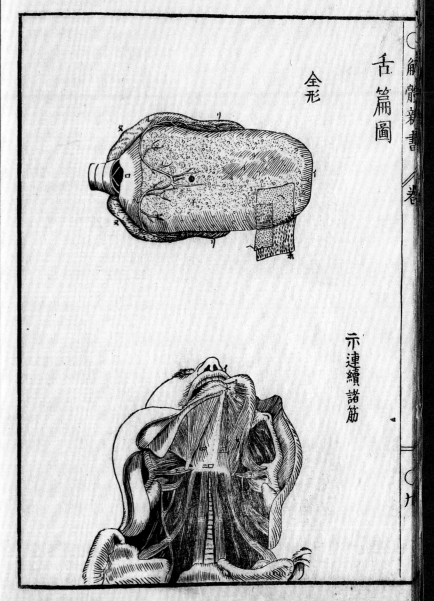

舌篇圖

全形

示連續諸筋

An Anatomical Essay on the Movement of the Heart and Blood in Animals (1628 and other editions)

William Harvey

Exercitatio anatomica de motu cordis et sanguinis in animalibus. Frankfurt-am-Main, Germany. 1st ed.; 72 pp. with etchings; 5½ x 7³⁄₁₆ in. (14 x 18.2 cm)

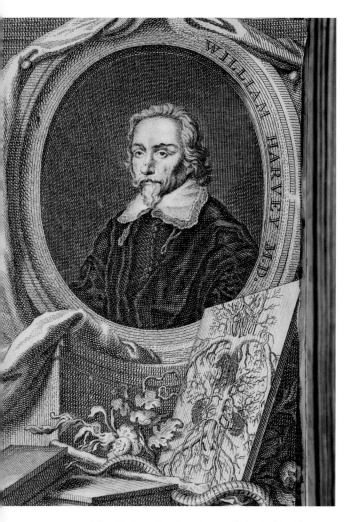

ABOVE: A frontispiece drawing of a very botanical looking human circulatory system, on a table with books, vines, and an Asclepius staff (with snake curled around), propped up against a portrait of William Harvey. *Anatomical Exercises of Dr. William Harvey...* (London, 1673)

OPPOSITE: In *De motu cordis*, chap. 13, using a ligature on the arm, Harvey demonstrates how the valves and arteries are interconnected, and how the valves in the veins allow blood to flow back toward the heart. *Exercitatio anatomica de motu cordis...* (Leiden, 1737)

William Harvey's *De motu cordis et sanguinis in animalibus* is the single most famous exercise in medical research to have come down to us from the premodern age. In just seventy-two pages of somewhat cumbersome Latin prose, Harvey (1578–1657), the personal physician of King Charles I, dismantled centuries of Galenic medical dogma to present a new image of the body. Drawing on the observation of the still beating hearts of vivisected frogs, fish, dogs, and pigs, together with mathematical calculation and an elegantly simple experiment involving ligatures tied around a human arm, Harvey showed how blood flowed through the arteries and veins via the lungs, propelled by the contractions of the heart in systole. *De motu cordis* thus represented the triumph of the "new science" of the seventeenth century, a science in which observation and experiment took precedence over classical textual authority, no matter how ancient.

Except that it didn't quite happen in that way. A conservative by nature, in setting out his ideas on circulation, Harvey was in some respects following well-trodden ground: the view that blood moved through the infamous "invisible pores" of the septum of the heart (a key element in the Galenic system) had been denied by the Paduan anatomist Realdo Colombo (1516–59) in the mid-sixteenth century; the pulmonary transit of the blood had been posited by Arabic authorities in the thirteenth century, and again by the Protestant heretic Michael Servetus (1511?–53) some seventy years before *De motu cordis* appeared. In fact, what Harvey believed he was doing was reasserting the primacy of Aristotle's biological views. As explained in the crucial eighth chapter of *De motu cordis*, Harvey's own Aristotelian view of the primacy of the heart and of the importance of circular motion rested, in the end, on a metaphorical view of the world, in which Nature ("who does nothing in vain") endlessly replicates herself. Blood circulates in the body, Harvey claimed, in much the same way that the planetary bodies move in circles, or that moisture, warmed by the sun, circulates in the atmosphere. The heart was much more than a mere pumping mechanism. Instead, its "fiery heat" represented a "store of life…the sun of our microcosm."

In restoring the heart to this quasi-mystical primacy Harvey, a Royalist, was also implicitly making a political statement. *De motu cordis* was extravagantly dedicated to King Charles, whom Harvey addressed as "the sun of his microcosm, the heart of the state." The function of kings, hearts, and the sun was essentially the same: to spread life and succor ("power…and grace") throughout their respective domains. In 1628, the year in which Harvey's treatise appeared, the king had already embarked upon his disastrous confrontation with Parliament, which would lead to the eleven years of "personal rule" in which Charles attempted to govern the macrocosm of the state in much the same way that Harvey believed the heart "ruled" the body: in splendid isolation.

—JONATHAN SAWDAY

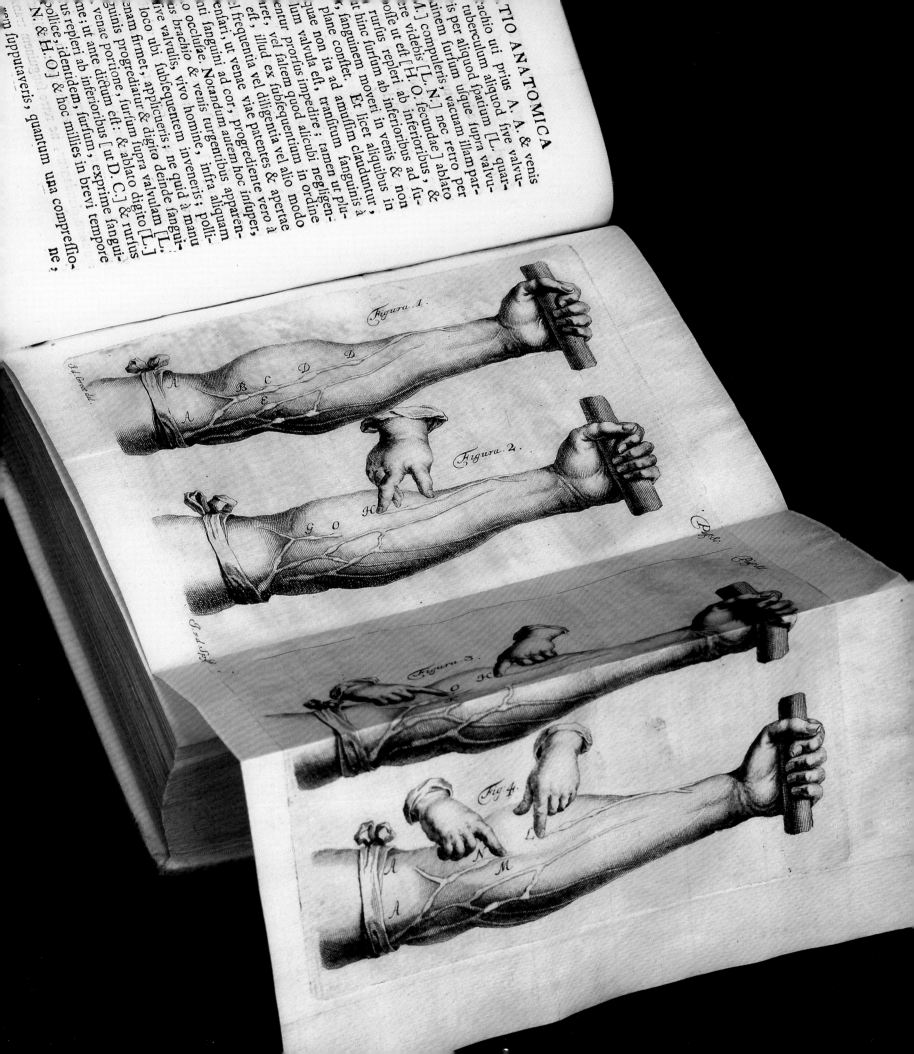

A. A. & venis
brachio ui prius A. A. & venis
tuberculum aliquod five valvu-
is per aliquod fpatium [L. quar-
quinem furfum ufque illam par-
M.] compuleris, vacuam illam par-
re videbis [L. N.] nec retro per-
offe ut eft [H. O. fecundae] ablato
rurfum ab inferioribus ad fu-
t hinc furfum moveri in venis & non
fanguinem moveri in venis & non
quae non ita ad amuffim fanguini,
plane conftet. Et licet aliquibus in
lum valvula eft, tranfitum ut plu-
quae non ita ad amuffim fanguinis à
centur, illud ex diligentia vel alio modo
ret, vel faltem quod alicubi in ordine
el frequentia viae patentes & apertae
ref, illud ex diligentia vel aperiae
enfari, ut venae diligentia vel alio à
ni fanguini ad cor, progrediente vero à
o occlufae. Notandum autem hoc infuper,
s brachio, vivo homine, infra aliquam
o occlufae, venis turgentibus appaen-
ive valvalis, applicueris; ne quid à manu
loco ubi fubfequentem inveneris; polli-
enam firmet, applicueris & digito deinde fangui-
nam firmet, furfum fupra valvulam [L.]
porione, furfum fupra valvulam [L.
guinis progrediatur & ablato digito [L.]
venae portione, furfum fupra digito [ut L.
ne; ut ante dictum eft: & ablato fangui-
us repleri ab inferioribus [ut D. C.] & rurfum
pollice, identidem, furfum, exprime fangui-
em fuppuraveris, quantum una compreffio-
N. & H. O] & hoc millies in brevi tempore
ne ?

Drawings of Arteries (ca. 1797)
Charles Bell

Edinburgh. Bound manuscript; ink and watercolors; 70 pp.; 7½ x 10⅝ in. (19.2 x 27 cm)

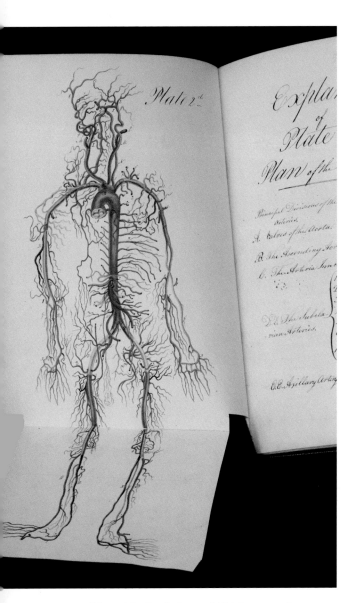

ABOVE: "Plan of the Aortic System." This image works at two levels: it is both a map of arteries and veins and a recognizable human form, yet without a clear outline—an absence that renders it somewhat surreal, especially the head. Drawings, pl. 2

OPPOSITE: Bell did not give this poignant plate a title. The "sketch," in Bell's own words, is from "the head of [a] black [showing] the most common and regular distribution of the branches of the Carotid Artery." Drawings, pl. 4

*S*ir Charles Bell (1774–1842) is a complex figure in the history of medicine. His name is associated with a number of achievements such as diagnosing Bell's palsy (a type of facial paralysis) and Bell's spasm (a facial tic), while his extensive engagement with the fine arts is well known and his work as an artist admired. In addition to his writings on anatomy, surgery, physiology, and facial expression, Bell also authored *The Hand* (1833), a work on natural theology designed to affirm the existence of God through the study of His works. Thus Bell has been treated both as a medical hero, especially for his work on the nervous system, and as a kind of marvel by virtue of being talented in both medicine and the visual arts.

His theological concerns fit less readily into conventional narratives of medical progress. Yet they remind us that Bell thought hard about a range of major intellectual issues—the nature of human will, for instance—and in examining any one of his works it is helpful to bear this breadth in mind. Equally vital is his background. He was born in Edinburgh during the Enlightenment, when the city possessed a culture of extraordinary vitality in philosophy and literature as well as in the visual arts and medicine. Talented as Bell undoubtedly was, the love he manifested for studying the human body both intellectually and aesthetically and the expression of it through the manual activities of dissection, drawing, printmaking, and painting were by no means unusual. These points help us to appreciate the exquisite work in this manuscript with its twelve colored plates.

This book is only attributed to Bell, since he nowhere signed or dated it; most likely it was produced before 1800, and hence by a young man. Many of the basic principles of illustrated anatomical works were well established by the end of the eighteenth century: a picture of a dissection, with specific parts identified by a letter, which in turn refers to an accompanying explanation. Bell's illustrations are intriguingly diverse, visually speaking. They range from those that show body parts severed from their context, such as plate 2 (left), to images where the humanity of the dissected subject is inescapable, as in plate 4 (opposite). The fact that all the images are colored certainly adds to their appeal, lending them an elegant vitality. While the palette is rich and vivid, the subject matter is distinctly somber.

Bell's aesthetic is difficult to define and does not fit easily into familiar style terms. No doubt it was driven, at least in part, by natural theology, which found visual evidence of God's design in His creation. Bell's networks included major contemporary artists such as the Landseer brothers, hence placing his images in such artistic contexts would be particularly productive. Until such scholarship is further developed, however, we can at least enjoy, honor, and reflect upon this unusual work by paying it careful attention.

—LUDMILLA JORDANOVA

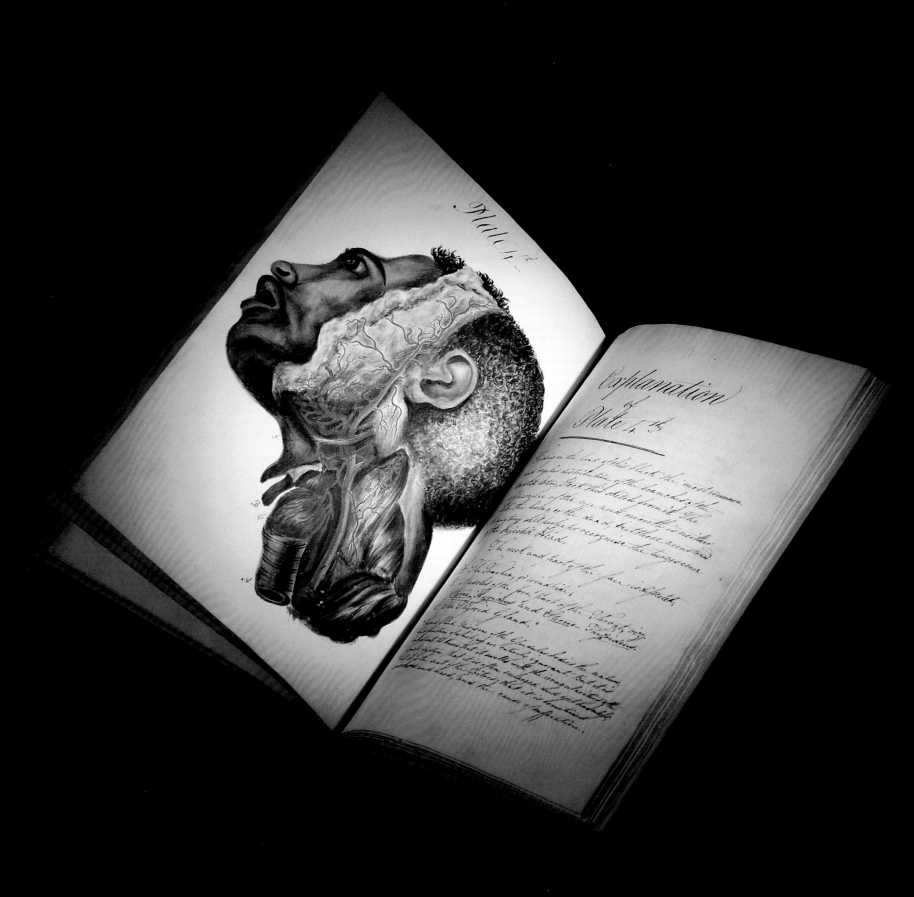

Atlas of Topographic Anatomy (1911)
Eugène-Louis Doyen with J.-P. Bouchon and R. Doyen; heliotypes by E. Le Deley

Atlas d'anatomie topographique. Paris. Printed book, 7 parts in 4 vols.; 12 x 8⅝ in. (30.5 x 22 cm)

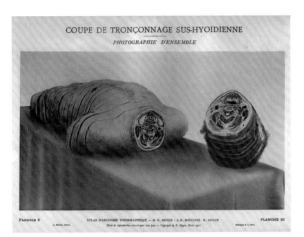

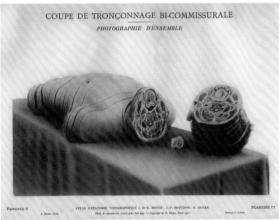

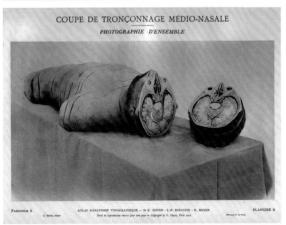

Issued in seven installments by the flamboyant Parisian surgeon Eugène-Louis Doyen (1859–1916), this atlas of 279 "heliotyped" photographic plates of cross-sectioned bodies was a radical departure from past practice. In the early twentieth century the use of photography in anatomy was rare—most anatomies featured lithographic or engraved drawings and paintings. Rarer still was the representation of the human body in such a starkly uncompromising and aggressive fashion, as if, one critic argued, it was "nothing more than slices of the most common tree." But more than that, Doyen's atlas was highly theatrical and provocative in its poses. Ostensibly designed to instruct students and serve as a reference for colleagues, it seemed deliberately to flout professional decorum.

It was created through a process he called megatomy, similar to the way microtomes were used to prepare histological slides but with much larger and thicker slices. Doyen preserved the bodies using a technique to harden the organs while maintaining their shape and color. After a series of injections with preserving fluids, the cadavers were left for two to six months, the length of time depending on levels of fat in the body. Having undergone this "veritable scientific mummification," the bodies were secured on a mobile trolley mounted on rails and fed through the megatome, a five-meter-long band saw running on a six-horsepower engine. The slices, mounted and sequentially photographed for reproduction in the *Atlas*, were then retained for use in lectures and displays. The photographic plates were heavily retouched, resulting in a strangely arresting hybrid of photography and painting.

During his career the enormously prolific Doyen devised many new techniques and inventions, including an electrical treatment for cancer. The first surgical filmmaker, he produced and starred in more than sixty motion pictures between 1898 and 1906 (including one of a surgery to separate conjoined twins). Variously described as brilliant, extravagant, and a charlatan, the self-promoting Doyen was politically active on the left, a philanthropist and controversialist celebrated across Europe and America, even as he was deplored and ostracized by the medical establishment.

His first attempt to display his anatomical slices ended in tumult. On April 19, 1910, more than two thousand students, professors, and socialites crammed themselves into the grand amphitheater at the Faculty of Medicine in Paris to see the opening of Doyen's course in topographic anatomy. Many came to protest. During the lecture, which was illustrated by colored lantern slide projections of the photographic plates, Doyen stood by as a chorus of boos and whistles went up; paper planes thrown from the audience gave way to stones and fistfights broke out. When the faculty suspended the course Doyen moved on to other venues and continued to give lectures featuring projections, films, and dissections performed on the spot for audiences of up to a thousand.

Doyen believed that photography and motion pictures would come to play a vital role in surgical pedagogy and research. Most of his photographs were destroyed during World War II, leaving copies of this fragile atlas as a rare material trace of his legacy.

—Lisa O'Sullivan

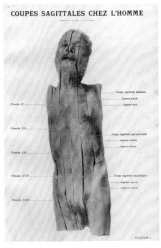
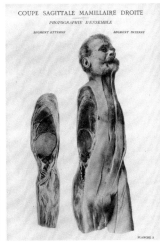
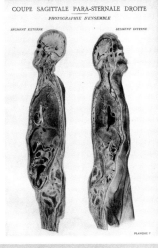
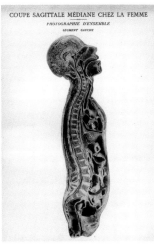
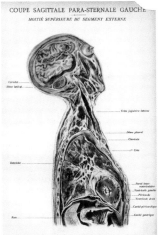
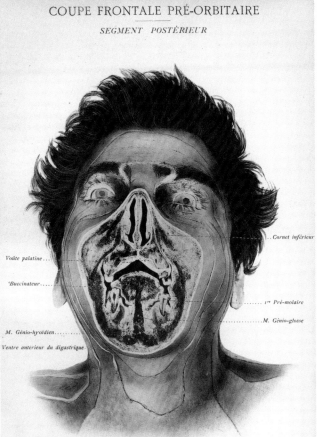

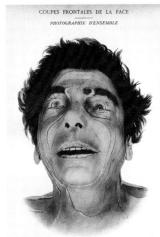
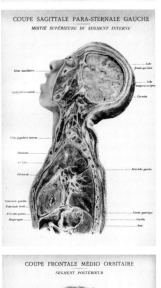
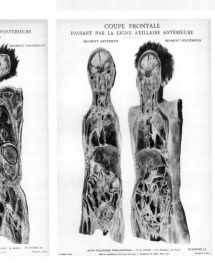
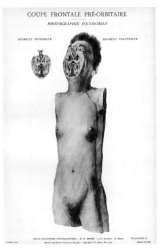
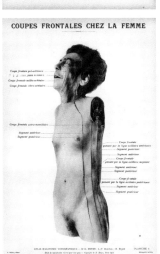

COUPE SAGITTALE MAMILLAIRE DROITE

MOITIÉ SUPÉRIEURE DU SEGMENT INTERNE

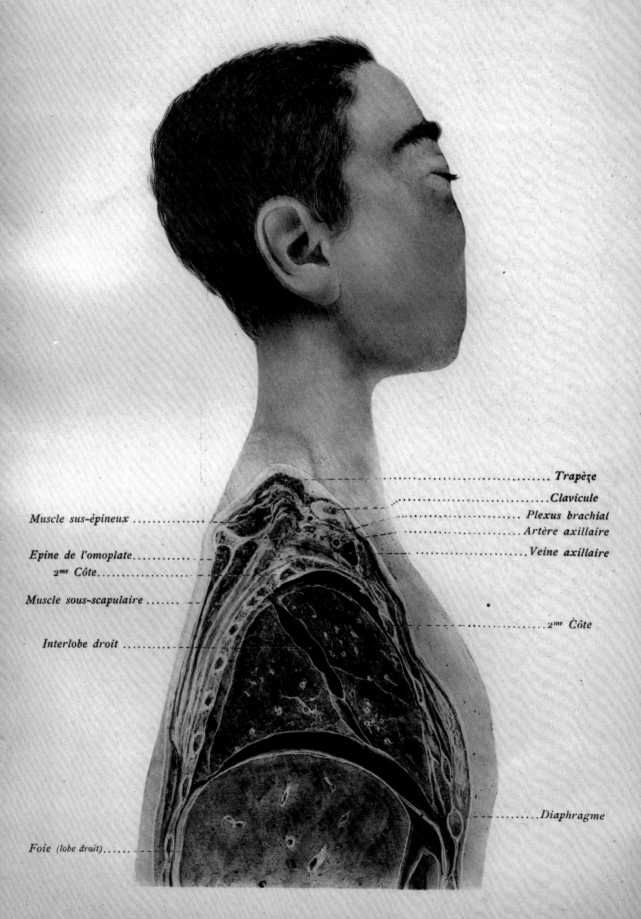

Trapèze

Clavicule

Muscle sus-épineux .... Plexus brachial

Artère axillaire

Epine de l'omoplate .... Veine axillaire

2me Côte ....

Muscle sous-scapulaire ....

2me Côte

Interlobe droit ....

Diaphragme

Foie (lobe droit) ......

ATLAS D'ANATOMIE TOPOGRAPHIQUE — Dr E. DOYEN - J.-P. Bouchon - R. Doyen   PLANCHE 2

A. Maloine, éditeur   Droit de reproduction réservé pour tous pays — Copyright by E. Doyen, Paris 1911   Héliotypie E. Le Deley

COUPE DE TRONÇONNAGE DU POIGNET
PASSANT PAR LA PREMIÈRE RANGÉE DES OS DU CARPE

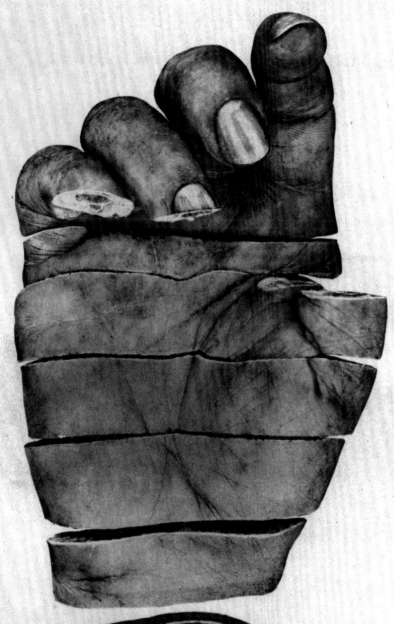

Extenseurs..Long extenseur du pouce
Cubital postérieur..Radiaux

Semi-lunaire...Court abducteur du pouce
Apophyse styloïde du cubitus..........................Scaphoïde

Muscles fléchisseurs superficiels
et profonds..........................Tendon du long supinateur
Cubital antérieur................................Artère radiale
Nerf médian.............................

Tendon du muscle grand palmaire

Tendon du muscle petit palmaire

ATLAS D'ANATOMIE TOPOGRAPHIQUE — Dr E. DOYEN - J.-P. BOUCHON - R. DOYEN

The Palmistry Entertainment of Praetorius, or The Treasury of Palmistry (1661)

Johann Praetorius with works by Robert Fludd, Nicolaus Pompeius, and Caspar Schott

Ludicrum chiromanticum Praetorii; seu Thesaurus chiromantiae... Leipzig. Printed book, 1,026 pp.; 6⅜ x 7½ in. (16 x 19.4 cm)

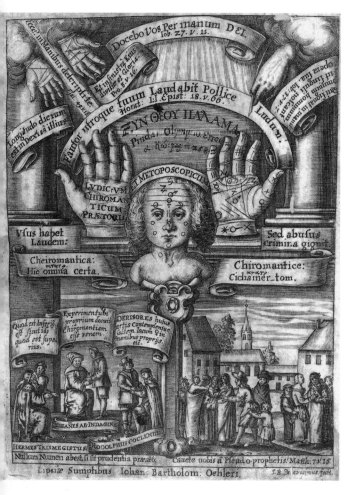

ABOVE: *Ludicrum chiromanticum Praetorii* engraved title page emblematizes chiromancy's practical and philosophical components. In the center of the page a pair of hands flank a face; planetary symbols adorn their key features.

OPPOSITE: Pompeius's *Chiromantiae praecognita* is supported by a foldout page listing the *nota*, symbols that are drawn by connecting the points in the hands.

Chiromancy, the art of palm reading, thrived in Renaissance Europe. It worked on the premise that the geography of the hand could be read. The three main lines, for instance, could be correlated with the principal organs: heart, brain, and liver. The geography of the hand—a "mountain" was formed at the base of each digit, joined by "plains"—could be read alongside a celestial map. Manuals of chiromancy circulated in manuscript from the fourteenth century and were printed in increasing numbers through the seventeenth century. Chiromancy was akin to astrology (divination from the stars) and physiognomy (the reading of the face). After around 1600, following a papal bull denouncing chiromancy and other forms of divination, some authors sought to explain chiromancy, like physiognomy, as wholly natural. Others, such as the English physician Robert Fludd (1574–1637), developed the astrological components of the art. Fludd was known for his elaborately illustrated tomes on occult philosophy and disputes with the French theologian and philosopher Marin Mersenne (1588–1648).

As more people began to practice the art its legitimacy was increasingly challenged, and questions about its principles and plausibility featured in debates about occult philosophies and the theological legitimacy of divination. Concerns about the operation of natural causes and the extent of free will were at the root of these debates. If the lines on the hand were caused by the positions of the planets at the time of one's birth, then one's hand could be read as accurately as, or more accurately than, one's nativity. Did a chiromancer read the natural signs of one's character, like a physiognomer? Or, like an astrologer, did he traffic with unnatural spirits and meddle in free will? Or was he simply a charlatan peddling causal implausibilities in the name of an ancient art?

The Palmistry Entertainment was assembled in 1661 by Johann Praetorius (1630–80), professor of philosophy at the University of Leipzig and a devoted student of divination, especially through the reading of hands. The nine works in this volume provided an up-to-date compendium of the major works on chiromancy by some of Europe's leading scholars. For instance, Praetorius reprinted chapters on chiromancy from Fludd's multivolume *Utriusque cosmi... historia* (History... of the Two Worlds) (1617–26), as well as an extract from a lost work of Nicolaus Pompeius (1591–1659), professor of elementary mathematics at the University of Wittenberg, where he lectured on chiromancy. Also represented in the *Ludicrum chiromanticum Praetorii* is the Jesuit scholar Caspar Schott (1608–66), who treated on chiromancy in his massive work about the magic of art and nature published in four volumes between 1657 and 1659. At the opposite end of the occult spectrum from Fludd, Schott explained chiromancy in natural terms and rejected any astrological associations. The longest work in the volume is by Praetorius himself.

By the end of the seventeenth century chiromancy, like other forms of divination, had been discredited as an intellectual system, even if it was explained naturally. Scholars ceased writing systematic expositions of chiromancy, but diviners continued to specialize in palmistry as a form of fortune-telling.

—LAUREN KASSELL

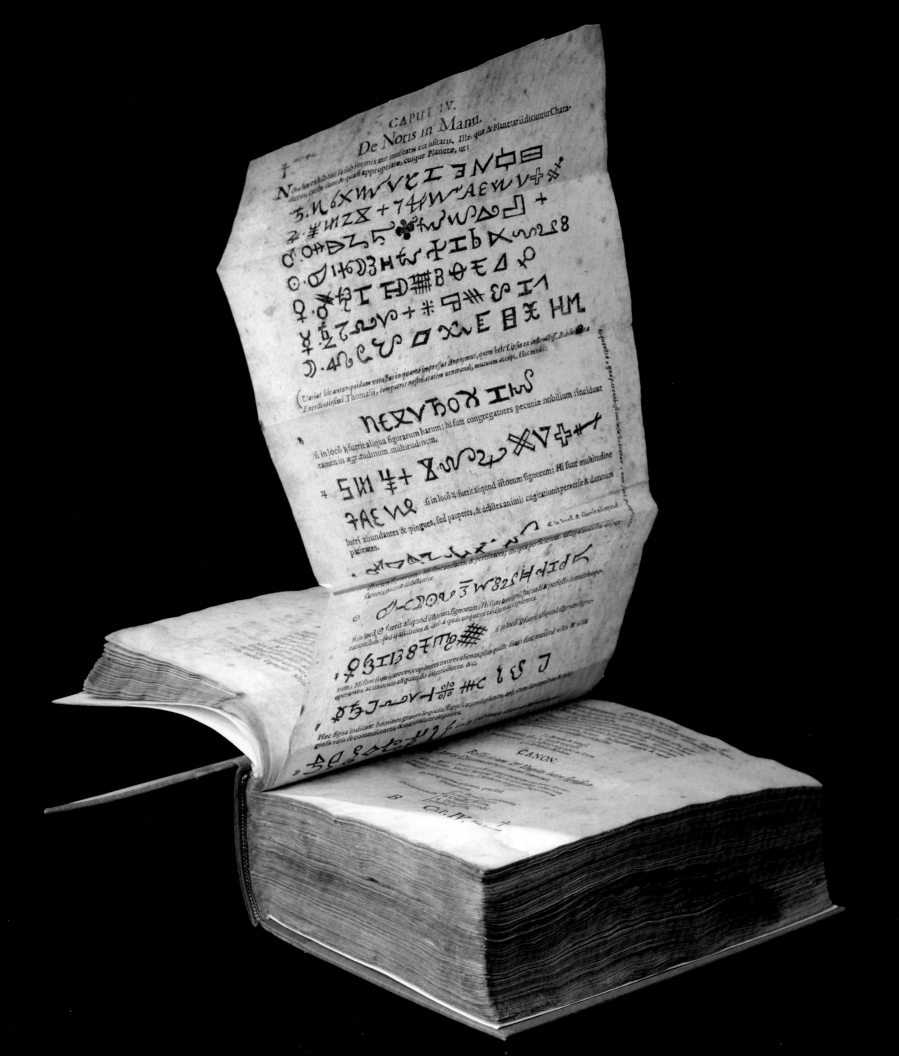

De Notis in Manu.

Notæ hæ exhibent se sub formis aut inusitatis aut usitatis. Illæ, quæ & Planetarii dicuntur Chara-
cteres, certæ sunt, & quasi appropriatæ, cuique Planetæ, ut:

(Variat hic autor quidam vetustus in quarto impressus Anonymus, quem hîc Lipsiæ ex instructiss. Bibliotheca
Excellentissimi Thomasii, compatris nostri ætatem venerandi, mutuum accepi, Hoc modo.)

si in loco ♄ fuerit aliqua figurarum harum; hi sunt congregatores pecuniæ nobilium: incidunt
tamen in ægritudinum multitudinem.

si in loco ♃ fuerit aliquod istorum signorum; Hi sunt multitudine
lucri abundantes & pingues, sed pauperes, & debiles animi: cogitationis perversæ & damnum
patientes.

istorum signorum; Hi sunt audaces & pertinaci, ih-que perfidiæ; utrsq.exercitatæ dispo-
sitiones pati sunt subsistantis.

si in loco ⊙ fuerit aliquod istorum signorum; Hi sunt benigni, jucundi & perfecti in multis ope-
rationibus, sed quibiles & ato à quâcunque re tædium accipiente.

si in loco ♀ fuerit aliquod istorum signo-
rum; Hi sunt fornicatores, cupientes uxores alienas, plus quâm suas; sunt maximè viles & villa
operantes, ac uxorum aliquando interfectores. &c.

Hæc signa indicant homines graves, loquela, significatione plenos, atq; cum familiaritate & reli-
giosis viris se comaniscentes, & naturaliter eligentes.

On Human Conception and Generation (1587)
Jakob Rueff, trans. Wolfgang Haller

De conceptu, et generatione hominis. Frankfurt-am-Main. Printed book with woodcuts, 92 pp.; 5½ x 7¾ in. (14 x 19.5 cm)

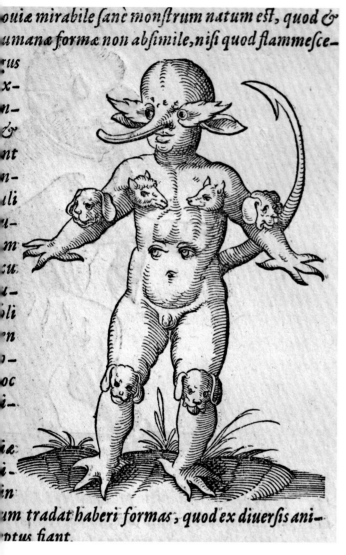

ouia mirabile sanè monstrum natum est, quod &
umana forma non absimile, nisi quod flammesce-
rus

um tradat haberi formas, quod ex diuersis ani-
ntus fiant.

ABOVE: The widely reported 1547 "Monster of Crackow," a child apparently born with a devilish face and tail, claws instead of hands, eyes on his stomach, and animal heads growing from his elbows, knees, and chest. *De conceptu*, fol. 43 recto

OPPOSITE: The left-hand page depicts a child born with the head of its unformed twin growing from its stomach; the date is not given. The right-hand page depicts conjoined twins born in Switzerland in 1543; the caption reminds the reader of a similar Swiss case from 1553. *De conceptu*, fols. 39 verso and 40 recto

Jakob Rueff (1500–58; also known as Ruf) was a surgeon who rose to the top of Zurich's medical profession, becoming the *Stadtartzt*, or chief city doctor. He came from a modest family background and did not have a university education, but his talent as a physician and humanist brought him to prominence. In addition to his interest in the history of physicians and astrologers, he was an enthusiastic playwright, drawing his themes from the Bible and folklore.

Rueff capitalized upon a burgeoning print culture to create and circulate medical and humanist knowledge in broadsheets, pamphlets, and books. His medical writing includes works on the eye and tumors, but his most successful publication was *De conceptu, et generatione hominis*. It was first published in 1554, in a German edition written by Rueff, and then immediately afterward in a Latin translation by Wolfgang Haller. (Dutch and English translations from 1591 and 1637 respectively indicate that there was a long-lived market for the work.) As the dual-language approach indicates, the book aimed at a wide audience and was intended to appeal to physicians, humanists, and also midwives. Rueff was responsible for the training and oversight of all midwives in Zurich and had a special interest in this group of readers. The book's broad content, conveyed in visual as well as textual form, contributed to its popularity and usefulness for training purposes. It addressed medical instruments and ingredients, impediments to conception, the development of the fetus, and also—in a series of lively images—the positions that the fetus could take in the womb. Rueff also examined more esoteric topics, such as the capacity of the Devil to generate children, while another chapter featured "monstrous births," the term used to describe physically deformed children. Giving full play to his medical and humanist interests, he described recent local births as well as others dating back to Roman antiquity.

The 1587 Latin edition was produced by the Feyerabend publishing house in Frankfurt-am-Main. It was based on the new Feyerabend edition of 1580, which was notable for its updated woodcut illustrations by the prominent printmaker Jost Amman (1539–91). While Amman closely followed the earlier woodcuts by Jos Murer (1530–80), he rendered many of the new figures more elegantly, and in the chapter on monstrous births, in particular, he featured a sequence of more animated, cherubic children's bodies. Amman added several new scenes, including one juxtaposing females assisting a woman giving birth with men pointing to the stars, apparently discussing the child's natal horoscope. Another striking new image depicts Adam and Eve standing beside the tree of knowledge. A skeleton has replaced the tree's trunk, with the serpent twisted around its shoulders. Death's presence reminds Rueff's readers of the fleeting nature of human life and closes the circle of human experience.

—JENNIFER SPINKS

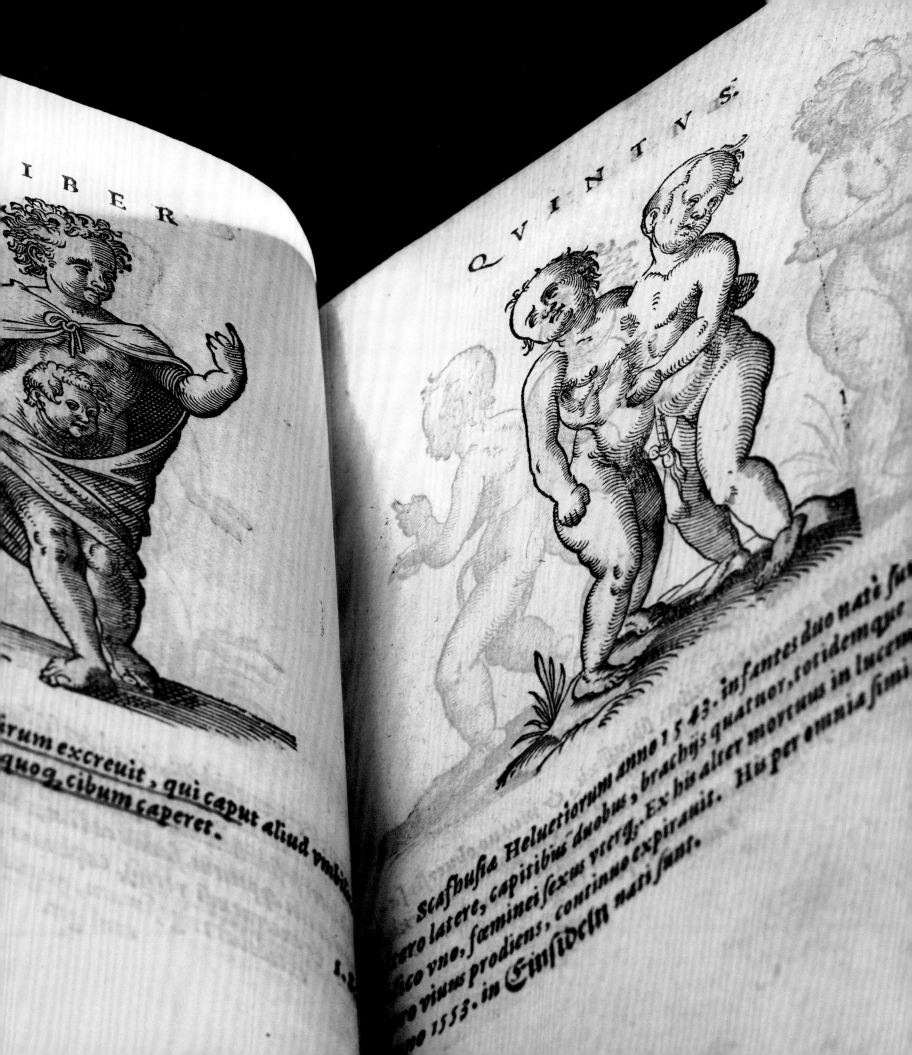

rum excreuit, qui caput aliud vmb...
...quoq; cibum caperet.

Scafhusia Heluetiorum anno 1543. infantes duo nati fu...
...tero latere, capitibus duobus, brachijs quatuor, totidemque...
...co vno, fœminei sexus vterq;. Ex his alter mortuus in lucem...
...ro viuus prodiens, continuo expirauit. Hu per omnia simi...
...no 1553. in Einſideln nati sunt.

Monstra: A Collection of Sixty-five Drawings, in Part Colored, Representing Monstrosities in the Museum of G. W. Klinkenberg (ca. 1820–40)
G. W. Klinkenberg

Leyden. Bound hand-drawn, colored plates; 50 sheets; 18½ x 21⅜ in. (47 x 54.3 cm)

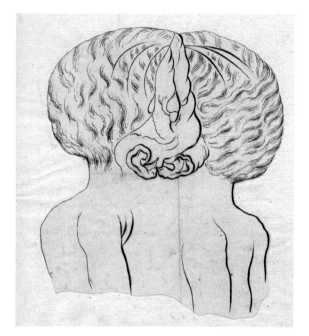

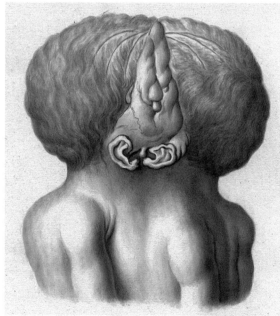

ABOVE AND OPPOSITE: Cephalothoracopagus conjoined twins

The word "monster" comes from the Latin *monstrare*, "to show," and from the derivative of *monare*, "to warn."

Two boys, one head. One boy, two heads. One woman, three breasts. One sheep, two heads. One pig, no head. *Monstra* ("monsters") is from the collection of G. W. (or G. J.) Klinkenberg, known to us only through this collection of original drawings.

(Left, opposite, and page 100, top) Cephalothoracopagus (twins conjoined at the head and thorax). Child or children? The caption, translated from the Dutch (by Willem Mulder), reads:

> *A human monster after a full-term pregnancy*
> *There are 2 boys fused at the breast and part of the abdomen*
> *There are 2 umbilicals and 2 heads that make a whole.*
> *They lived for 2 days…*

A profile pressed against a fun-house mirror—a fictional monster. It is as if two beings, in turning toward each other, melted inward so that half of each intended face is now deep inside the skull. Is there room in the dark for inner faces and one brain? Topped by uneven brows and a full mop of hair, the face we see gazes downward with a scowl of worldly disdain. If these eyes opened at all, perhaps each glimpsed a scene neither much liked.

On the back of the head a pair of vestigial ears has squeezed out at the base of the skull. Pieces of the missing features have begun to form, but there is no chance that there will be a second face on the backside of this skull, as in an ancient Janus.

> *Of the fused Heads, here one can see the 2*
> *ears are situated close to each other*
> *Above there is an oblong form with*
> *a narrow little growth to be seen.*

The "narrow little growth," is it another face? I turn the drawing upside down, a face appears. Elongated, the extra folds and ears turn into a fleshy nose, beard and horns curl like ram horns. Did anyone at the time of this birth also see this devil in the nape of the neck?

(Page 100, bottom) Bicephalus (double-headed conjoined twins).

> *Two fused to another*
> *in Normandy*
> *Born in Havre de Grace at Honfleur*
> *Boys.*
> *Being of 9 months pregnancy*
> *lived for 3 days and there*
> *baptized*
> *Henrij and Jaque*

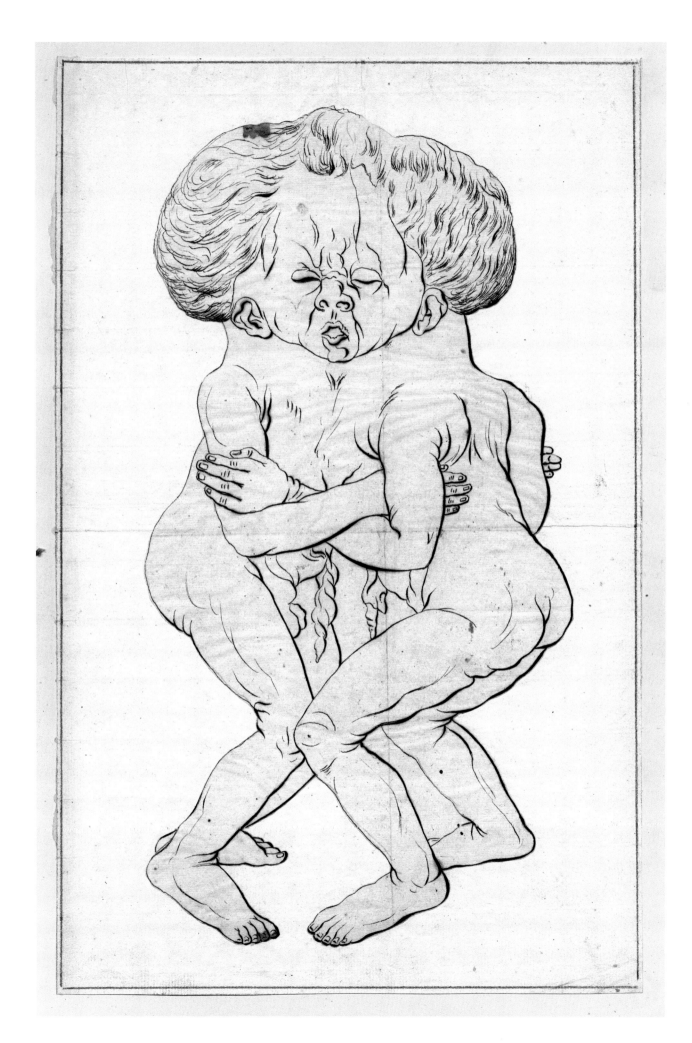

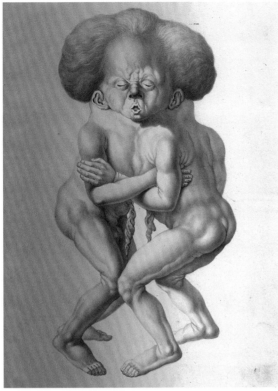

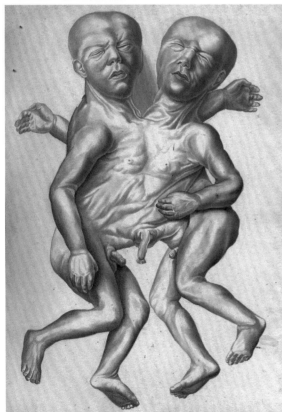

ABOVE, TOP: Cephalothoracopagus conjoined twins

ABOVE: Bicephalus conjoined twins

Jasseau
(1829)
Original
Is in the museum
of G. J. van Klinkenberg

The legs, feet, arms, hands, necks, heads of these brothers seem perfect and complete. The center of their bodies, strained and warped: incomplete division, commingled organs. If only they had been able to pull away from each other, become unstuck before birth.

In a flip book of conjoined twins how anatomies change! Arms flail, embrace, legs kick, entwine, a dance step is executed.

(Opposite) A SEQUENTIAL DISSECTION OF A HEADLESS FETUS. This lumpish sack with vestigial hooves is a pig with no head and no labels. The skin is unbroken, the dome smooth between the shoulders. The drawings of the crooked skeleton and sausage-like body lack charm. But the artist has turned the creature inside out, pulled the glistening organs out of the animal's interior, hanging one of them (heart? liver? spleen?) from string pinned above, where it dangles, like a blood-filled medallion or badge of honor, around the headless neck. Lacy tissues, gelatinous sacks, beautifully coiling intestines. The boundary between artistic spectacle and pathological specimen is thin. Opened-up, translucent bags, views of internal perfection, lacking all external charm, but delicate, magical.

(Page 102) THREE-BREASTED WOMAN.

Picture of a woman with three
Breasts. She let her Child suck at
my house pictured by
painter Banting in request of Professor Suerman
Signed in the year 1833
G. J. Klinkenberg
this woman was married to a
bricklayer

Consider the drawing of the woman's torso in pastel shades, soft and haunting. We expect bilateral symmetry in our external parts: nostrils, eyes, ears, legs, arms, breasts—two of each—there must be some mistake. What did the neighbors of the bricklayer's wife think? Was her condition a wonder or a curse? If she gives birth, does she nurse a litter? It is said that Anne Boleyn, second wife of Henry VIII, besides having six fingers on one hand also possessed a third breast.

(Page 103) THE SHEEP WITH TWO HEADS. Rough but lush, curling hair, furry conjoined ears, lolling tongues. Did it live in a sideshow, or on a farm where you could pay the farmer to take a look?

Centuries ago (and throughout the world today) doctors, scholars, priests, and ordinary citizens have asked simple questions about anomalies, trying to wrestle the nature and numbers into line. Was this kind of birth caused by human behavior? Did the mother sleep with a bear? Was she a witch? How do you determine the number of human beings? Is it by the number of legs, arms? How many souls, one or two? Mystery and much sorrow…

—ROSAMOND PURCELL

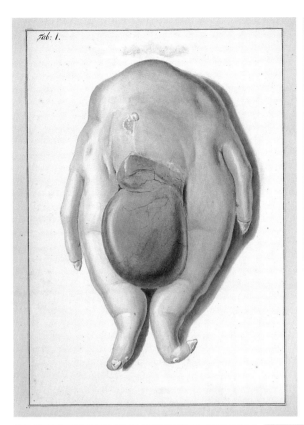
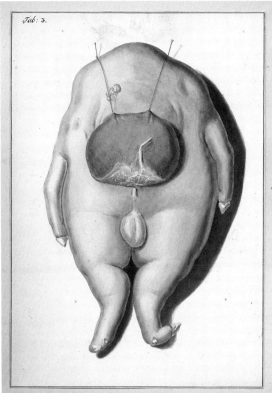
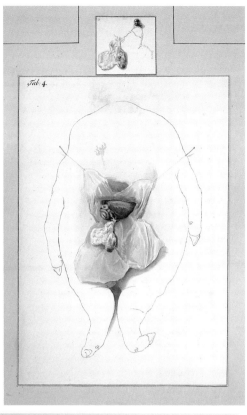
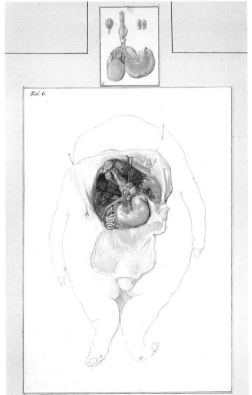
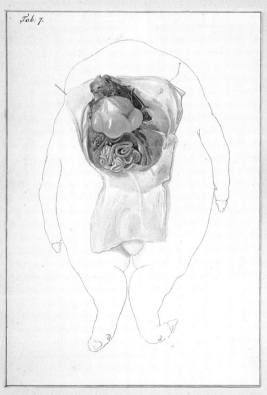
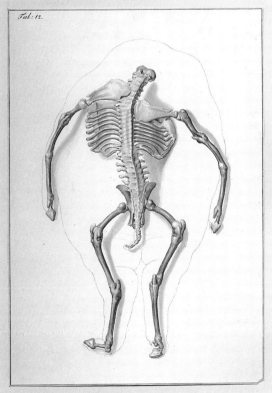

ABOVE: Progressive dissection of a headless pig

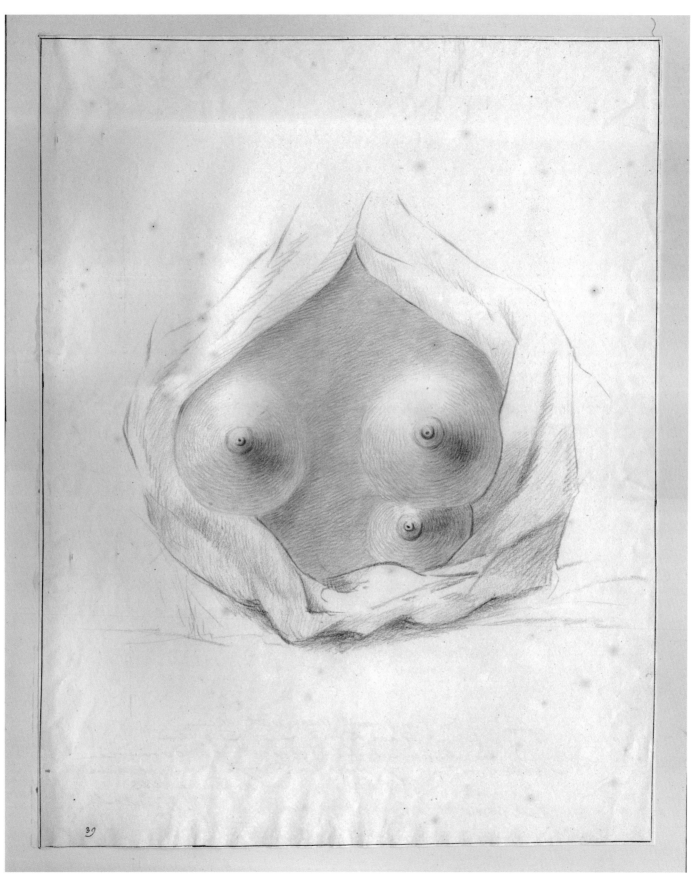

ABOVE: The three-breasted woman

OPPOSITE: The sheep with two heads

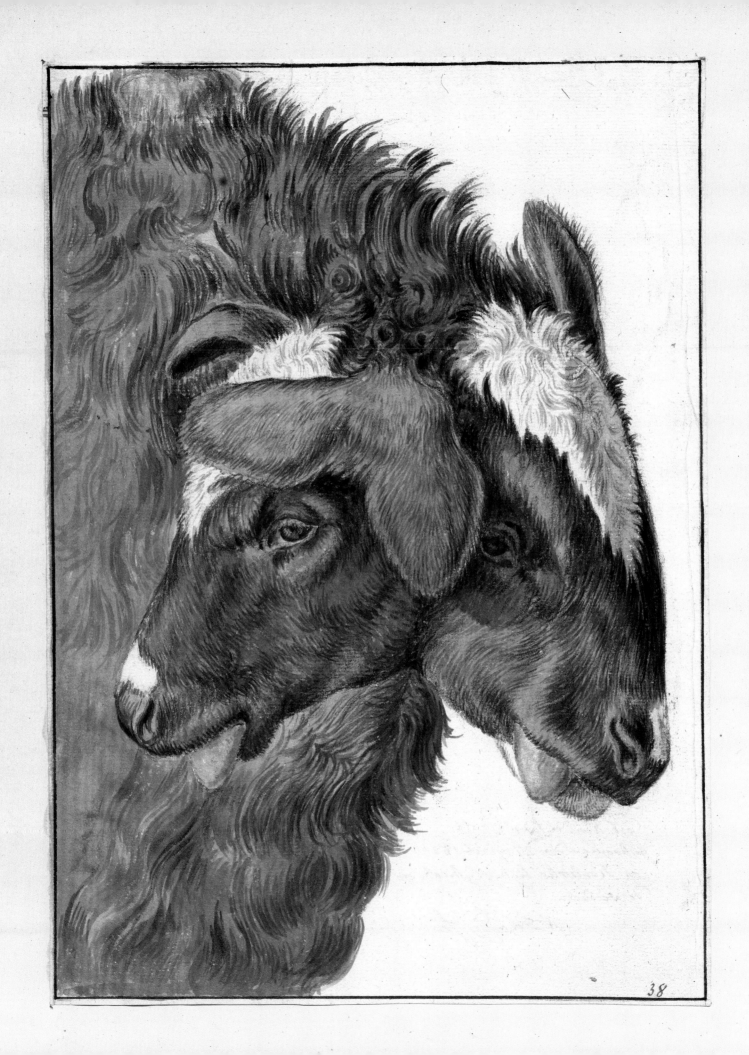

38

On the United Siamese Twins (1829–31, 1874)
Compiler unknown

England. Scrapbook, unpaginated; 10 x 12⅝ in. (25.4 x 32 cm)

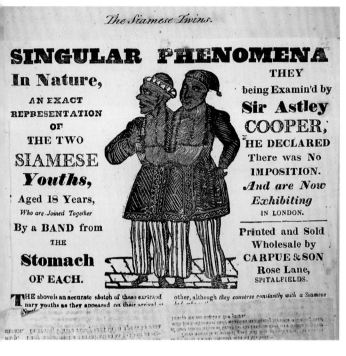

ABOVE: One of the many posters, souvenir booklets, tickets for shows, letters, news clips, magazine articles, lithographs, political cartoons, and testimonials collected in the National Library of Medicine's Chang and Eng scrapbook. *On the United Siamese Twins*

OPPOSITE: In grammar a "copulative conjunction" is the connection of linguistic units (words, clauses, or sentences, by words such as *and*, *plus*, or *also*) that have an additive or causal relation. A greater meaning arises, a whole greater than the sum of its parts, when the related ideas are conjoined. The print's title indicates that the twins' connection was of just such a type.

OVERLEAF: A typical spread of pages from the scrapbook.

One of the most notable show-business acts of the nineteenth century was the ten-year run of Chang and Eng Bunker, the original Siamese Twins, who shared a liver via a small band of tough flesh. Brought from their native Siam by an English sea captain in 1829, they toured the United States (for a time, under the aegis of P. T. Barnum), England, Europe, Canada, Cuba, and South America.

Their English tour of 1829–31 inspired an anonymous collector to make this scrapbook, with the words "The Siamese Twins" written in ink on the top of each page. Pasted neatly into the book are tickets, handbills, articles, satirical prints, news clippings—a hodgepodge of paper shards relating to the twins and their stay in England. Like most "prodigies" (as they were known in that era) Chang and Eng had to do more than simply satisfy the curiosity seekers. To draw a large audience of ticket-paying customers, prodigies had to put on a show, and the more varied the better. The brothers performed feats of strength, somersaults, and gymnastics and topped competing acts by playing the badminton-like game of battledore and shuttlecock. The scrapbook holds five illustrations of Chang and Eng with rackets in their hands. (Did they play singles or doubles? Their opponents are never depicted.)

Chang and Eng were relentless merchandisers. Classified ads, posters, and handbills in the scrapbook tout the sale of keepsakes from the twins and souvenir pamphlets. And the promotional material always comes with a claim: the twins have been examined and authenticated by "many scientific men." In an era filled with humbug and hokum (no less so than now) the brothers were the real McCoy, and it paid constantly to remind everyone of it. You saw the brothers, you saw the two and only.

The medical examinations were also staged as shows. One such "performance," at Egyptian Hall, a large theater in Piccadilly, is the subject of a lengthy pamphlet (also included in the scrapbook). The examination featured this experiment: The attending physicians, "on the suggestion of Doctor Roget" (he of the *Thesaurus*), placed "a silver teaspoon…on the tongue of one of the twins, and a disk of zinc on the tongue of his brother; when the metals thus placed were brought into contact, the youths both cried out 'Sour, sour.'" Their bodies had made a complete electrical circuit.

The nineteenth century prided itself on willful individuality, on extraordinary men rising from the mob, but here was a stunning example of that and, well, something else: an "inseparability" that was single and double. And a consciousness that was private and shared.

On the United Siamese Twins revels in the display of their conjoined twinness and follows them more than forty years, to their double death in 1874. A few hours after Chang died of a blood clot in his brain, Eng is said to have died of shock. The scrapbook is a reliquary of the promotional haze of entertainment, commerce, and science that surrounded the twins. Chang and Eng didn't invent that cultural stew but they nearly perfected it.

—JAMES TAYLOR

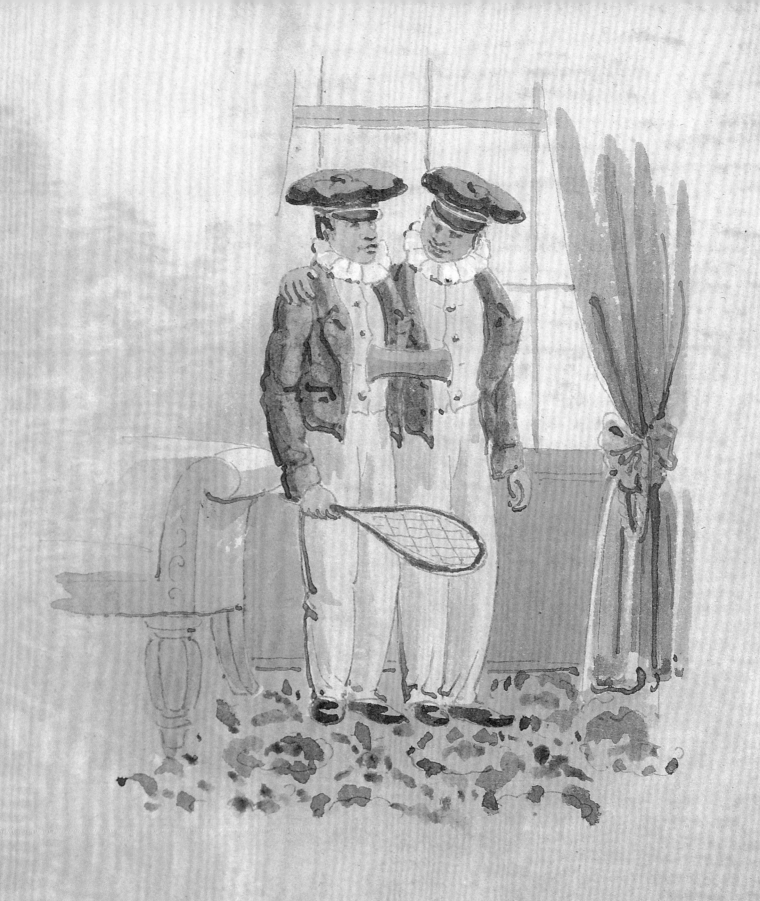

A Copulative Conjunction

SADLER's WELLS.

SKIMMER of the SEAS.

GOLDEN PIPPIN.

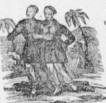

Wednesday, Thursday, Friday, and Saturday,
January 5, 6, 7, and 8. *1831.*

ONLY!!

THE

Siamese Youths

Will have the honor of appearing upon the Stage, in the
popular Pantomime of

Mother Goose

Or, *The Golden Egg,*

Previous to their departure for SIAM, which is positively
fixed for *Sunday Morning* next.

N. B. It is respectfully intimated that an opportunity
now offers to behold these Astonishing Youths, (with the
whole of the Entertainments of the Evening) at less ex-
pence than the original Exhibition of these prodigies of
nature cost to view.

W. Glendinning, Printer, 25, Hatton Garden.

SADLER'S WELLS.
Under the immediate Patronage of His Most Gracious Majesty.
Immediately on the opening of the doors every part of the theatre
was crowded to an excess, in all the avenues leading to the theatre
hundreds were anxiously waiting to obtain admission. On the
Siamese youths appearing upon the stage, the most deafening
shouts of applause followed on their entering the boxes. This
evening, To-morrow, and Saturday will be a repetition of the
Juvenile Fêtes, on which evenings the Siamese youths will appear.
THIS EVENING, To-morrow, and Saturday, to commence with
THE SKIMMER OF THE SEAS; or, The Water Witch. After
which, a Ballet Divertisement by Mrs. Searle and pupils,
be succeeded by the introduction of the SIAMESE YOUTHS.
To conclude with HARLEQUIN AND MOTHER GOOSE; or,
The Golden Egg. Pantaloon, Mr. Morton; Harlequin, Mr. Gay;
Clown, Mr. Matthews; Columbine, Mrs. Searle; Mother Goose,
Mr. Andrews.   *Jan. 1831.*

GARRICK'S SUBSCRIPTION THEATRE, LEMAN-STREET,
GOODMAN'S FIELDS.
THIS EVENING will be presented the historico-nautical and
domestic melodrama, called THE MUTINY AT THE NORE,
or, British Sailors in 1797. Principal characters by Mr. Freer, Mr.
W. J. Simpson, Mr. Gann, Mr. Conquest and Mrs. Mangean. After
which, a new ballet, entitled THE NEW YEAR'S GIFT; or, The
Bonny Broom Girls and the Merry Corn Thrashers. To conclude
with an entirely new grand national melodrama, entitled TWM
JOHN CATTY, THE WELSH ROB ROY.

FOUR JUVENILE NIGHTS.

SIAMESE
These interesting Youths
being about to leave En-
gland for their native
country on Sunday next,
the proprietors have pre-
vailed upon Capt Coffin
to exhibit them on the
Stage of this Theatre on
Wednesday, Thursday,
Friday, and Saturday
next, being the last times
they will ever be seen in
this country.

YOUTHS.
The Boys will exhibit
their various manœuvres
with which they gene-
rally amuse themselves,
their history, and the
various particulars con-
nected with it will be
given to the Audience
from the Stage, by Mr.
Hale, their interpreter
and conductor.

SADLER's WELLS.

Admit the Bearer & Party to

THE BOXES,

On payment of 1s. 6d. each Person,
From January 3 to 31, 1831.

Boxes may be secured of Mr. PARKER, at the Box Office, from 10 till 4.
Private Box for Eight £1 1s.
Doors Open at 6.   Begin at Half-past 6.   *T. Dayus.*

Sadler's   **Wells.**

Admit   Bearer

And Party to the BOXES

On payment of 1s. 6d. each Person,
From January 3 to 31, 1831.

Boxes may be secured of Mr. PARKER, at the Box Office, from 10
Private Box for Eight £1 1s.
Doors Open at 6.   Begin at Half-past 6.   *T. Dayus.*

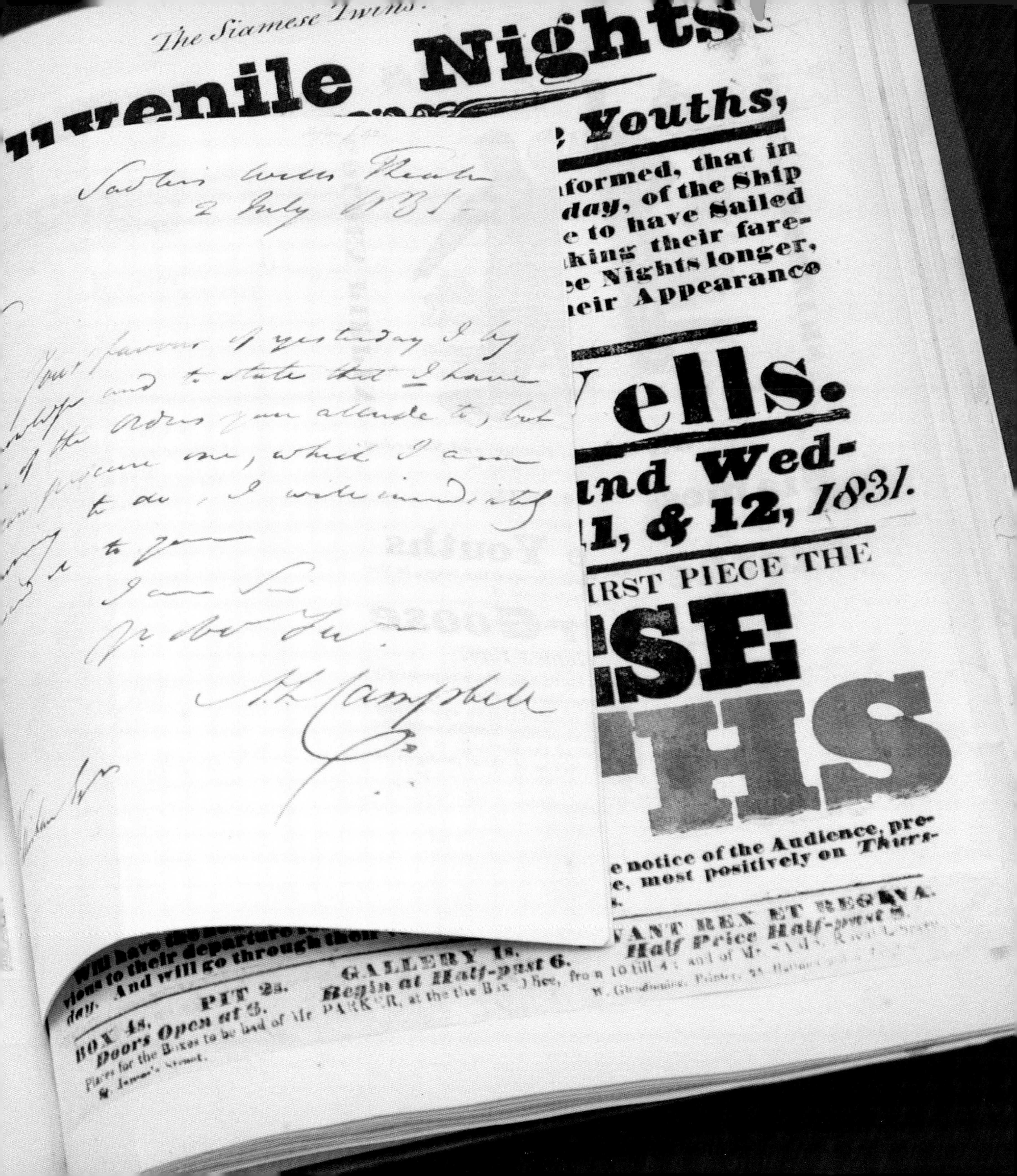

The Siamese Twins.

venile Nights!

Youths,

Sadlers Wells Theatre
2 July 1831

Your favour of yesterday I by
...ledge and to state that I have
... of the Order you allude to, but
... procure one, which I am
... to do, I will immediately
... to you

I am Sir

Jr &c &c

N.L. Campbell

...formed, that in
...day, of the Ship
...e to have Sailed
...king their fare-
...ee Nights longer,
...heir Appearance

ells.

nd Wed-
1, & 12, 1831.

IRST PIECE THE

SE
HS

...e notice of the Audience, pro-
...e, most positively on Thurs-
...s.

...VANT REX ET REGINA.
Half Price Half-past 8.
...from 10 till 4; and of Mr SAMS, Royal Library

W. Glendinning, Printer, 25 Rupert...

Will have the honour...
...vious to their departure...
...day. And will go through their...

BOX 4s.
PIT 2s.
GALLERY 1s.
Doors Open at 5.
Begin at Half-past 6.

Places for the Boxes to be had of Mr PARKER, at the the Box Office
St. James's Street.

Facts Connected with the Life of James Carey (1839)
James Akin

Philadelphia. Printed pamphlet with lithographs, 8 pp.; 5¼ x 7¾ in. (13.5 x 19.5 cm)

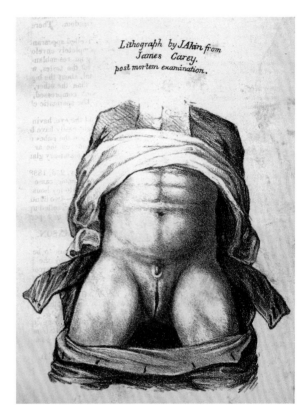

ABOVE: James Akin made this illustration at Carey's postmortem examination in Philadelphia on June 5, 1838. It bears Akin's attestation that attending physicians approved his anatomical representation of Carey's ambiguous genitals. *Facts*, after p. 8

OPPOSITE: James Carey driving his coach. *Facts*, frontispiece and title page; lithographs by James Akin

When James Carey died in 1838 his secret was laid bare. People had always been born with atypical anatomies, but in the nineteenth century a new scientific, medical discourse emerged. Doctors thrilled to confront unusual cases such as Carey's, debating whether "true hermaphrodites" existed in the human species. Earthworms, snails, and some reptiles could be hermaphrodites, these experts argued, but not humans. The author of this pamphlet, the engraver and caricaturist James Akin (ca. 1773–1846), believed otherwise: he hoped that the postmortem examination of James Carey's body would "elucidate if not confirm the hypothesis that hermaphroditic characters exist."

Much more than an autopsy report, Akin's pamphlet shows, in style and tone, the excitement that anomalous bodies generated. Audiences liked to read about oddities of various sorts, scientists were keen on collecting unusual specimens, and physicians yearned to dissect extraordinary cadavers. In addition to the account of Carey's autopsy, *Facts Connected with the Life of James Carey, Whose Eccentrick Habits Caused a Post mortem Examination by Gentlemen of the Faculty to Determine Whether He Was Hermaphroditic* includes a witty poem ("Carey's life, outré and strange! / Illustrates nature's freaks in change"), lithographic illustrations, and a sentimental biography ("Conscious that busy intermeddlers might surprise him sleeping, and when in a state of nudity, discover his strange malconformation [*sic*], he continually girded his pantaloons securely about his loins").

"Hermaphrodite" was the term most frequently used in the eighteenth and nineteenth centuries to designate ambiguously sexed individuals. Pejorative labels were also frequently applied. Though Akin's pamphlet employs terms such as "unfortunate monstrosity," it also includes an empathic narrative of Carey's life.

Akin begins by portraying Carey as more beast than man, a stooped hunchback who exhibited "features of a grotesque melancholy aspect" and emitted "preternatural discharges from his nasal vessels" that could cause vomiting among onlookers. But later in the pamphlet Carey is presented as a human being, a moral creature. Whether working at a foundry or driving a stagecoach, Akin tells us, Carey maintained a "firm and manly deportment," despite his "effeminate appearance," and was honest, loyal, and punctual in attending to his duties.

The sentimental account of Carey's relationships with his employers and others who befriended him was designed to elicit sympathy. Just as readers could be titillated and horrified by the descriptions and images of Carey's extraordinary genitalia, they might also be moved by his spiritual redemption: he was a human being with a soul capable of salvation.

Upon death Carey's body became available for observation and dissection, his secrets flayed open for sensationalist pamphleteering and, more than a hundred years later, historical scholarship. But the living Carey never confronted the surgeon's knife. Surgical intervention to "normalize" bodies became standard practice later in the nineteenth century. So it remains today, though increasingly challenged by bioethicists and the intersex-rights movement.

—ELIZABETH REIS

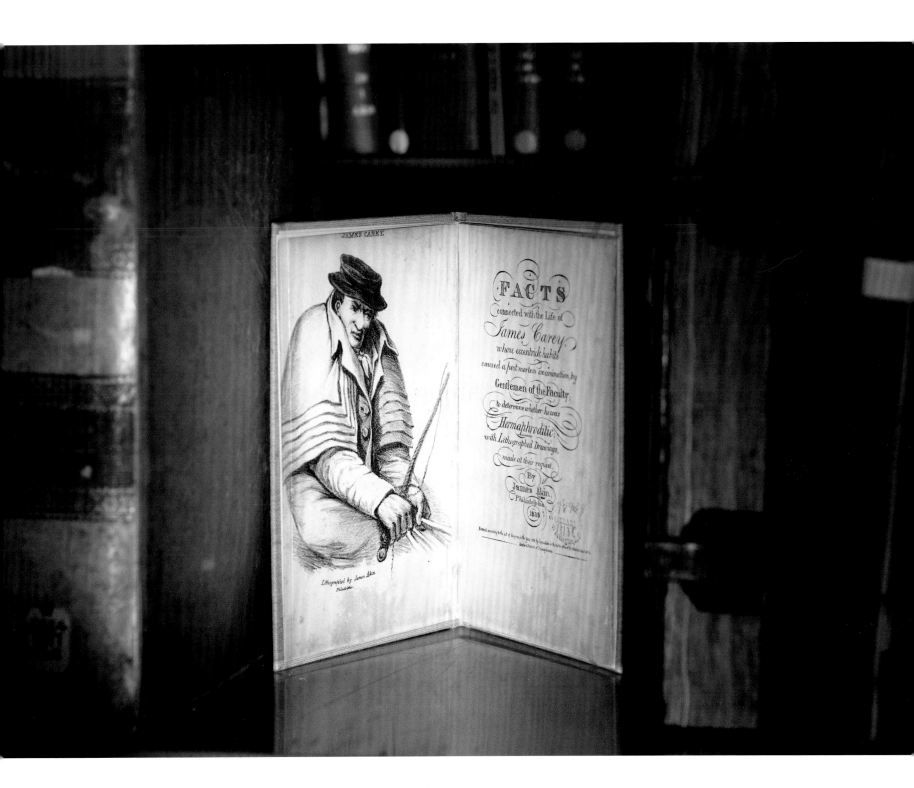

JAMES CAREY

Lithographed by James Akin.
Philadelphia.

FACTS
connected with the Life of
James Carey
whose eccentrick habits
caused a post-mortem examination, by
Gentlemen of the Faculty,
to determine whether he was
Hermaphroditic:
with Lithographed Drawings,
made at their request.
By
James Akin,
Philadelphia.
1838

Entered according to the act of Congress in the year 1838 by James Akin in the Clerks Office of the District court of the
Eastern District of Pennsylvania.

Symptoms in Schizophrenia (ca. 1930)
James D. Page

Rochester, New York. Motion picture, black-and-white, silent, intertitles, 16mm; 12:00

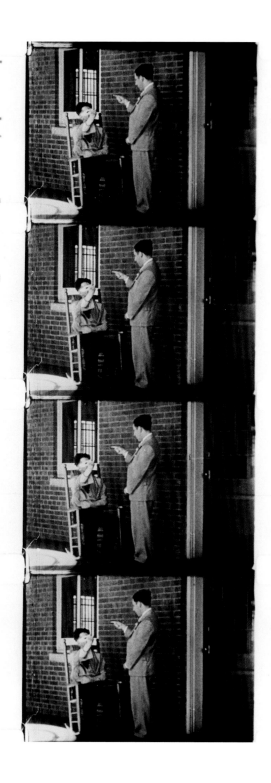

chizophrenia was a new diagnosis in interwar American medicine. Invented in 1911 by Swiss psychiatrist Eugen Bleuler (1857–1939), after World War I the term gradually supplanted "dementia praecox," which was associated too closely with German psychiatry. When *Symptoms in Schizophrenia* was shot, roughly twenty years later, the nature and origins of schizophrenia remained wholly unknown (as they still do today): the film's intertitles declare the disorder "chronic" and make no reference to treatment, recovery, or cure. As a consequence schizophrenia could be "defined" only by observing and describing a set of diffuse psychic symptoms, none of which could be found in all cases.

James Daniel Page, professor of psychology at the University of Rochester, supervised the filming. Shot with only a stationary camera, his silent, twelve-minute film records eighteen patients in scenes of fifteen to forty-five seconds. The inmates, white adults of both sexes, stand or sit, mostly outdoors, at a redbrick institution with porches and well-kept lawns. An opening sequence depicts a large gathering of men socializing on park benches on hospital grounds.

Each patient performs a single symptom. Extravagant bodily symptoms predominate: gestures, tics, and postures. The longest scenes almost take the form of vaudeville skits: in "motor catatonia," a staff member arranges the arms of patients in amusing poses (opposite, bottom center); in "echopraxia," a patient reflexively mimics the movements of the interviewing doctor (left). Page presumably made his film to provide in-house instruction about schizophrenia and its subtypes. A few written sentences are interspersed throughout, but there is no narrative coherence. The hospital and suited authority figures are unidentified. No patient names or pseudonyms are given. Viewers learn nothing about the cases or about schizophrenia as a psychological process. Eerily, the faces of many inmates are obscured: in some segments a blindfold blocks the patient's sight, as if he had been placed before a firing squad; in others holes have been cut out for the patient's eyes. The patients perform for the camera and seem less crazy than comical. Their jerky, exaggerated movements are almost Chaplinesque.

During the second quarter of the twentieth century the asylum was the preferred destination for those deemed insane; more than four hundred thousand people accumulated in mental hospitals across the country. A generation later, anti-psychiatric sentiment and the patients' rights movement led to the emptying of the asylum: patients were "decarcerated" onto streets and into prisons and flophouses. Did Page's subjects suffer this fate? How many underwent insulin coma therapy or were surgically sterilized for eugenic reasons, two widespread practices at state asylums in the 1930s? How many were given electroshock or lobotomized in the 1940s and 1950s? And how many of them would endure until the advent of chlorpromazine (1950), the first antipsychotic compound, and the era of modern psychopharmacology?

This remarkable film, silent, mysterious, disjointed, and disturbing, doesn't ask or answer these questions. Its abrupt ending—without credits, commentary, or closure—only adds to the feeling of psychic fragmentation it so powerfully documents.

—MARK S. MICALE

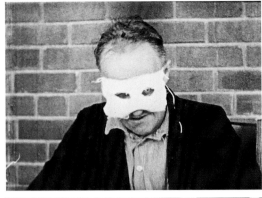 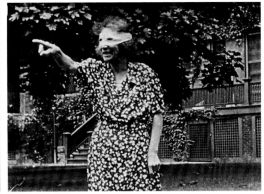 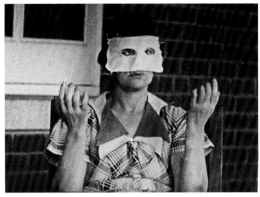

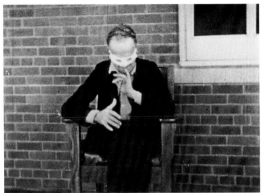

Schizophrenia (dementia praecox) is the most prevalent of mental disorders. About one per cent of the population eventually develop it.

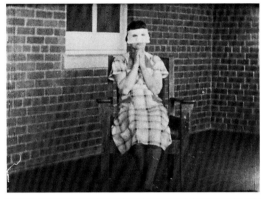

It is essentially a chronic disease of unknown origin, characterized by marked personality disintegration.

In general appearance schizophrenics resemble normal individuals. All body types are represented. Distinction lies in their mental content and behavior.

Schizophrenics are divided into four clinical groups: simple, paranoid, catatonic and hebephrenic.

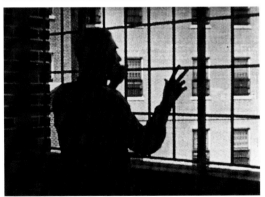

Delusions and hallucinations occur in most hebephrenic, catatonic and paranoid patients. The latter often give evidence of these symptoms by conversing or arguing with imaginary individuals.

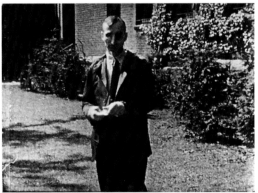

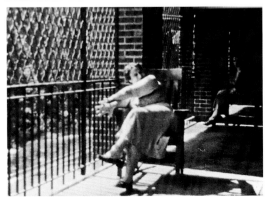 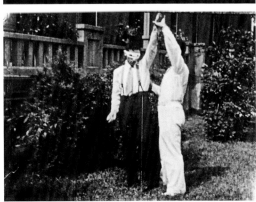 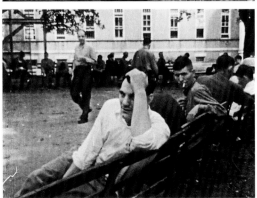

Clinical Collection on Dermatology and Syphilology (1886–90)
Nikolai Porfir'evich Mansurov

Klinicheskiĭ sbornik po dermatologīi i sifilologīi. Moscow. Printed journal, 4 vols. in 1, with wood engravings
and original, tipped-in albumen photographic prints, 386 pp.; 6⅜ x 9½ in. (16.3 x 24.3 cm)

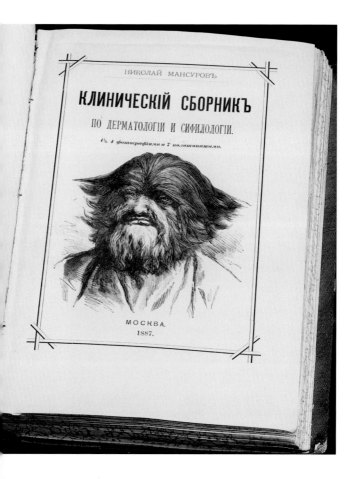

ABOVE: *Clinical Collection* 2 (1887) carried an article on "hairy people" inspired by Mansurov's encounter with an actual case of polytrichia. Its cover featured a wood engraving of a "hairy man."

OPPOSITE: The article on hairy people includes a photograph of Mansurov's patient Adr. Evtikhiev (lower left) and a photograph of "the Bearded Lady" Julia Pastrana (1834–60), who toured Europe and North America in the 1850s (upper left). Pastrana died in childbirth while in Moscow in 1860. Anatomy professor Ivan M. Sokolov performed the autopsy and embalmed her body, along with that of her stillborn son, who was delivered by caesarean section. Apparently a colleague alerted Mansurov to the autopsy photographs preserved at the Anatomy Institute of Moscow University Medical School, and he included two (upper and lower right) in a follow-up article on differences between "acquired" and "hereditary" polytrichia. *Clinical Collection* 2 (1887), facing pp. 24 and 40; 3 (1889), facing pp. 12 and 14

Nikolai Mansurov (1834–92) was the first dermatologist in Russia (and one of the first anywhere) to use photography systematically in medical illustration. "Photography," he wrote, "provides a particular visual aid," allowing "comprehensive and absolutely true" representations of skin diseases, "which could hardly be achieved in other fields of medicine." Since Russia lacked specialized periodicals in dermatology, Mansurov began to issue (at his own expense) an annual *Clinical Collection on Dermatology*. Begun in 1886, the *Collection* consisted of Mansurov's reports on new diagnostic techniques, therapeutic treatments, and interesting cases encountered in his practice, as well as occasional clinical lectures. In five years he issued four volumes. What made Mansurov's *Collection* unique was the use of high-quality photographic illustrations of his patients, five to eight per volume. Since no technology yet existed that could reproduce photographs, each one had to be printed in numerous copies and then glued by hand to a special paper insert with handwritten captions. Notwithstanding the resulting high cost of the volumes, *Collection* enjoyed wide popularity among Russian dermatologists.

Mansurov had graduated with honors from Moscow University Medical School in 1858 and joined the staff of a clinic run by Fedor Inozemtsev (1802–69), the school's star professor of surgery. The next year Inozemtsev arranged for Mansurov to travel abroad for advanced training in dermatology, particularly syphilis. Mansurov spent almost three years studying with the field's foremost authorities, including Philippe Ricord (1800–89) in Paris and Ferdinand Hebra (1816–80) in Vienna. Then he went to Turin, where he began work on "syphilization," a controversial new treatment for syphilis invented by the French physician Alexander Auzias-Turenne (1812–70) and propagated by Casimiro Sperino (1812–94). Modeled after smallpox vaccination, the new method involved injecting patients with material from their own syphilitic ulcers. Mansurov conducted extensive investigations and wrote his dissertation on syphilization, which he defended upon his return to Moscow in 1862. Although his examiners were skeptical they could not deny the quality and intensity of his research, and they awarded him the doctor of medicine degree.

The next year Mansurov opened Russia's first systematic course on "syphilis and skin diseases." It was not required in the curriculum, but given the enormous spread of syphilis and other skin diseases in Russia there was no shortage of students. However, teaching was difficult. There were no Russian textbooks on the subject and no specialized clinics where students could study dermatology and treat patients. Although Mansurov was not paid for teaching and had to earn an income through an extensive private practice that occupied much of his time, in 1864 he published the first Russian textbook on skin diseases, compiled from the latest German and French manuals and monographs. At his own expense he created a large collection of colored wax models of various skin lesions and arranged for students to visit his private patients.

Mansurov's considerable efforts did not advance his career. In 1869, when the Medical School finally established a separate department of venereal and skin diseases, the position

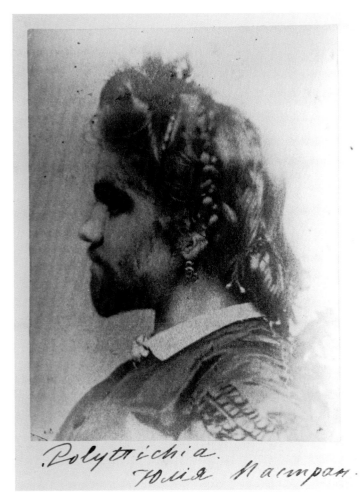

Polytrichia.
Юлія Пастран.

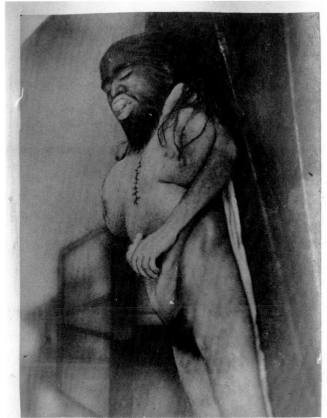

Polytrichia
(Julia Pastrana)

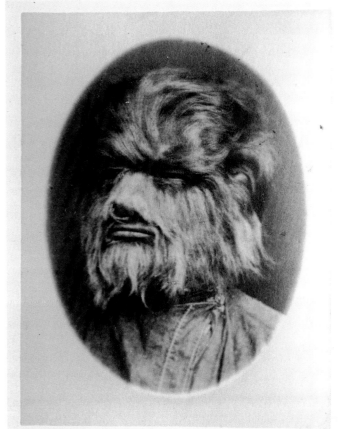

Polytrichia s. Homo pilosus. Агр. Евтихіевъ

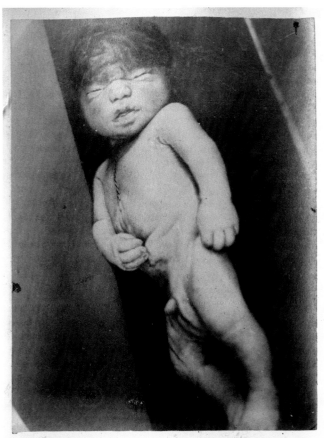

Polytrichia
Ребенокъ Юліи Пастраны

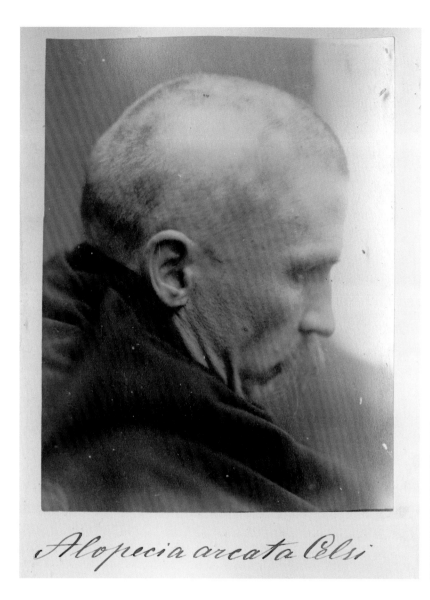

Alopecia areata Celsi

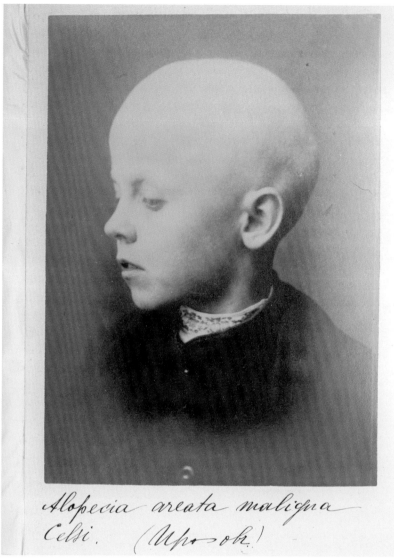

Alopecia areata maligna Celsi. (Uproh.)

ABOVE: Two patients (a grown man and nine-year-old boy) suffering from "malignant baldness," alopecia areata. *Clinical Collection* 3 (1889), facing p. 20; 1 (1890), facing p. 52

of professor and chairman went to his former classmate Dmitrii Naidenov (1835–84), who had distinguished himself only by courting Moscow's rich and powerful. Undiscouraged, Mansurov continued his teaching and research, publishing regularly in Russian and foreign medical periodicals. In 1875 he produced a voluminous monograph on tertiary syphilis, focusing on brain damage and psychoses and their treatment. He maintained close contacts with colleagues in Europe and became a corresponding member of dermatological societies in Paris, Berlin, and Vienna.

Mansurov finally obtained a professorial position at the Medical School in 1884, and the next year he became chairman of its department of venereal and skin diseases. His appointment coincided with important developments that enabled him to advance his specialty. In 1884 the Russian government adopted a new university statute that made venereal and skin diseases a required course for medical students. Almost simultaneously Moscow University expanded its medical school with a new "clinical town" that consisted of several large specialized hospitals attached to corresponding departments such as pathology, surgery, and internal

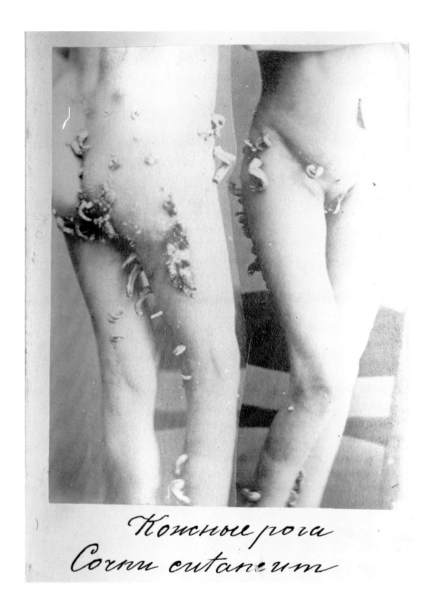

Кожные рога
Cornu cutaneum

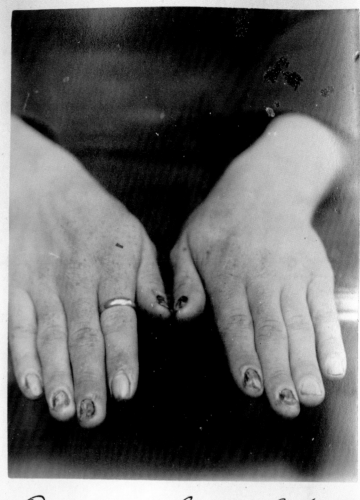

Onychia Syphilitica

ABOVE LEFT: A patient with a very rare disorder, "skin horns" (cornii cutanum). Note the "collage" technique of combining, in one illustration, two photographs of the same patient taken from different angles. *Clinical Collection* 3 (1889), facing p. 8

ABOVE RIGHT: A patient with syphilis-induced loss of fingernails (onychia syphilitica). *Clinical Collection* 3 (1889), facing p. 24

diseases. Unfortunately the university did not afford Mansurov's department its own clinic, only a ward with twenty beds in an old city hospital. Determined to create a solid clinical base for research and teaching, Mansurov turned to private patrons and in a few years raised more than 200,000 rubles to build Moscow's first hospital for skin disease.

Mansurov's appointment also provided him with his own laboratory and easy access to patients at the university's numerous hospitals. He published "Bacteria in Syphilis" (1885), a lengthy paper that described new bacteriological research methods and discussed the role of bacteria in infectious diseases, particularly syphilis. In 1890 Mansurov issued a second edition of his popular *Collection*. But that was its last year of publication. The next year, the Moscow Dermatological and Venereological Society (established with Mansurov's active involvement) began issuing its own journal. Late in 1892 a large building for his dermatological hospital was finally completed. But in November, at the peak of his career, Mansurov died from "influenza, complicated by pleuritis."

—NIKOLAI KREMENTSOV

One Hundred Case Histories Concerning the Origin, Course, Treatment, and Cure of the Falcadina Disease (1826)
Giuseppe Vallenzasca

Cenni Istorici Concernenti l'Origine, l'Andamento la Cura e la Cessazione della Malattia Falcadina. Milan, Italy. Bound manuscript on paper, 184 + 20 pp.; ink and watercolor illustrations; 6⅞ x 9½ in. (17.5 x 24 cm)

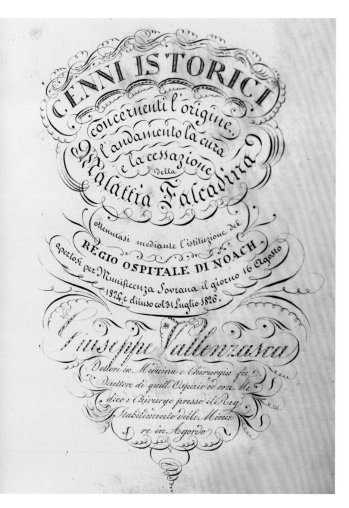

ABOVE: *Della Falcadina*'s title page is a swirling extravaganza of calligraphic ornaments and festoons. Note the whirlpool curlicue at the bottom of the page. Dedicated to a viceroy of the House of Hapsburg, the calligraphy is reminiscent of the diplomatic minuscule based on Carolingian script—appropriate for an imperial presentation text.

OPPOSITE: Martino Micheluzzi, a young boatman, was hit in the face by a piece of lumber. Inflammation followed and he lost his nose, both eyes, uvula, and hard palate. *Della Falcadina*, pl. 3. Many of the cases report that the onset of Falcadina was initiated by trauma to the face.

In 1826 Dr. Giuseppe Vallenzasca presented an extravagantly illustrated and embellished manuscript—written with florid penmanship on gilt-edged paper—to His Imperial Highness, the Most Serene Prince and Lord Ranieri, the viceroy of Lombardy and Veneto. Vallenzasca was a man of many parts: physician; hospital administrator; member and correspondent of scientific and medical societies in Vienna, Bologna, Venice, Treviso, and Rovigo; recipient of the Grand Gold Medal for Civil Merit (with ribbon) from the imperial court in Austria; as well as a skilled artist and an adroit diplomat and courtier. The manuscript was an account of a mysterious and terrible disease, *la Falcadina* (probably a strain of syphilis), which had long afflicted a mining district in the Tyrolean Alps.

The magnificent lettering and embellishments came from the hand of a talented professional scribe. The illustrations, perhaps from the hand of Vallenzasca himself, and reproduced from an original source at half their actual size (Vallenzasca tells us), are a strange, stunning blend of Golden Book and DC Comics with a soupçon of Poussin. The patients—miners, milkmaids, humble people—display their inflammations and ulcerations in disturbing, brightly colored portraits, often with ghastly smiles.

Prince Ranieri, to whom the manuscript is dedicated, was a Hapsburg archduke who presided over the imperial court in Milan when Stendhal lived there. He laid the first stone in the railroad bridge over the lagoon from terra firma to Venice. He presided over the brutal suppression of the 1848 uprising in northern Italy.

The town after which the disease was named, Falcade, stood midway between Milan and Salzburg, in the mountains northwest of Venice, not far from Trieste, the Austro-Hungarian empire's seaport. Through Ranieri's beneficence, in 1824 a hospital was set up in neighboring Agordo, under Vallenzasca's superintendency. At that time, Falcadina (which Vallenzasca compares to the Hungarian *skerlievo*, the Scottish *sibbens*, and Canadian *lue*) had afflicted the region for thirty-six years. Vallenzasca vanquished it in two years, through the imposition of quarantines, forty days of isolation in a hospital ward. (The Italian *quarantena* is related to the Italian name for the forty days of Lent, *quaresima*.) The tactic was so effective that Vallenzasca was able to shut down the hospital in 1826. The question of whether Falcadina was a miner's disease, or a sexually transmitted disease, or something else, became moot.

In the pages of the manuscript, Vallenzasca presents the lives of the lowborn to the potentate. Domenica Strim, daughter of a certain Matteo, lived the life of a rootless wayfarer for many years until, in 1790, she returned to her native Falcade from Trieste. She became stricken with venereal ulcerations and "condylomatous excrescences," and through her "dishonest behavior" spread the disease to others. That was the first known case of Falcadina.

The cases are told with fine-grained attention to the manifestations and causes of the disease. Martino Micheluzzi (opposite), a strapping young boatman working the Cordevole River, was hit in the face by a piece of lumber. Inflammation soon followed. He quickly lost his

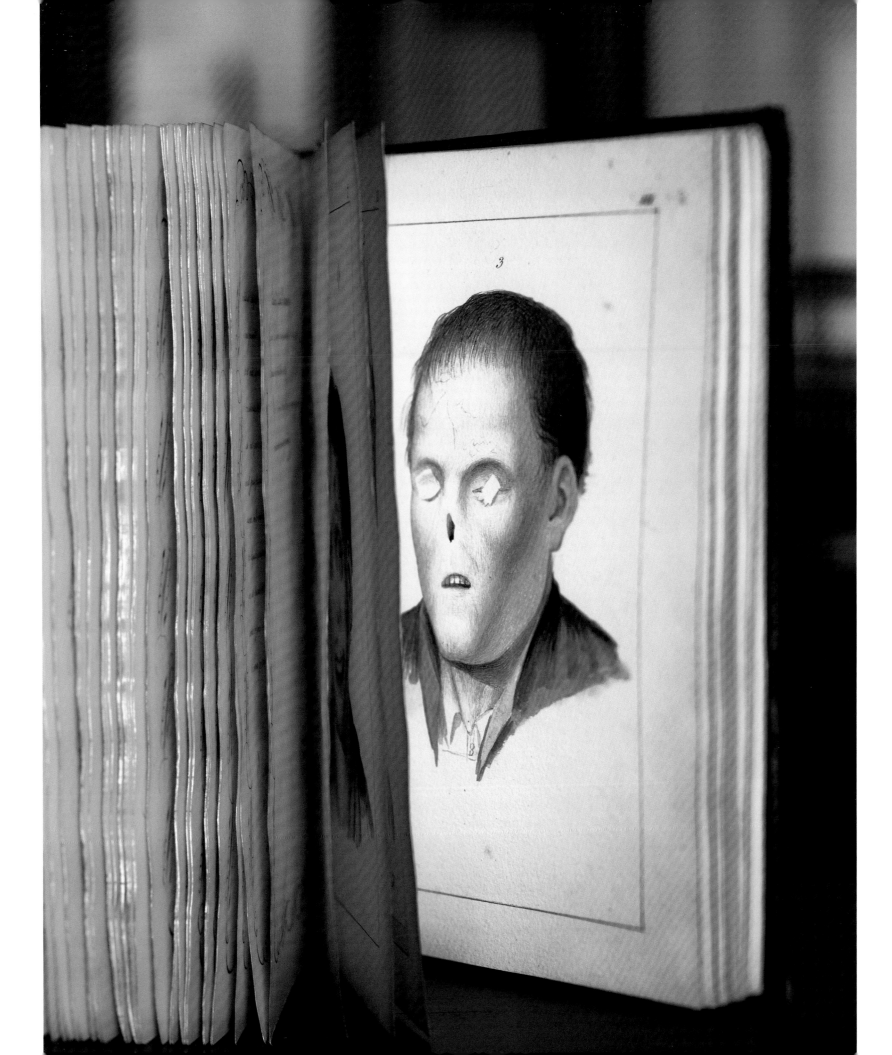

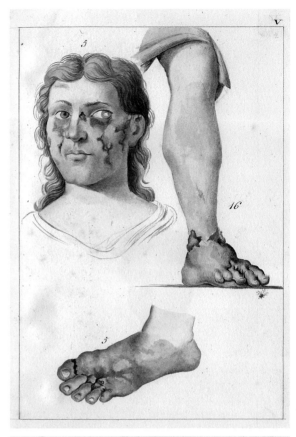

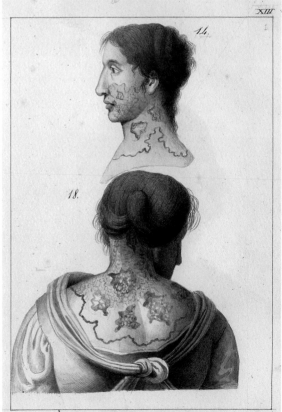

nose, both eyes, uvula, and hard palate. (In many cases Falcadina seems to have been induced by trauma.) The severe scarring that followed caused his mouth to shrink. He could eat only soft food, and that no larger in size than a walnut. Micheluzzi's stay in the hospital of Noach cured his inflammations but couldn't reverse the damage. Vallenzasca drily notes that he left the facility "less miserable than before."

Agata Lapieruz (opposite) lost her nose, upper lip, and bottom half of eyelids after she was afflicted by "reddish patches covered with tiny blisters that soon dry up and flake off," changing form and location with "protean" rapidity. The sores eventually formed crusts and attacked the soft flesh of the face.

Maria Gossuin (top left) was just fourteen when she first received treatment at the hospital but had ignored the steadily worsening symptoms for years. Vallenzasca notes that had the "beneficent Sovereign not interposed his care," her family likely never would have been able to embrace her again.

The entire family of Adriana De Rocco, age fifty-five (bottom left), succumbed to Falcadina until she, last of all, contracted the disease from her grown, married daughter. By the time she was admitted to the hospital, a "herpetic ulceration" covered with dense purulent scaling had spread across her shoulders, covering both shoulder blades. The treatment involved mercuric oxide, decoctions of burdock root and holywood, *Ethiops Mineral* (black sulfide of mercury), and sulfur fumigations. She gradually recovered and returned home.

The manuscript paints a grim picture of poverty and filth in the mountain villages. The peasants of the region are the "lowest of the low, notably shiftless." The spread of the disease between male roommates or within a single family, Vallenzasca surmises, can occur through skin-to-skin contact or dirty sheets. The "rustic indolence" of the inhabitants of the region, combined with poor nutrition and insalubrious residences, along with the habit of wearing "greasy and unwashed" woolen clothing, results in dermatological conditions that turn into deeper, internal disorders.

The book then is an odd concoction—a beautifully crafted manuscript of distressing case histories and shocking illustrations. It may have served Vallenzasca's purposes. He was a skilled rhetorician, who looked to the imperial viceroy for patronage, advancement, and help for the patients under his care. But presented and read may be two different matters: when Lorenzo de' Medici was presented with *The Prince* by Niccolò Machiavelli, he barely glanced at it in his delight at another gift, a pair of stud dogs he received that same day.

—ANTONY SHUGAAR

TOP: Maria Genuin was fourteen years old when she first received treatment at the hospital but had ignored the steadily worsening symptoms for years.

BOTTOM: Adriana De Rocco, age fifty-five, had a "herpetic ulceration" across her shoulders, covered with dense purulent scaling.

OPPOSITE: Agata Lapieruz lost her nose, upper lip, and bottom half of eyelids after being afflicted by "reddish patches covered with tiny blisters that soon dry up and flake off." Rapidly changing form and location, the sores eventually formed crusts and attacked the soft flesh of the face.

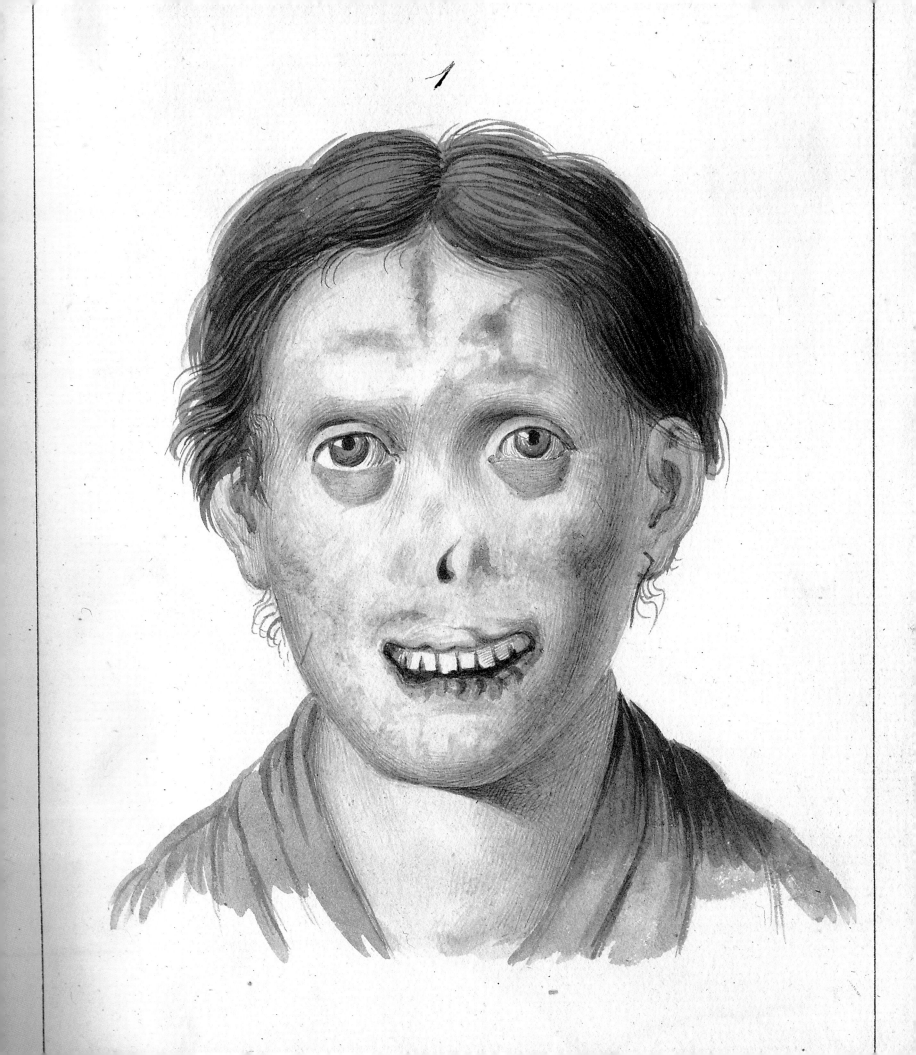

An Inquiry into the Causes and Effects of the Variolæ Vaccinæ, a Disease...Known by the Name of the Cow Pox... (1798)

Edward Jenner

London. Printed book, with etching in colored ink, with watercolor, 80 pp.; 7½ x 9¹⁵⁄₁₆ in. (19 x 25.2 cm)

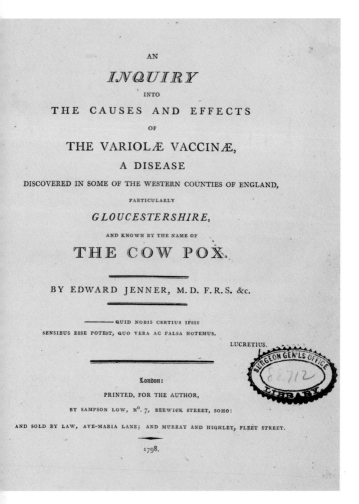

ABOVE: Title page, Edward Jenner, *An Inquiry into the Causes and Effects of the* Variolæ Vaccinæ, *a disease discovered in some of the western counties of England, particularly Gloucestershire, and known by the name of the cow pox* (London, 1798). After this first edition, the book quickly went through many other editions and was translated into many languages.

OPPOSITE: A color etching, delicately touched up with watercolor, of pox lesions. *Inquiry* (1798), facing p. 32

Much was at stake when, in 1798, Edward Jenner (1749–1823) self-published his method for preventing smallpox. With its characteristic pustules on the skin, smallpox spread in waves throughout Africa and Asia in ancient times, then into Europe in the Middle Ages and, after European contact, to the Americas and Oceania. By the eighteenth century smallpox was a global pandemic, causing the death, suffering, and disfigurement of millions. Jenner, an obscure, London-educated physician who practiced medicine in rural Gloucestershire, saw the effects of the disease firsthand and took to studying it.

It was common knowledge among Gloucestershire residents that dairymaids who contracted cowpox could not get smallpox. Jenner documented some of these incidents and conducted his own experiments, validating and transforming folk knowledge into scientific discovery, through the methods and rhetoric of science. In perhaps Jenner's earliest experiment (*Inquiry*, case 17), dairymaid Sarah Nelmes contracted cowpox from a cow named Blossom. Jenner applied Nelmes's cowpox matter to the arm of eight-year-old James Phipps. When Jenner later exposed the boy to smallpox, Phipps showed no sign of the disease. Jenner applied this method to a number of children, most famously his own son (*Inquiry*, case 22). The illustration accompanying Phipps's case (opposite) is a composite of two cowpox infections, from Nelmes and another dairymaid. As Jenner explained, he wanted to visualize on one arm the stages of cowpox from its early blistering to its later dimpled rupture.

The Royal Society refused to publish Jenner's findings on the grounds that the evidence for his claims was insufficient. But it was not simply the small number of case histories in his treatise on smallpox prevention that led the formidable institution to reject him, it was the unlikeliness and novelty of his suggested safeguard. "The Cow-pox protects the human constitution from the infection of the Small-pox," Jenner claimed. How could infected fluid from a beast prevent disease in humans?

Before Jenner, variolation was the principal method of protecting against smallpox. With variolation, pus from an infected victim is transferred to a patient who—by getting a mild infection—gains immunity to a more severe reinfection. But introducing smallpox intentionally sometimes led to the mutilation and death of previously healthy patients. By using the less virulent cowpox, such results could be avoided. Jenner coined the term "vaccination" after "variolation," taking as its root the Latin word for cow, *vacca*. He also named "cowpox" and its Latin term *variolae vaccinae* after the human smallpox (*variola major* or *minor*) to link the two diseases and so, by name and analogy, argue for cowpox's power to immunize against smallpox.

Jenner hoped his findings would become "essentially beneficial to mankind" and that his pamphlet would serve as a guide to help physicians identify cowpox and administer vaccination properly. The British government publicly recognized his work in 1802 by awarding him £10,000, and another £20,000 in 1806. It also helped him to found a National Vaccine Establishment. Within a decade of publication Jenner's method began to spread worldwide.

—RON BROGLIO

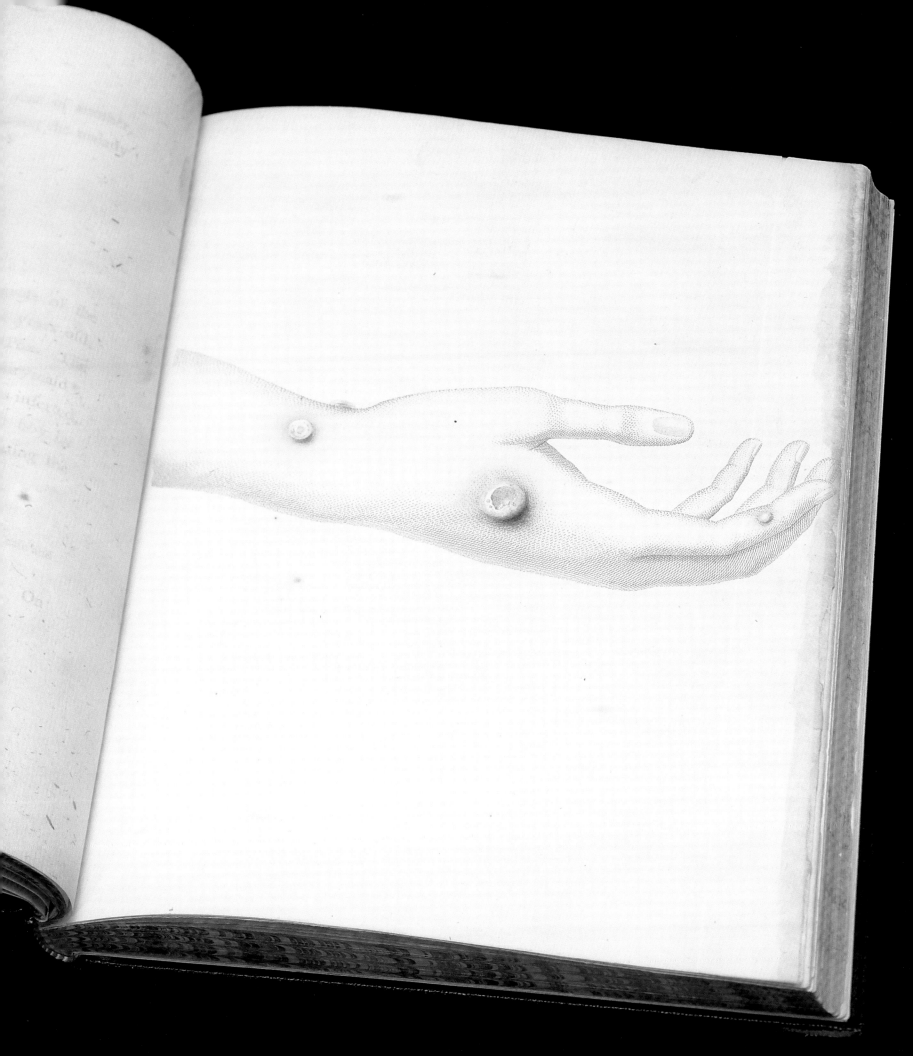

Atlas of Skin Diseases (1856–76)
Ferdinand Hebra; drawings and lithographs by Anton Elfinger and Carl Heitzmann

Atlas der Hautkrankheiten. Vienna. Printed book with chromolithographs, 10 parts in 2 vols.; 17¾ x 23¼ in. (45 x 59 cm)

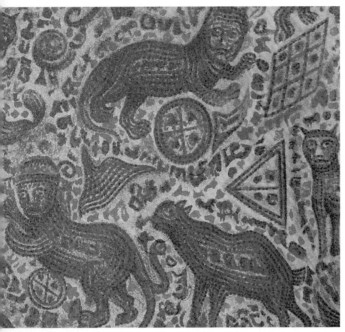

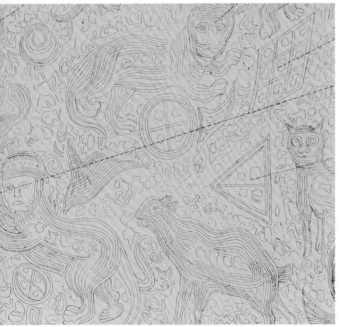

ABOVE AND OPPOSITE: "A tattooed man" with details of chromolithograph showing a section of the breast and related outline drawing. *Atlas* pt. 8 (1872), pls. 9–10

This grand atlas of skin diseases is a striking example of the richly illustrated publications that distinguished nineteenth-century dermatology. Beginning with Robert Willan's *Description and Treatment of Cutaneous Diseases*, published in London between 1798 and 1808, and Jean-Louis-Marie Alibert's 1806 *Description des maladies de la peau*, based on his observations at the Hôpital Saint-Louis in Paris, modern dermatology established itself as a discipline intrinsically tied to the use of colored images. Unlike other branches of pathology, dermatology is concerned with diseases showing on the outermost organ and is thus dedicated to the visual scrutiny of the body's surface. Ferdinand Hebra (1816–80) stressed the significance of the eye for dermatological diagnosis and teaching. Diseases of skin can be taught only if the students have the "objective view" of what they are being lectured about. Hebra accordingly advertised his atlas as a clinic in book form, with the life-size images standing in for the sick and the texts for the words of the teacher. His clinic on paper, Hebra claimed, has the additional advantage of always providing a typical example of even the most uncommon skin condition.

The folio volumes were issued by Vienna's court printing press in ten installments, using the then recently developed technique of chromolithography. While the earlier atlases authored by Willan and Alibert had been illustrated with hand-colored engravings, this technique allowed the artist to draw directly onto the lithographic stone, and also to print in color. The result, according to Hebra, was hitherto unseen "truth to nature." The mostly life-size illustrations in his atlas were initially produced by Anton Elfinger (1821–64) and completed after his death by Carl Heitzmann (1836–96), both simultaneously draftsmen and medics, and each lithograph is described as having been "painted from nature and chromolithographed" by one or both of them.

Each of the ten issues is dedicated to a group of disorders displaying symptoms on the human body's surface: from lupus to eczema to various kinds of skin cancers. The images focus on body parts such as legs, arms, genitalia, face, and neck and not only elaborate on the skin lesions but also render dress or hairdo with care. Viewers accustomed to the traditions of modern portraiture might be tempted to regard them as empathically rendered likenesses of individual persons. However, these images oscillate between portraits of diseases and effigies of patients. The image of the two children with a pigment deficiency known as albinism, for instance, lacks any accompanying case description (p. 125). They are generic Austrian children, and the suggestion that they are siblings mainly stresses the fact that their condition is a hereditary one, independent of an otherwise good state of health. Another image depicts a father and son with hirsutism (pp. 126–27). They are treated like medical curiosities; the text relates them to portraits of a seventeenth-century family with a similar condition initially collected for the cabinet of curiosities at Ambras castle.

An oddity within the atlas, a cultural rather than physical anomaly, is the tattooed man in the section on pigment anomalies (opposite and details left). Hebra says that this is a rare case of a man of "Caucasian race" who had an "artistically accomplished full body tattoo," acquired

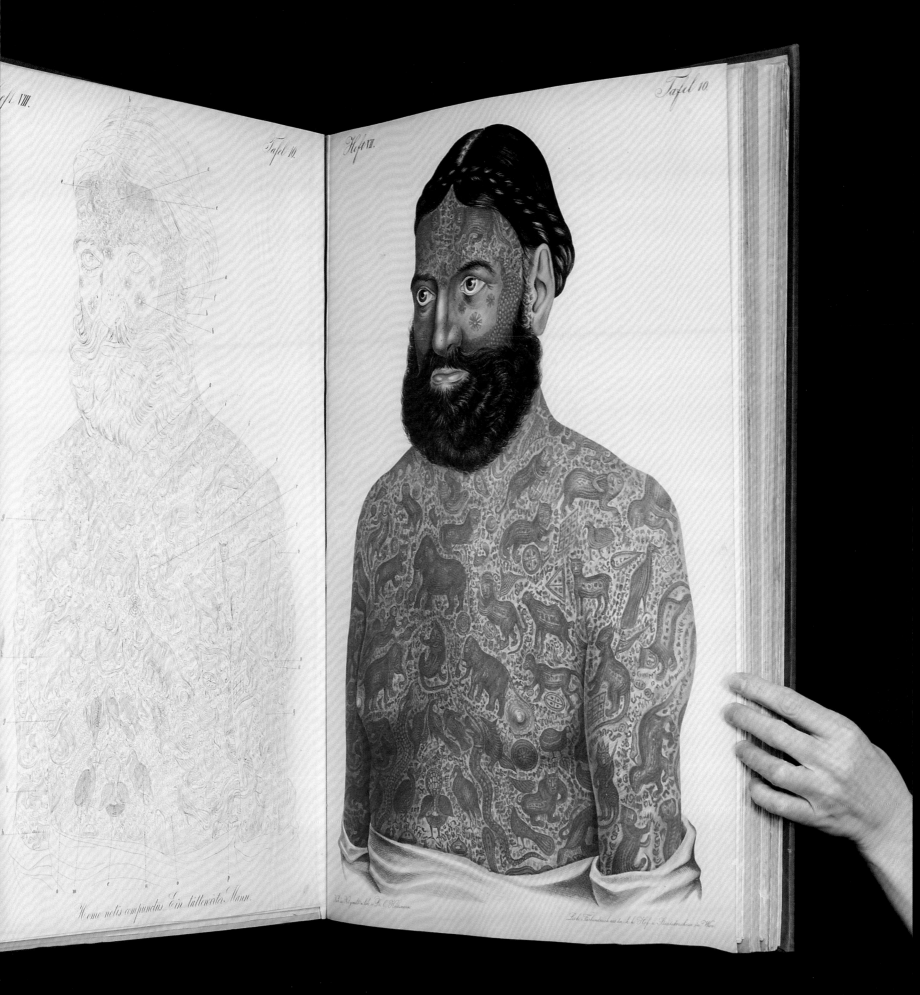

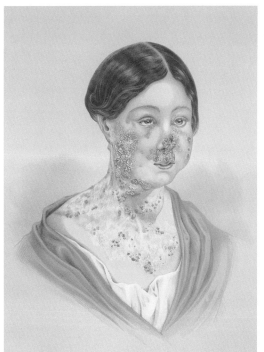 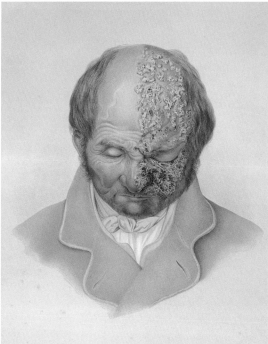 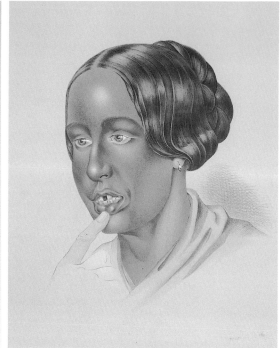

ABOVE, LEFT TO RIGHT: Woman with advanced lupus vulgaris; man with herpes zoster (shingles) at face and pate; woman with bronze tan caused by intake of silver-bearing medicaments. *Atlas* pt. 1 (1856), pl. 4; pt. 6 (1866), pl. 7; pt. 8 (1872), pl. 7

on his travels in Burma. The tattooed man, unlike the other figures presented in the atlas, is introduced as an individual, a "handsome and robust Albanese of forty-three years by the name of Georg Constantin, whose skin is, in the parts spared by the tattoo, beautiful, smooth, and fair despite the fact that his beard and hair are of a shiny black." He was familiar to many readers as a famous circus performer who traveled through North America and Europe.

A distinctive device of Hebra's atlas is the use of two versions of each image. As demonstrated here for the depiction of the tattooed man, each lithograph is accompanied by a print restricted to an outline drawing into which numbers are inserted, mapping the disease, or, in this case, the pictures tattooed on his body. Text and images are closely linked, and individual symptoms are often detailed as representing various stages of a disease. The intermediate prints thus bring the progression of time to the otherwise static image without destroying the integrity of the clinical picture established in the color lithographs.

—MECHTHILD FEND

RIGHT: Hands and forearms showing herpes iris. *Atlas* pt. 6 (1866), pl. 6

OPPOSITE: Children showing a hereditary form of albinism. *Atlas* pt. 8 (1872), pl. 1

OVERLEAF: Father and son displaying hirsutism, increased growth of facial hair. *Atlas* pt. 10 (1876), pls. 7–8

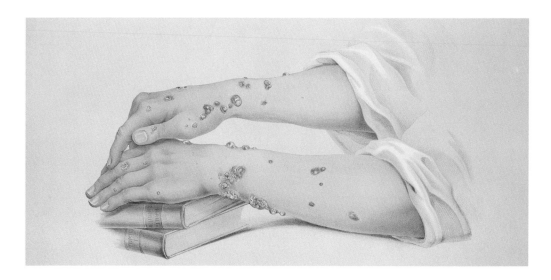

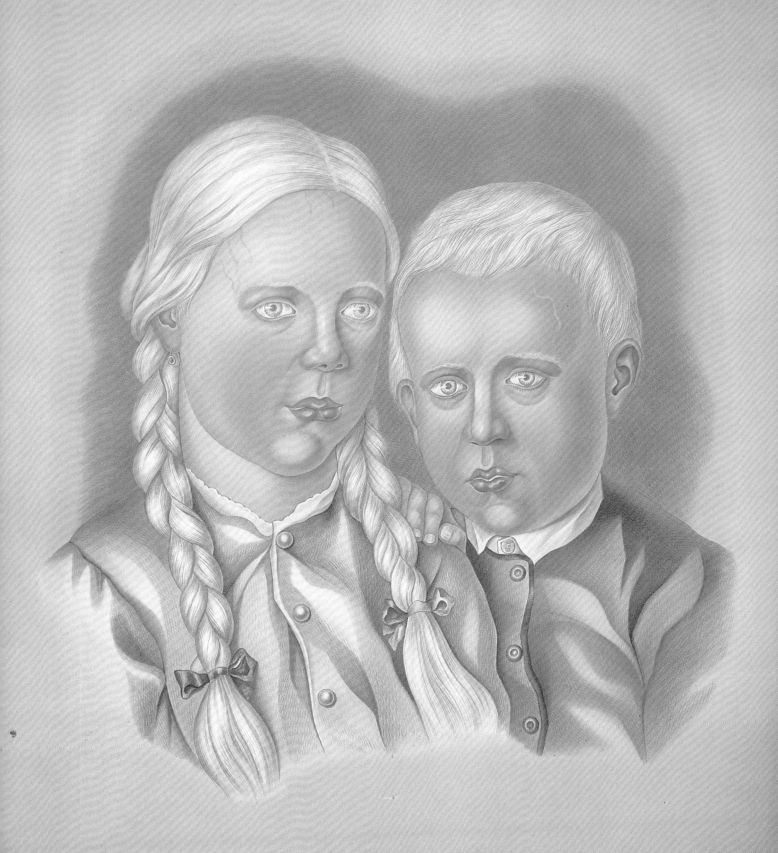

Nach der Nat. gemalt u. lith. v. Dr. C. Heitzmann.

Lith. Farbendruck aus der k. k. Hof- u. Staatsdruckerei in Wien.

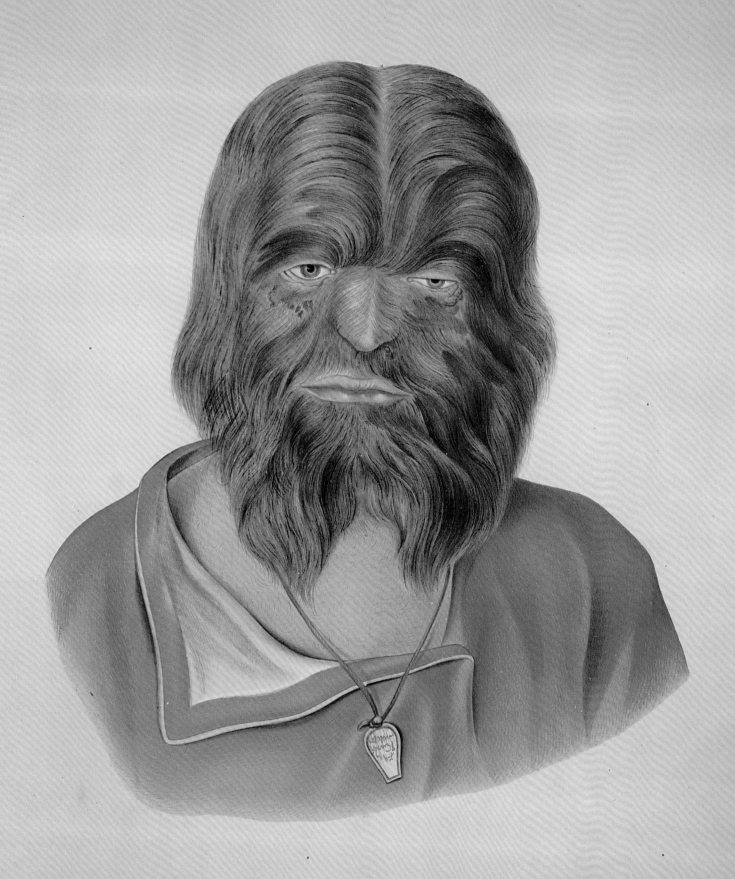

Nach der Natur gemalt u. lith. v. Dr. C. Heitzmann.

Lith. Farbendruck aus der k.k. Hof- u. Staatsdruckerei in Wien.

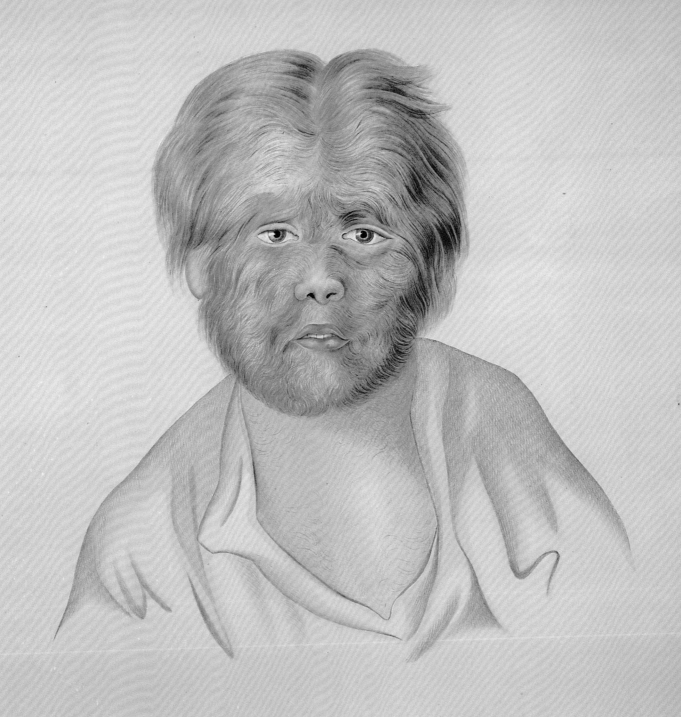

Nach der Nat. gemalt u. lith. v. Dr. C. Heitzmann.

Lith. Farbendruck aus der k. k. Hof- u. Staatsdruckerei in Wien.

The Stereoscopic Skin Clinic (1910)
Selden Irwin Rainforth

New York. Boxed set: handheld viewer (copper, wood, glass); 128 stereograph cards (colored photographs); 5 x 5¾ in. (12.7 x 14.8 cm)

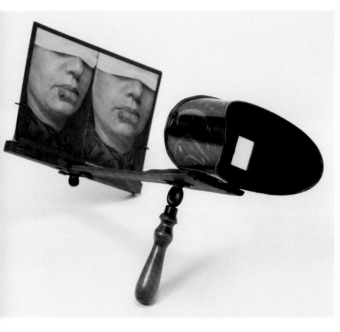

ABOVE: Stereoscope (copper, wood, and iron hinges, with glass lenses and felt lining) included in the box with viewing cards. The device faithfully follows the design of the celebrated essayist and anatomy professor Oliver Wendell Holmes Sr. *Stereoscopic Skin Clinic*

TOP, LEFT TO RIGHT: *Eczema erythematosum facei:* A chronic rash of the face commonly seen in adults. "The excoriations caused by scratching and rubbing alter its appearance." *Cicatrices palate mollis post ulcerationes syphiliticas:* "A circumscribed or diffused gummatous infiltration of the soft palate" that occurs in the tertiary stage of syphilis.

MIDDLE, LEFT TO RIGHT: *Trichophytosis unguium:* In most instances, ringworm of the nails affects only three or four fingers. "Untreated, the malady persists for years, with no tendency to spontaneous recovery." *Naevus pigmentosus:* Pigmentary moles may be "present at birth and undergo various development later.... Growths smaller than a pea are best removed by electrolysis"; larger growths should be destroyed by an "application of solid carbon dioxid."

BOTTOM, LEFT TO RIGHT: *Zoster:* Also known as "shingles," *Herpes zoster* is "an acute, self limited, probably specific, infectious disease of the nervous system," marked by lesions, "slight fever and neuralgic pains." *Sarcomatosis cutis:* "Malignant connective tissue tumors ... may have their origin in any organ of the body," including the skin. "Nodes develop in various regions but rarely reach any considerable size because death soon ensues."

The wooden handle of the viewer feels well worn. Grasping it with your fingers, you press your face against the rim of the felt-lined device and attempt to focus on the image. You see a patient—child, woman, or man—with three-dimensional, brightly colored pustules, welts, roughness, scars, birthmarks, moles, eruptions. This is New York physician Selden Rainforth's early-twentieth-century effort to harness the power of three-dimensional viewing technology (stereoscopy) to present a "clinic" of more than a hundred different kinds of skin lesions.

Rainforth (1879–1960), who also invented the "self-threading needle and holder," was not the first doctor-stereographer. In 1862 Harvard professor Oliver Wendell Holmes Sr. invented a handheld stereographic viewer so that Americans sitting in their parlors could peer at images of far-off lands and natural wonders. Rainforth's efforts were part of a craze for medical stereoscopy, which was seen as a technology of modernity that might supplant two-dimensional photography and make available to physicians, in their offices, clinical presentations of the vivid, dramatic, and disfiguring effects of skin trauma and disease. His dermatologic atlas contained 128 rectangular cards, each five inches wide and seven inches tall, with two photographs that, when placed in the handheld viewing device, displayed the dimensionality, texture, and extent of various dermatological conditions. Originally black and white, the photographs were hand tinted to display the range of colors in skin disease. On the back of each card Rainforth provided synonyms for the condition and a capsule summary of diagnosis and treatment.

The images are disturbing—tuberculous affections of the skin, keloids, smallpox, cancers, and especially syphilis in its infinite variety. (Early-twentieth-century medical schools typically had a Department of Dermatology and Syphilology.) In the cards shown here, fingertips (middle left) display the result of ringworm of the nails, the fungal distortion of the nailbed and its lingering effects. A woman's face (bottom left) illustrates the effects of shingles (*Herpes zoster*), which covers her eye, the eruption of the vesicles, and the drying yellowish and brownish crusts that fall off after several days. A child's face (middle right) displays a pigmented mole (*Naevus pigmentosus*), which Rainforth suggests may be removed with electrolysis, if small. Larger moles, he suggests, can be destroyed with solid carbon dioxide (dry ice). A blue-eyed man's chest (bottom right) displays sarcoma, or, in Rainforth's words, "malignant connective tissue tumors." An older man's face (top left) illustrates erythematous eczema, the redness of the skin, the thickening of the outer layer, the dryness and itching it produces. Although calamine lotion and zinc oxides may relieve the trouble, Rainforth advises doctors to instruct patients to avoid anything likely to produce facial congestion. The dark-faced man (top right) displays the stigmata of tertiary syphilis—a "gummatous infiltration" that eats away at the jaw and soft palate. Rainforth warns that ulceration, pain, and discomfort may intensify as the deformation of the mouth progresses. Unlike other skin conditions and diseases, he offers no treatment for this sexually transmitted disease.

—SUSAN E. LEDERER

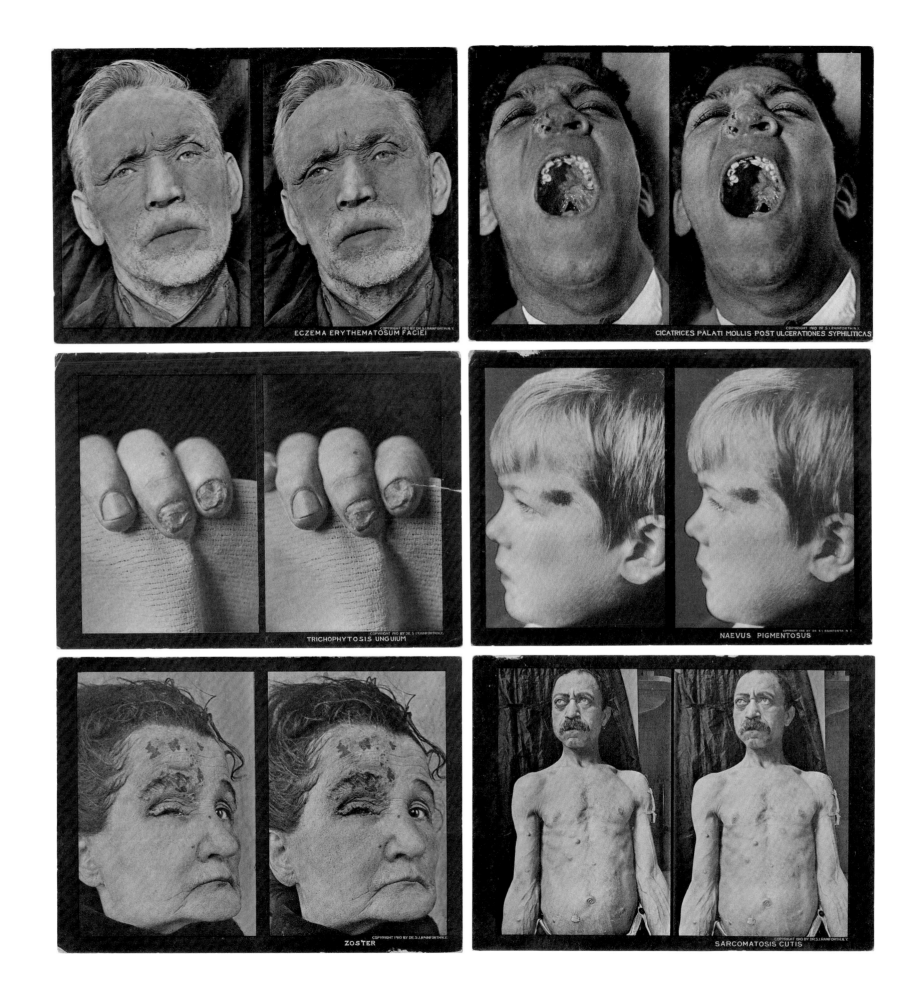

ECZEMA ERYTHEMATOSUM FACIEI

CICATRICES PALATI MOLLIS POST ULCERATIONES SYPHILITICAS

TRICHOPHYTOSIS UNGUIUM

NAEVUS PIGMENTOSUS

ZOSTER

SARCOMATOSIS CUTIS

Stereoscopic Pictures for Cross-Eyed Children (1942)
Carl Hubert Sattler

Stereoskopische Bilder für schielende Kinder. Verlag von Ferdinand Enke, Stuttgart, Germany.
Printed booklet, 24 pp., 6¼ x 3⅛ in. (16 x 8 cm); 108 cards, 2 x 2⅞ in. (5 x 7.3 cm)

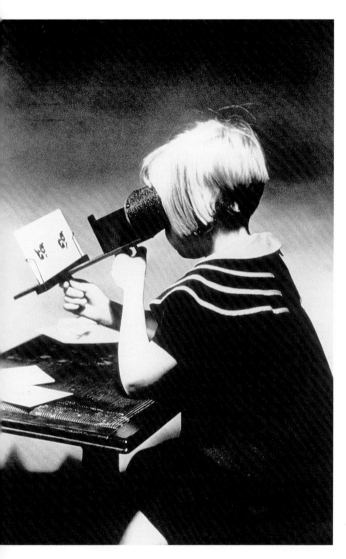

ABOVE: A young girl does corrective exercises for strabismus, using a stereoscope, ca. 1940 (place and source unknown).

OPPOSITE: Selected pairs of strabismus diagnostic and exercise cards. *Stereoskopische Bilder*

Most people have two eyes directed forward. In ophthalmology textbooks one is asked to imagine a line drawn from each eye to an object on the horizon: two parallel lines representing two lines of sight are blended by muscular and neural processes into a single image—binocular vision with depth perception. When the lines are askew, both eyes do not fix on the same point. It is hard to live with the ensuing double vision; the image from one of the eyes is suppressed by the brain, and instead of seeing double the person literally sees single. Thus "strabismus": deviation of one visual axis in the normal visual act, also referred to as "squint" and other colloquial terms that manifest the cosmetic dismay that has always accompanied the condition—lazy eye, boss-eyed, cross-eyed, walleyed, cockeyed.

Pavlov's influential work on acquired conditioned reflex suggested that the eye and brain could be retrained with repetitive exercises, particularly in young children. In 1927 Carl Hubert Sattler (1880–1953?), a Königsberg physician, produced an inexpensive set of stereoscope cards for the diagnosis and treatment of juvenile strabismus at home, subsequently widely translated and reprinted. This edition was published in 1942.

The cards come in pairs that, viewed through a stereoscope, make a composite picture. An umbrella handle is bereft of its canopy. The strabismatic child will see only the handle or the canopy. Asking her what she sees will indicate which eye is fixing on an image and which is suppressed. Bringing the images together—seeing the umbrella whole—is the therapy. According to Sattler, other stereoscope cards, featuring abstract shapes, were hard for children to relate to or describe. Thus the sad moon, the chick following the rooster, etc., were designed to make these exercises *fun*—though generations of children struggling to put the broom in the snowman's hand might testify differently. An accompanying booklet told parents and physicians what to ask with each pair, often beginning with the phrase "What do you see?"

British stereoscope cards produced during World War II show airplanes with parachutists descending from them. Sattler's cards, designed in the 1920s, betray no hint of the historical circumstances of the year of their reprinting: the duck still opens its beak, the frog still jumps through a hoop. Nonetheless ophthalmology was profoundly changed by National Socialist policies regarding Jewish doctors and scientists; by 1942 Sattler was one of the few strabismus specialists left in Germany. Debates over the causes and etiology of strabismus often mentioned hereditary factors and neurotic instability—the very terms "lazy eye" or "boss eye" suggest constitutional failure. To have such a condition was profoundly dangerous; under the Nazis, hereditary conditions associated with undesirable character, even eminently correctable ones, were grounds for sterilization or worse.

When these charming cards were issued, German armies were occupying much of Europe, Hitler had convened the Wannsee Conference to coordinate the Final Solution, and trainloads of Jews and other "enemies" were beginning to arrive at Auschwitz and other death camps.

"What do you see?" The question hangs in the air of historical time with quiet intensity.

—HANNAH LANDECKER

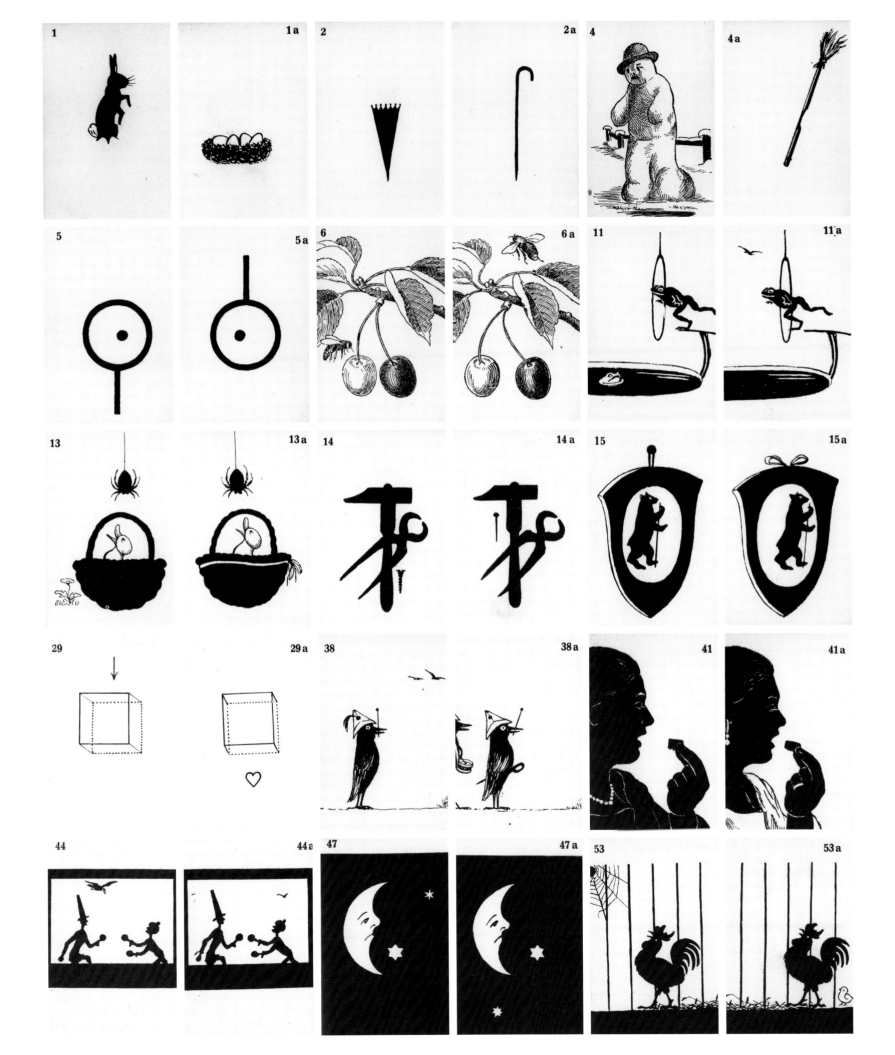

Biomicroscopy of the Eye: Slit Lamp Microscopy of the Living Eye (1943–49)
Milton Lionel Berliner; illustrations by J. McGuiness Myers

New York and London: Paul B. Hoeber, Inc.; © 1943, 1949 Hoeber Medical Division, Harper & Row Publishers, Inc.
Printed book with color illustrations by J. McGuiness Myers, 2 vols.; 1,512 pp.; 6½ x 10 in. (16 x 25.4 cm)

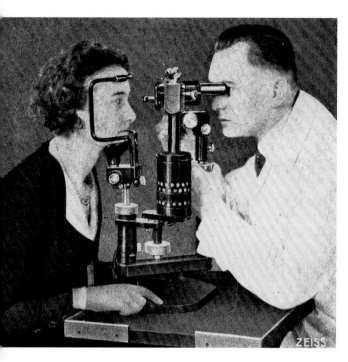

ABOVE: Eye examination with a Zeiss biomicroscopic apparatus. *Biomicroscopy of the Eye*, vol. 1, p. 35

*A*n intense light that seems to shine directly into your brain, the quelling of the strong impulse to pull away, a professional stranger breathing so close by. Anyone who has gone forehead-to-forehead with an ophthalmologist will have some familiarity with biomicroscopy. But few of us have much sense of what might be seen in the depths of our own eyes with that devastating beam.

In 1943 Milton L. Berliner (1895–1981) published the first half of a two-volume compendium of biomicroscopy in clinical practice. The first volume of *Biomicroscopy of the Eye*, with 512 images—40 pages of color plates—was followed in 1949 by the lavish second installment, with 1,233 illustrations, 503 in color. Given the lights and lenses that constitute the technique, one wonders why the camera is so little involved. There is no angst here about the dubious objectivity of Berliner's hand-drawn images of the living eye versus precise photographic transcription, merely a matter-of-fact statement of the impossibility of attaining adequate photographs.

Consider these drawings (opposite) of changes to the aqueous humor, the watery space between the lens and the cornea: "A residual veil (diffuse illumination), floating like a sail, in the anterior chamber." Delicate layers of tissues and their liquid ruptures are drawn in a sinuous style; that these are living eyes is communicated in the use of shocking color. Without the imprimatur of medicine this might appear a quintessential example of outsider art, an obsessive cataloguing of fantastic images of the diseased inner eye cut by light. Yet volume 1 was greeted by reviewers as "one of those rare books that profoundly influence clinical practice." Volume 2 was similarly welcomed for its lack of esoteric abstraction from day-to-day clinical practice—a hinted comparison to earlier, less-accessible compendia of such material. Berliner's books were seen to present not only the technique but the difference the technique made in the clinic.

Biomicroscopy couples a microscope with a focused beam of light; its history is entwined with that of the lightbulb. It originated in the 1910s with Allvar Gullstrand (1862–1930), ophthalmologist and Nobel Prize winner, who made a controllable beam of very intense light using a slit opening and a condensing lens (which came to be called a slit lamp), rather than shining a light directly on the eye. The biomicroscope works, Berliner tells us, like a searchlight in a night sky, or sunlight entering a darkened room through a crack. Objects in the path of the searchlight beam are illuminated, or suspended particles of dust become visible as they scatter the sunlight. Similarly, the transparent tissues of the cornea, lens, and aqueous, being gels, scatter the intense "pencil of light" projected into the eye. This evocation of the light of knowledge in the darkened room of the body—applying the illuminatory focus of science to make even the transparent visible—is here made poignant by the systematic elaboration of the clouding of sight. Exudations, inflammations, coal particles, lacerations, vascularization, sclerosis, opacities, scarring: portraits of a thousand ways in which the eye can be the seat of blindness.

—HANNAH LANDECKER

OPPOSITE: Drawings of the eye's innards as seen through the biomicroscope. *Biomicroscopy of the Eye*, vol. 1, pl. XL

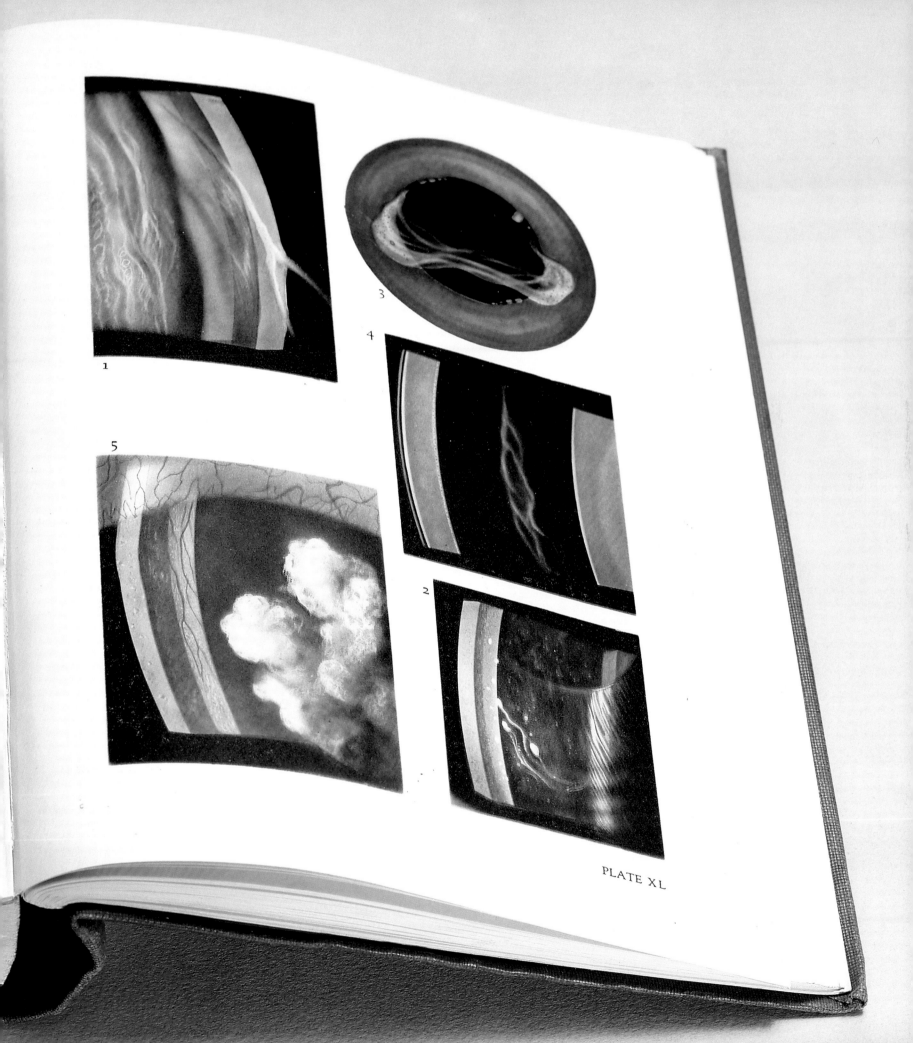

PLATE XL

The Life and Education of Laura Dewey Bridgman, the Deaf, Dumb, and Blind Girl (1878)
Mary Swift Lamson

Boston. Printed book, 373 pp. with plates; 4⅞ x 7⁹⁄₁₆ in. (13 x 19.5 cm)

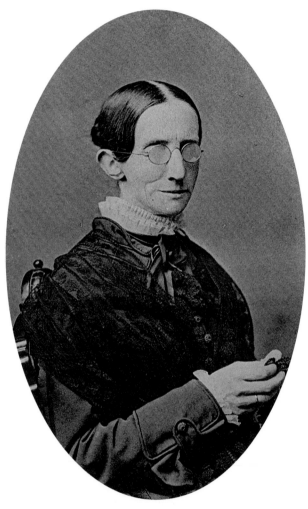

ABOVE: Laura Bridgman in her late forties, engaged in crochet work that she sold to visitors for pocket money. *Life and Education of Laura Dewey Bridgman*, frontispiece

OPPOSITE: The elegantly bound volume, which includes a signed holograph facsimile of Bridgman's widely circulated religious poem "Holy Home." Bridgman transcribed it by folding paper over a tablet with grooved lines, a method of lettering commonly used by the blind in this period, and which appears in the facsimile signature on the book cover.

This biography of Laura Bridgman (1829–89), the first deaf-blind person ever to read, write, and converse in the finger alphabet, attracted little interest when it appeared in 1878. Consisting largely of extracts from the journal of Bridgman's teacher Mary Swift Lamson (1822–1909) and other teachers at the Perkins Institution for the Blind, Lamson's narrative lacks the drama of Helen Keller's famous autobiography, published twenty-five years later. Lamson's timing was also unfortunate. In the 1840s and '50s thousands of admirers had flocked to see Bridgman on "exhibition days" at Perkins, and Charles Dickens's touching depiction of her in *American Notes* (1842) had made her an international celebrity. But as she aged and lost her girlish charm public attention faded. By the time *The Life and Education of Laura Dewey Bridgman* appeared, few remembered the "fair young creature" rescued, as Dickens said, from her "dark prison" and brought into the light of human community.

Bridgman's rescuer was Samuel Gridley Howe (1801–76), director of Perkins, who recognized the bright seven-year-old as the ideal subject for scientific and pedagogical experiments he hoped to undertake—experiments that would not only establish the educability of the deaf-blind but also prove the innateness of ideas, including the idea of God. If Bridgman, cut off from most sense data since the age of two, could learn language, develop a natural conscience, and ultimately reason her own way to the existence of a Divine Creator, she would stand as a living refutation of both Calvinistic pessimism and the Lockean view of the child's mind as a blank slate, dependent for knowledge on the sensory apprehension of external objects.

To preserve his experiment's integrity Howe, a Unitarian, had ordered the female teachers who oversaw Bridgman's daily instruction to insulate her from all religious doctrine. Nevertheless, when he embarked on a European tour in 1843 he gave sole charge of his prize pupil to Lamson, who like many Perkins teachers was an orthodox Congregationalist concerned about Bridgman's soul. Upon his return sixteen months later, he was dismayed to find Bridgman throwing tantrums and parroting orthodox doctrine. Ignoring Lamson's insistence that she had not violated his trust, he publicly blamed her for ruining his experiment by filling Bridgman's head with frightening Calvinist notions and disciplining her too harshly. Lamson left Perkins shortly thereafter, married well, and devoted herself to philanthropy.

Lamson's memoir, published two years after Howe's death, was her long-delayed response to his accusations. Howe's daughters dismissed the book as a "dry record of facts," but it is better understood as a subtle challenge to both Howe's philosophy and his portrayal of Lamson as the willful, punitive teacher who force-fed Calvinist doctrine to an uncomprehending deaf-blind girl. With the support of eminent theologian Edwards Park, whom she enlisted to write the introduction, Lamson argued that Howe had misunderstood his own pupil. While Bridgman's "highly nervous temperament" gave her mind its "unusual power," it also agitated and irritated her. She needed the religious consolations that Howe deliberately withheld; once freed from his control she could overcome anger and fear and declare to Lamson: "God gives me strength."

—ELISABETH GITTER

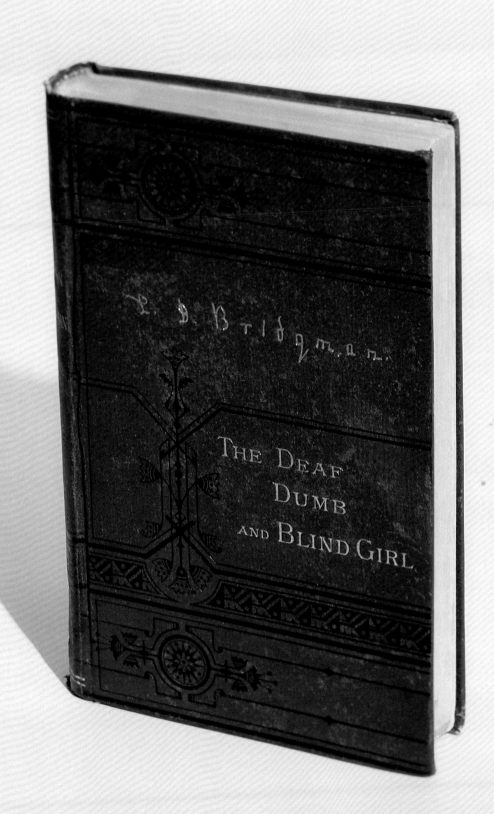

Mayerle's Lithographed International Test Chart (1907)
George Mayerle

San Francisco. Lithograph with hand-colored swatches on cardboard; 27¾ x 22 in. (71.1 x 55.8 cm)

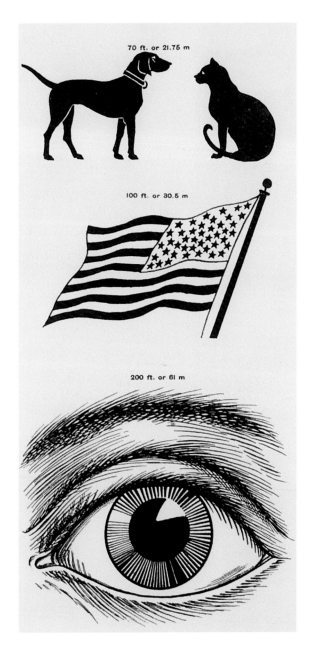

ABOVE AND OPPOSITE: Optometrist George Mayerle combined an array of eye tests on a single chart that, he boasted, was "accurate, artistic, ornamental, practical and reliable." Marketing the chart to fellow practitioners, he promised that it "makes a good impression and convinces the patient of your professional expertness."

This multilingual eye-test chart, published in 1907, was the creation of the optometrist George Mayerle (ca. 1870–1929), a "Graduate German Expert Optician" who set up shop in San Francisco in the mid-1890s. Optometry was professionalizing at the time, and Mayerle was on board. A charter member of the American Optometric Association at its founding in 1898, a decade later (not long after the eye chart appeared) Mayerle delivered a lecture on "The Progress of Optical Science" at a national conference of opticians. Typically, professionalizers were anxious to make a distinction between certified, licensed expert practitioners and undiplomaed marketers of nostrums and products. But Mayerle straddled the line. If he saw himself as a scientific practitioner, he was also right at home in optometry's peddler tradition, selling a variety of products to a national market, including "Mayerle's Diamond Crystal Eye Glasses" and "Mayerle's Eyewater," which he pitched as "the Greatest Eye Tonic" and sold by mail order and in drugstores.

His eye chart, which he claimed to be "the result of many years of theoretical study and practical experience," combined four subjective tests done during an eye examination. Running through the middle of the chart, the seven vertical panels test for acuity of vision with characters in the Roman alphabet (for English, German, and other European readers) and also in Japanese, Chinese, Russian, and Hebrew. A panel in the center replaces the alphabetic characters with symbols for children and adults who were illiterate or who could not read any of the other writing systems offered. Directly above the center panel is a version of the radiant dial that tests for astigmatism. On either side of that are lines that test the muscular strength of the eyes. Finally, across the bottom, boxes test for color vision, a feature intended especially (according to one advertisement) for those working on railroads and steamboats. The chart measures 22 by 28 inches and is printed on heavy cardboard; a positive version of it appears on one side, a negative version on the reverse. It sold for $3.00 or for $6.00 with a special cabinet designed to reveal only those parts of the chart needed at the time ("thus avoiding many unnecessary questions").

The "international" chart is an artifact of an immigrant nation—produced by a German optician in a polyglot city where West met East (and which was then undergoing massive rebuilding after the 1906 earthquake)—and of a globalizing economy. One advertisement promoted it as "the only chart published that can be used by people of any nationality," such as might be needed by a practitioner in almost any American city. Another ad, which appeared around the same time, touted it as "the only chart...that can be used equally well in any part of the world." Mayerle's internationalism was part of a marketing strategy, but when it suited him he could patriotically claim that his wares contributed to the project of American imperial expansion. A 1902 advertisement, for instance, boasted that a pair of his eyeglasses was used "at Manila, during the Spanish-American War," by none other than Admiral Dewey himself.

—STEPHEN P. RICE

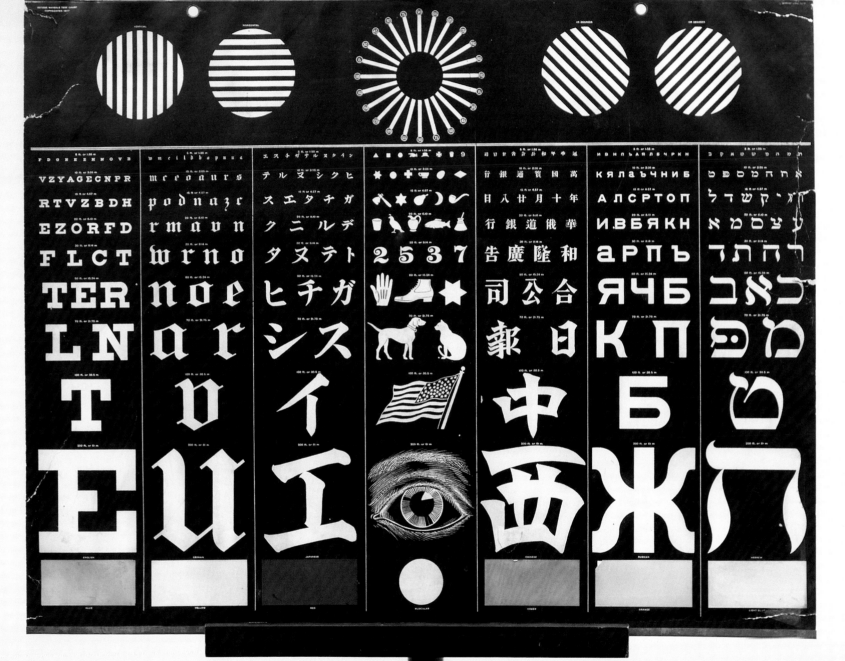

Experimental Surgery Drawings (1929–30)
William P. Didusch

Baltimore. Ink and pencil drawings on card stock; 1929: 7 x 8¾ in. (18 x 22 cm); 1930: 7⅜ x 11⅛ in. (18.9 x 28.5 cm)

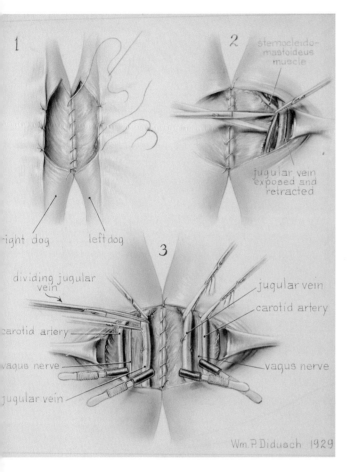

ABOVE: William Didusch's drawing (1929) of W. M. Firor's operation to suture two dogs together at the neck, connecting the jugular vein of one to the carotid artery of the other, and vice versa.

OPPOSITE: William Didusch's drawing (1930) of W. M. Firor's procedure to remove the pituitary gland from the head of a monkey.

In 1929 Warfield Monroe Firor (1896–1988), a young surgeon, commissioned William Didusch (1895–1981), an equally young medical illustrator, to make drawings for an article on his surgical experiments. Both were rising stars at Johns Hopkins Medical School in Baltimore. A student of the renowned medical illustrator Max Brödel (1870–1941), Didusch was already recognized for his accuracy and encyclopedic knowledge of anatomy. His illustrations, like those of his teacher, had a hyperrealistic shine, a gloss that gave his drawings of living tissue the luster of commercial magazine art.

But why did Firor prefer hand-rendered illustrations for his article? Before 1930, limitations in halftone printing technology made photographic reproductions appear gray and muddy. By contrast reproductions of drawings were highly legible. An artist, far more selective than a camera, could omit well-known or superfluous anatomical features, highlight "at-risk" elements (like the 1929 drawings of the vagus nerve shown here at left), and include—or exclude—the surgeon's hands and instruments as required. The illustrator showed what the surgeon wished to demonstrate. No more, no less.

Firor's operation went like this: he sutured together two dogs, under ether, at the neck, connecting the jugular vein of one to the carotid artery of the other, and vice versa. Placid animals were best. According to Firor, "Mongrels with…hound ancestry are particularly good." The goal was to find out "how long it is possible to cross the circulations of dogs and to ascertain the effects of a continuous exchange of blood between two animals." Why Firor thought this might be useful remains a mystery.

The operation resulted in a massive drop in blood pressure and, later, a fatal transfusion reaction from mixing the blood of unrelated animals. Firor repeated the procedure on forty pairs of dogs. All died, he noted, but some survived, unanesthetized, for as long as six days.

A year later, in another experiment also illustrated by Didusch, he used a specially designed suction tube to remove the pituitary gland, an essential, hormone-producing part of the brain, from monkeys. The monkeys survived the procedure but without hormone replacement died shortly after.

Was Firor a monster? Far from it. He was a family man whose young son likely had a pet of his own. He wrote articles for theological journals in his spare time. He was the author of influential research papers, the recipient of awards, and the subject of a *Time* magazine profile. Ingenious, creative, and dedicated to his patients, he became one of the country's most eminent surgeons.

Today such procedures would be prohibited. Firor, however, adhered to the ethical values of his time: animals were legitimate "subjects," to be freely exploited for the progress of medicine and the benefit of humanity. They were as disposable as candy wrappers. People too, if poor, black, imprisoned, disabled, or mentally ill, were used without their knowledge or consent for potentially lethal experiments.

I wonder if Didusch, a famously warm and gentle soul, lost any sleep over this commission. I did.

—MARK KESSELL

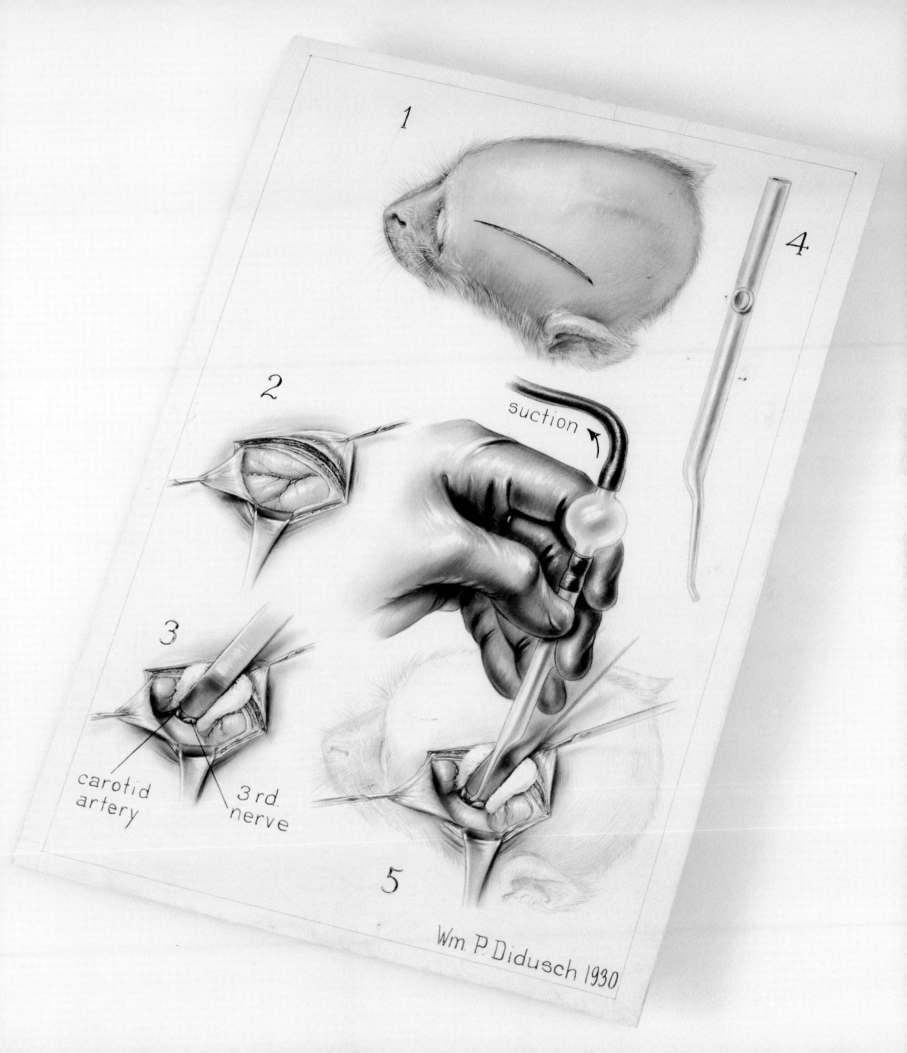

1

2

3

carotid
artery

3 rd.
nerve

4

suction

5

Wm. P. Didusch 1930

Atlas of Colored Plates Illustrating Features of Anatomy, Surgery, Deformities... etc. (1889)

Elias Smith

Peoria, Illinois. Printed book with chromolithographs; 30 plates; 14¾ x 10⅛ in. (37.5 x 25.7 cm)

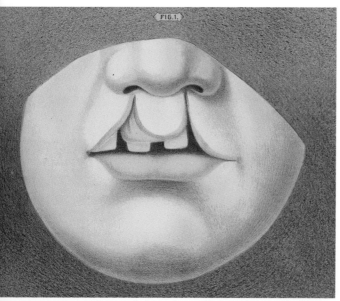

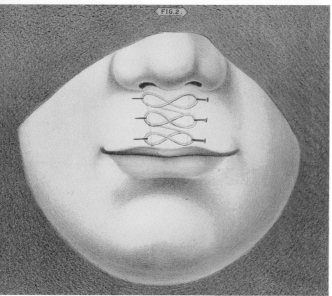

ABOVE: Double harelip with an idealized repair and post-operative sutures. *Atlas of Colored Plates*, pl. 7

OPPOSITE: Rhinoplasty. "The figure shows the kind of bandage which the patient will have to make up his mind to endure." The flap of arm skin will need to acquire a blood supply from the vessels of the face toward the formation of a new nose. *Atlas of Colored Plates*, pl. 10

"Deprived of the advantages of the dissecting room, the ideas once so thoroughly acquired soon begin to fade, and the images, once so distinct, become confused and mixed." So argues a blurb on the title page of Dr. Elias Smith's *Atlas of Colored Plates Illustrating Features of Anatomy, Surgery, Deformities, Displacements, Strictures, Fistulas, Cancer, Syphilis, Glanders etc., etc.* Yet the atlas itself is a bizarre admixture. Tracheotomy shares a page with disarticulated fingers. A charming series of hands applying scalpels, as though they were pens meeting paper rather than knives laying skin bare, gives way to horrifying illustrations of "operations upon the penis," of "catheters fixed" in a urethra, gangrenous buboes, and a disease passed from horse to human called glanders (which today, outside veterinary medicine, is studied in connection with biological warfare). Portraits appear, as when the scourge of syphilis invents a type of person—the so-called syphilide (a far cry from its near homophone "sylphide"). Another head turned to profile is a conglomeration of bends, folds, and impossible torsions of skin amounting to a type that could be termed a convolute.

Skin is what matters most, but not real skin. Instead, Smith's *Atlas* stages a dream about skin. The dreamer is an illustrator or surgeon for whom skin tears like paper, in whose hand, and through whose eye, bodies can be cut from the swath of their environment like paper dolls. We aren't sure if what we are looking at is part of a human face or a cloth snipped with a ragged-edged pair of scissors: the images here recall the theater's ritual draping of cloths and masking (off) of parts.

Devoid of 1890s accoutrements, as if by magic, a blue cuff (trimmed in gold) thrusts, darts, and points in many of Smith's illustrations. Suddenly we're in a marionette theater or puppet show. (Fittingly the *Atlas*'s publisher was the American Manikin Co.) I imagine our artist to be a sign painter by day and a dauber of syphilitic chancres by night. We see forms, mostly pink on ocher-colored backgrounds. Free floating, three hands detached at the wrist perform a ballet of fingers in a macabre parade of missing thumbs. Suddenly, noses struck off are reapplied to a face.

In ancient India, Brahmins developed a remedy for deformities that had been caused by "punishment for crime" by taking skin from the forehead to repair the partial or total loss of a nose. In fifteenth-century Italy, Antonio Branca and Gaspare Tagliacozzi (whose name means "mussel cutter") devised a nose-forming method that required the patient's face to be rigged to a flap of arm skin for weeks on end. Though the technique usually resulted "in deformity more hideous than that which it had been intended to cure," a statue honoring the great Tagliacozzi shows him holding a human nose. Neither Gogol's famous literary nose nor Freud's equally famous shine on the nose as the site of a patient's obsession, Elias Smith's *Atlas* features the refashioned nose of the amateur-professional, of masks now tragic, now comic, in a world where the distinction between the two is never clear cut.

—MARY CAPPELLO

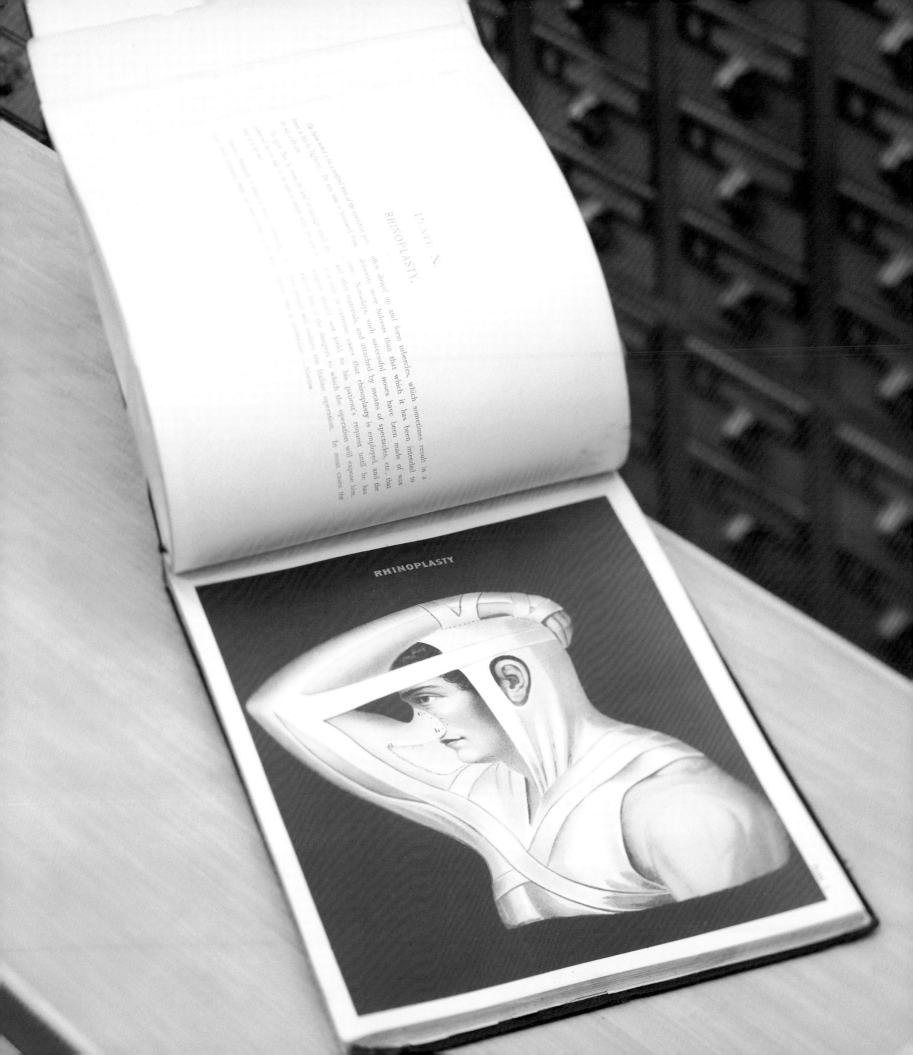

PLATE X

RHINOPLASTY.

RHINOPLASTY

Mesmerism Scrapbooks (1842–54)
Theodosius Purland

London. Scrapbook, with extra illustration, fancy section pages. 4 vols.; 8½ x 10¾ in. (21.6 x 27.3 cm)

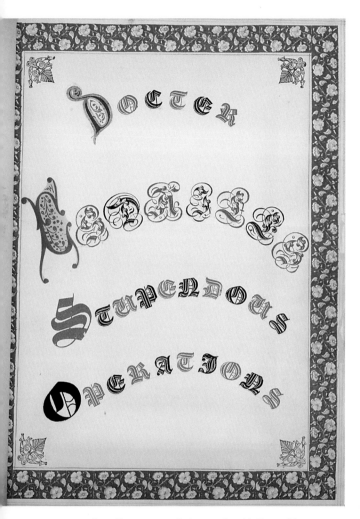

ABOVE: A section page made from cut-out letters of fancy typography, "Doctor Esdaills Stupendous Operations," begins a chapter of letters and reports about the Calcutta Mesmeric Hospital, India, directed by Dr. James Esdaile (whose name is spelled variously in the documents). Scrapbook, vol. 4

OPPOSITE: Esdaile claimed to have removed a ninety-pound tumor from a man "without his knowledge." Using a specially designed knife, he excised it in three minutes, reporting that the patient "had no difficulty in recovering from the shock, and is doing perfectly well." Letter (with drawing) from Esdaile to Dr. Elliotson, ca. 1850, Scrapbook, vol. 4

What was mesmerism? A mesmeric trance, according to one mesmerist, was induced by "the operation of the nervous force or power of one individual in a certain degree of activity upon the nervous system of another in a certain degree of passivity." Such trances could be established without even touching the subject, which seemed to indicate "the operation of some subtle but physical agency"—an invisible fluid that pervaded everything. Whatever the cause, the result was unusual intimacy between mesmerizer and mesmerized. Asked if "the minds of the mesmerist and the patient become one," Harriet Martineau replied "sometimes, but not often," specifying that when such unity occurs, the two people "taste, feel &c. the same things at the same moment."

The age of mesmerism (1775–1890s) was one of almost limitless possibility. People in trances communed with distant minds. They saw through solid objects and even bodily tissues to identify illnesses. Those most caught up in mesmerism (also called "animal magnetism") were "visionary enthusiasts," according to an article in *Punch*, "people like Theodosius Purland [1805–81], a dentist who energetically used mesmerism for tooth extractions as well as surgical operations." Alfred Russel Wallace, the evolutionary theorist, described Purland as "one of the most interesting, amusing, and eccentric men I became acquainted with during my residence in London, and with whom I soon became quite intimate." Purland had "immense energy and vitality—one of those men whose words pour out in a torrent, and who have always something wise or witty to say." He was also "a very powerful mesmerist" who "could succeed in sending patients into the mesmeric trance when other operators failed."

Purland documented mesmerism in four fascinating scrapbooks. Lovingly glued onto the now brittle pages are pamphlets, posters, letters, drawings, sermons, ticket stubs for séances. The scrapbooks also document the mesmeric hospital that Purland helped found for the alleviation of pain during amputation, tumor excisions, tooth pulling, and the like.

Mesmerism seemed to enable its subjects to transgress boundaries. In the mesmeric trance patients spoke and acted in ways that challenged their gender and class positions. They would dance, sing, assume familiarity with their superiors, commit other improprieties. In some cases a completely new character appeared, a phenomenon that was labeled double consciousness. Who *was* that person? What exactly *was* the nature of the self that allowed for such a fractured subjectivity?

Purland insisted that mesmerists were scientists. But the medical profession ignored the more than three hundred cases where mesmerism had some proven benefit and instead championed anesthesia. Why? Perhaps it was an unsettling sense of boundary transgression. Anesthesia uses impersonal gas to put a person to sleep and does not depend on a doctor's spell. The anesthetist's authority is not threatened by dangerous sympathies with his patient. The ideal of a community of sensation with strangers near and far is undone.

What a pity that mesmerism's dreams of openness and intimacy had to be buried along with its more outlandish fantasies!

—MARIANNE NOBLE

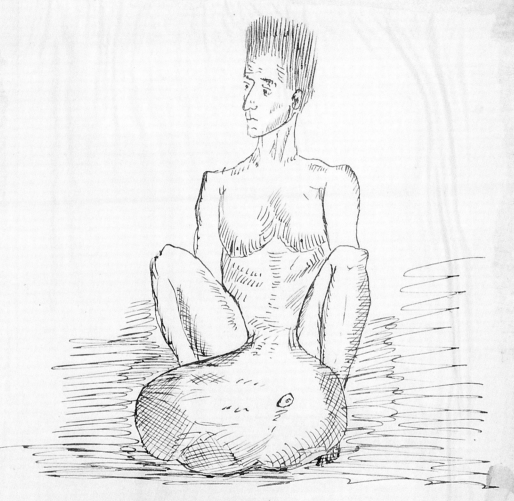

Boleram Ghose — aged 45

Tumer 6 feet in circumference

2 ft round the neck

weight 90 lbs.

Removed in the mesmeric sleep, in 3

minutes, by Dr Esdaile.

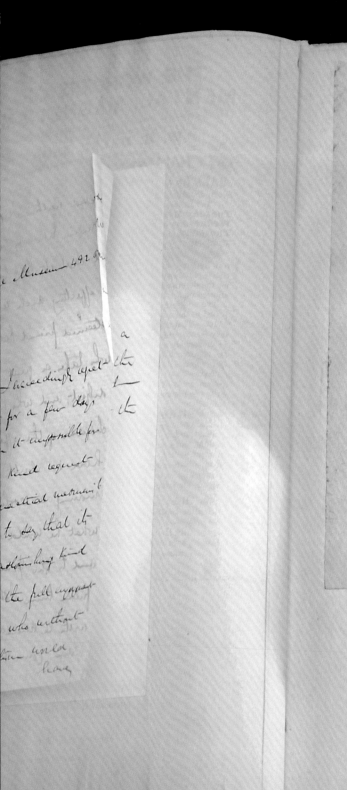

THE WONDERS OF MENTAL MAGNETISM.

1842

This new science, commonly called **Animal Magnetism**, will be practically illustrated by

W. H. HALSE, ESQ.

And three Young Ladies, on four successive Evenings, at the

CITY HALL, 110, CHANCERY LANE
AND
HALL OF SCIENCE, CITY ROAD, FINSBURY,

Seven doors from Featherstone Street, south; at Eight o'clock in the Evening. Admission ~~One Shilling each.~~

Tuesday Evening,	December 14	. . Hall of Science,
Wednesday do.	ditto 15	. . City Hall,
Thursday do.	ditto 16	. . Hall of Science,
Friday do.	ditto 17	. . City Hall.

N. B. As Mr. Halse finds that Lecturing and Discussion disturb his magnetizing powers, he will reserve himself for the illustrative parts, and call in the talented aid of his relative, Mr. Carlile, for the description and defence. Two triers or objectors will be allowed on the Platform, and a chairman appointed.

The following important and most interesting facts are established in this science.

1st.—That the primary physical sensations of the human being may be suspended, by the magnetizing power of the will of another, as thoroughly as under their state of death, *verified by the test of the monster Electrical Battery, at the Adelaide Gallery*, on one of the ladies; and by the electrical eel.

2nd.—That under the complete paralysis, prostration, or temporary death of the primary physical sensations, they may be recalled to life and health at the will and pleasure of the operating magnetizer.

3rd.—That while the primary sensations are in sleep, as deep as death, a new class of internal, secondary or mental sensations are called into life, exhibiting the most perfect memory of past life and action, and a purer or brighter intellectual power than in common life, presenting a sight without the eye, and a hearing without the ear; a taste without the palate, and a smell without the nostrils' power! and a touch without contact. A magnetic fluid performing all the intermediate offices.

Mr. Halse is open for engagement to illustrate before any Scientific Institutions or private parties, and to receive patients in his profession of Medical Galvanism, from Eleven to Four daily, at the City Hall, 110, Chancery Lane; leaving town on the 18th instant, over the holidays.

Alfred Carlile, Printer, Water-lane, Fleet st.

Mesmerism & Mesmero-phrenology.

AN EXHIBITION
OF
MESMERIC PHENOMENA,

Will take place every WEDNESDAY EVENING, at Mr. J. N. BAILEY'S Apartments, 63, Hatton Garden, COMMENCING AT 8 O'CLOCK PRECISELY.

ADMISSION, ONE SHILLING.

...tory of Mesmerism...Objections to Mesmerism---Experiments demonstrative of the truth of Mesmerism.

LECTURE II.

Spontaneous Catalepsy---Artificial Catalepsy induced in the waking state---Catalepsy in the Mesmeric state---Increase of Physical strength by Mesmeric Agency---Curative powers of Mesmerism---Demonstrations and Experiments.

LECTURE III.

Division of the Mesmeric state into Stages---Phreno-Mesmerism---Hypothesis of suggestive Dreaming---Mesmeric Thought-reading---Sympathy of taste and feeling---Clairvoyance---Illustrations and Experiments.

To commence at half-past Eight o'clock precisely.

ADMISSION to the Body of the Hall, 2d.; to the Gallery, 3d.

MASON, PRINTER, CLERKENWELL GREEN.

...M!
...1843,
...URSE OF
...ociation,
...6th, and the

...RSM
...Y!
...RES
...rds,
...20th Inst.
...ion,
...OLBORN,
...to Preside;
...e Evening
...tained,
...ING.
...d, although
...l.
...Exercise
...erved Seats,
...ng Acre; and 16,
...e, Waterloo-rd.;
...Hinckly's Coffee
...n, 167, Fleet-st.;
...O'CLOCK.
...High Holborn.

July 1843.

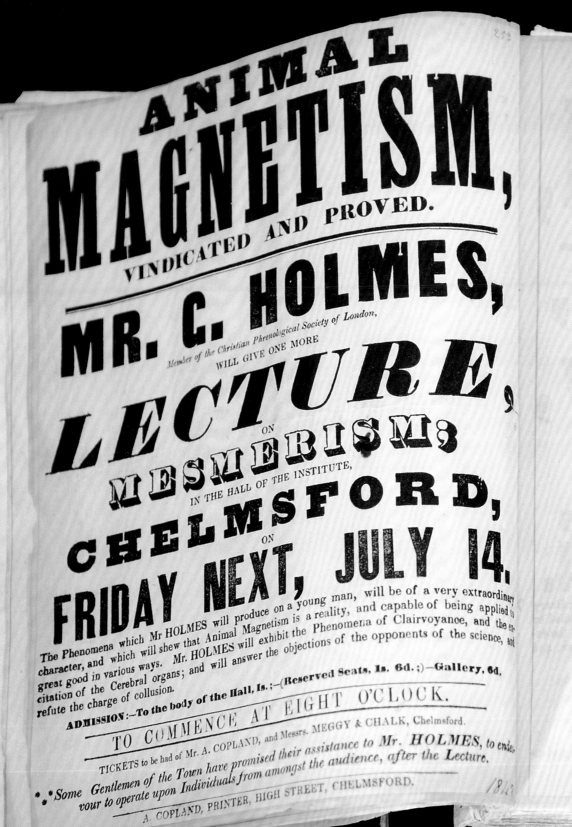

ANIMAL MAGNETISM,

VINDICATED AND PROVED.

MR. C. HOLMES,

Member of the Christian Phrenological Society of London,

WILL GIVE ONE MORE

LECTURE,

ON

MESMERISM;

IN THE HALL OF THE INSTITUTE,

CHELMSFORD,

ON

FRIDAY NEXT, JULY 14.

The Phenomena which Mr HOLMES will produce on a young man, will be of a very extraordinary character, and which will shew that Animal Magnetism is a reality, and capable of being applied to great good in various ways. Mr. HOLMES will exhibit the Phenomena of Clairvoyance, and the excitation of the Cerebral organs; and will answer the objections of the opponents of the science, and refute the charge of collusion.

ADMISSION:—To the body of the Hall, 1s.;—(Reserved Seats, 1s. 6d.;)—Gallery, 6d.

TO COMMENCE AT EIGHT O'CLOCK.

TICKETS to be had of Mr. A. COPLAND, and Messrs. MEGGY & CHALK, Chelmsford.

* *Some Gentlemen of the Town have promised their assistance to Mr. HOLMES, to endeavour to operate upon Individuals from amongst the audience, after the Lecture.

A. COPLAND, PRINTER, HIGH STREET, CHELMSFORD.

MESM

On Wednesday

Mr. J.

WILL DELIVER T

THREE

MES

In the Hall of th

242, HIG

The Second Lecture will
Third on W

SYLLABUS

LE

Introductory remarks---
merism---Modes of Mes
nambulists---Objections
strative of the truth of M

LE

Spontaneous Catalepsy
waking state---Catalepsy
Physical strength by M
Mesmerism---Demonstrat

LE

Division of the Mesme
rism---Hypothesis of sug
reading---Sympathy of t
trations and Experiments.

To commence at h

ADMISSION to the Body

MASON, PRIN

Dental Cartoons (ca. 1945)
Otto Elkan

Paris. Hand-drawn and painted cartoons on paper; 10⅝ x 9 in. (27 x 23 cm)

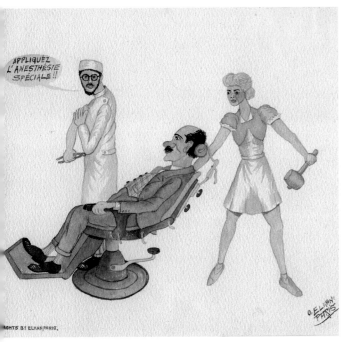

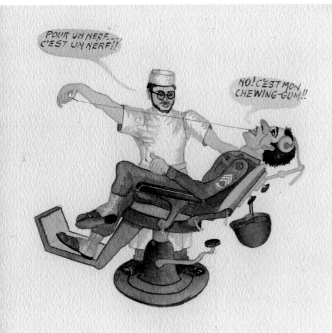

*W*ill you be able to find a good dentist when you need one? This question bedeviled mid-twentieth-century dentists and patients. And these wry cartoons play with this perennial problem.

We don't know for sure, but it seems likely that the man who made them was the Hungarian artist Otto Elkan, who was born in Budapest in 1884 and immigrated to France in December 1935. In 1943 Elkan (recorded as "Catholique—r. juive") was detained in a Nazi war camp in Chateau Tombebouc.

There are two series. One features pen-and-ink, black silhouetted figures and scenes, with patches of color and dialogue. The other, on textured paper, features watercolored drawings—and memorializes an American GI and a dental chair with all the attributes of a Weber Model D (patented in the United States in 1931 and widely distributed abroad). It was undoubtedly drawn sometime shortly after the Allied liberation of Paris.

Elkan's work documents not only the international spread of American dental technology in this period, but also a transatlantic cultural preoccupation with access to good professional dental care, particularly in wartime. In the late nineteenth century, people in need of a dentist faced a marketplace of practitioners with diverse levels of educational attainment, professional certification, technological sophistication, and practical competence. The early twentieth century brought a dramatic increase in standards of dental education and professional practice: luminaries within the field strove to endow dentistry with the scientific authority and social and economic status of medicine.

During World War II—when nearly all of Europe's professionally trained dentists had entered military service, been forced to flee, or been put in concentration camps—access to good dental care was severely restricted. At the same time dentists' increasing success in persuading the public of the importance of good dental care raised the demand for their services. And potential patients felt this lack quite keenly.

One of Elkan's scenes hints at the shortage of dentists by portraying the self-care attempt of a patient who fastens his aching tooth to a railroad car in an effort to accomplish extraction.

Elkan's substitution of cats and dogs for dentists and patients is of a piece with a long antic tradition in which animals stand in for human beings. But it is also part of a larger genre of dental slapstick fixated on the notion that the individual holding the forceps might not be a trained professional dentist—and that a hapless patient might not be able to discern the difference.

In the United States the same concerns were reflected in a 1943 short featuring the Three Stooges in which Larry, Moe, and Curly—window washers who accidentally slop soapsuds into the open window of a dentist's office, causing the proprietor to storm off—assume the dentist's role and extract a patient's tooth. In a related 1951 episode, *The Tooth Will Out*, the three—dressed in Victorian-era waistcoats as if to historicize the persistence of the problem of dentists' incompetence—are fired from their jobs and pay $500 to a huckster to become dentists instead.

As in Elkan's cartoons, hilarity ensues.

—ALYSSA PICARD

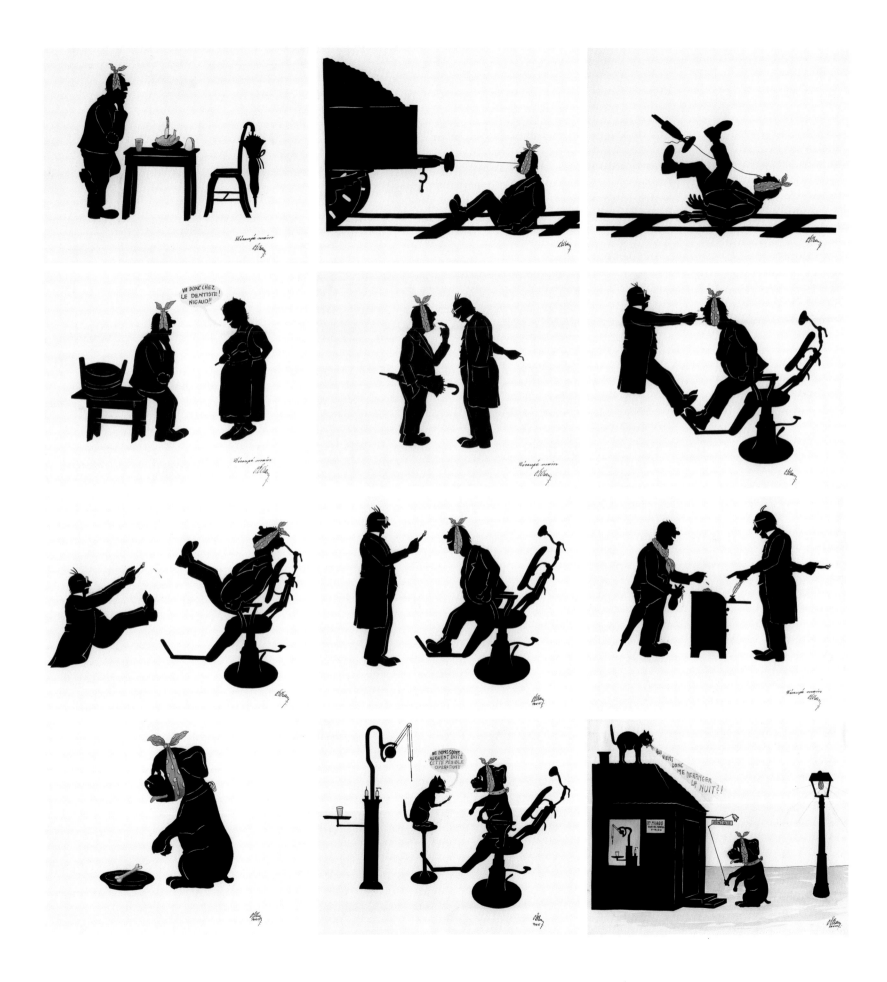

Dental Hand Silhouette Gift Album (ca. 1908)
W. H. Whitslar

Cleveland, Ohio. Album of gelatin silver photographs; 33 leaves; 5¾ x 8 in. (14.5 x 20 cm)

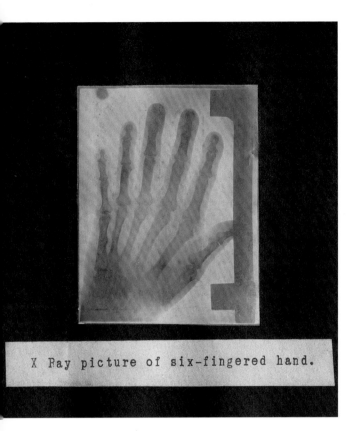

ABOVE: "X Ray picture of six-fingered hand," Dental Hand Silhouette Gift Album

OPPOSITE: (Top and bottom rows) "Noted Dentists" with autographed hand silhouettes. (Middle row) Chirognomic hand types: square (or useful), spatulate (or active), mixed, philosophic, psychic, and artistic (or emotional); unidentified source. Dental Hand Silhouette Gift Album

Photographs and hand silhouettes from the collection of Dr. W. H. Whitslar presented to his friend Dr. Burton Lee Thorpe" reads a typewritten label on the first page of this battered black album from sometime around 1908.

The book opens with a procession of images that is almost surrealist in its dream logic—illustrations based on the pseudoscience of chirognomy (the "Seven Typical Forms of Hands": "Elemental, Square, Spatulate, Mixed, Philosophic, Psychic, Artistic"); an X-ray of a six-fingered hand (the most common form of polydactyly); a "U.S. government finger-print identification record"; photos depicting "the influence of profession on the shape of the hand" (smith, shoemaker, typesetter, tailor, pianist); and finally a palmistry diagram.

After this free-associated introduction, another typed label—"Noted Dentists"—ushers us into a portrait gallery of Gilded Age and Progressive Era medical men in somber suits and starched collars, wearing their Vandykes, box beards, and walrus mustaches like badges of office. Each is paired with a white silhouette of his hand. Most are presented without comment, though there are exceptions: J. Taft's page includes the notation "Eloquent hand."

Dr. Will H. Whitslar (1862–1930), the "W. H. Whitslar" of the commemorative label, was a second-generation Ohio dentist and M.D., a professor of dentistry, anatomy, and pathology at Western Reserve University in Cleveland, "highly respected by his brethren in the profession," according to a contemporary source. His journal articles, on subjects ranging from the vexations of neurasthenic patients to ether's tendency to induce "erotic sensations" in female patients, reveal a searching mind, inclined toward flights of poetic fancy.

Whitslar's greatest hits at dental-society meetings were lectures such as his talk on "Chirognomy in Dentistry" (chirognomy being "the science of deducing the characteristics of a man from the shape of his hands"). He extolled the virtues of "chirognomical" tests in singling out students best fitted (social Darwinian allusion very much intended) for the dental profession. For example, the thick-palmed, stubby-fingered "elementary" hand offers evolutionary evidence of "the low grade of human intelligence," and those possessed of such hands, such as "the Laplanders and the lower class of Tartars and Slavs," are hereditarily unfit to be dentists.

Writing in the long shadow of the eugenicist Francis Galton (1822–1911), whom he quoted with approval, Whitslar was a product of his times, a medical man and devout Darwinian who nonetheless regarded palmistry, chirognomy, and physiognomy (the inference of a person's inborn character from his facial features) as sciences. In Gothic fiction, atavistic hands gave shape to social Darwinian anxieties about racial degeneration: Mr. Hyde, the good doctor's bestial alter ego in *The Strange Case of Dr. Jekyll and Mr. Hyde* (1886), has "corded, knuckly" hands "of a dusky pallor, and thickly shaded with a swart growth of hair." Likewise, in the eugenic theories of Galton's disciples polydactylic or brachydactylic (stubby fingered) hands were a sure sign of mental deficiency. Visual echoes of Dr. Jekyll's "large, firm" hands, "professional in shape and size," the eloquent hands in Whitslar's little black gift book speak volumes about the medical unconscious in the early twentieth century.

—MARK DERY

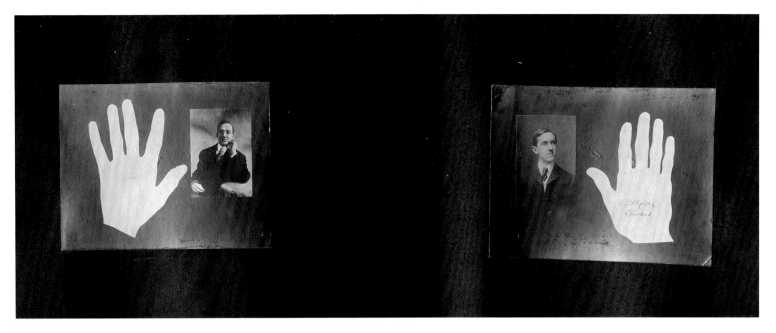

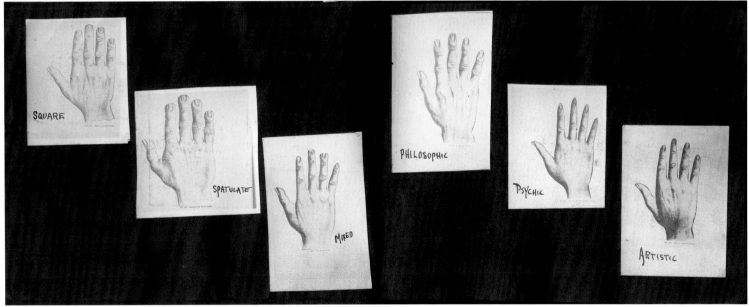

SQUARE

SPATULATE

MIXED

PHILOSOPHIC

PSYCHIC

ARTISTIC

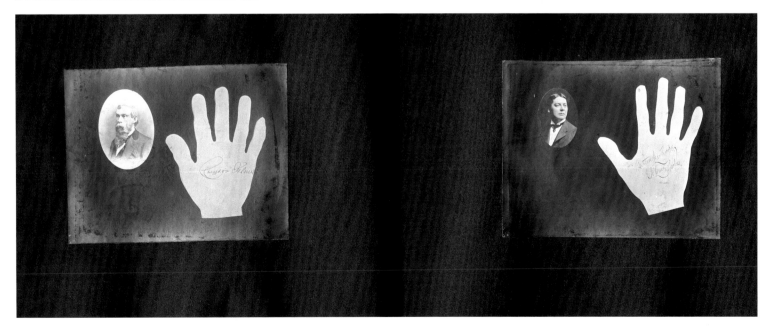

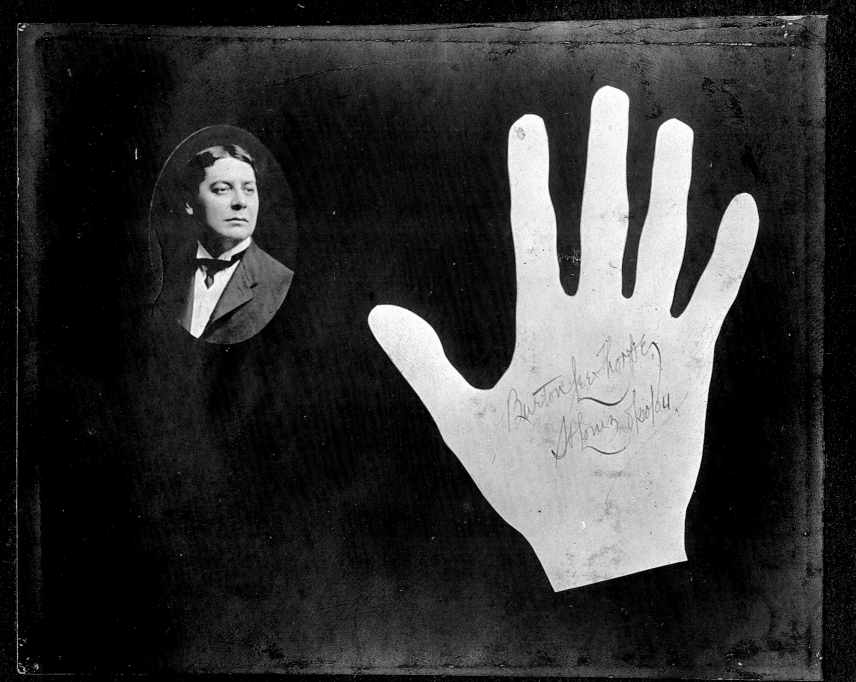

Burton Les Hoppe,
Howard ftoo/o4

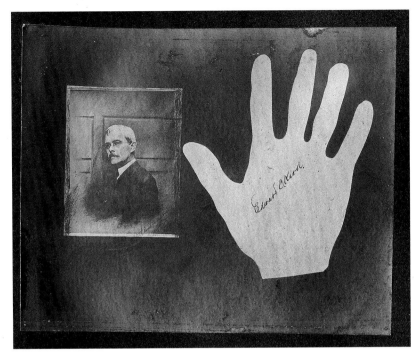

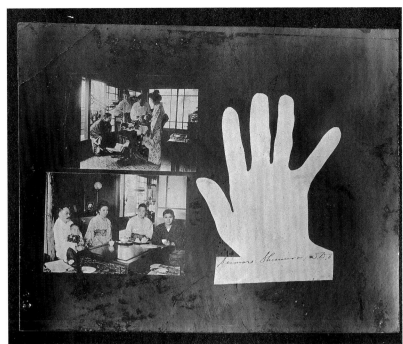

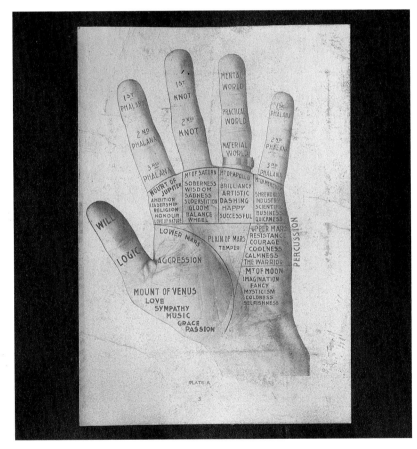

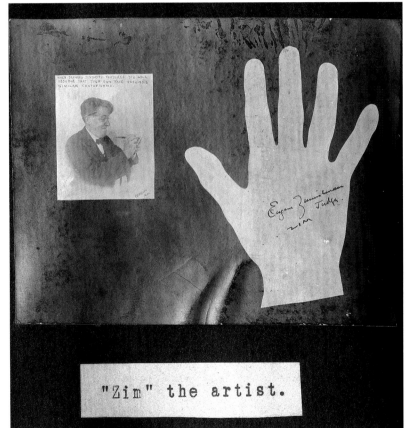

"Zim" the artist.

OPPOSITE: Burton Lee Thorpe, D.D.S., president of the National Dental Association, and his autographed hand silhouette. Dr. Thorpe was Whitslar's friend and recipient of the gift album. Dental Hand Silhouette Gift Album

ABOVE, CLOCKWISE FROM TOP LEFT: Photograph of Edward C. Kirk [Church?] and autographed hand silhouette. Scenes from Japan: a patient undergoing dental treatment and people having a meal, with autographed hand silhouette of Japanese dentist [Seimori?] Shimura. Photograph of "'Zim' the artist" (Eugene Zimmerman,

a political cartoonist and caricaturist for *Puck* and *Judge*, the most prominent late-nineteenth-, early-twentieth-century American satirical weeklies), with autographed hand silhouette. Zim is the only nondentist featured in the gift album. Above his photograph, a quote: "When drawing distorted features, you will observe that your own face assumes similar contortions" (from Zim, *This and That About Caricature* [New York, 1905], p. 25). Palmistry diagram; unidentified source. Dental Hand Silhouette Gift Album

Marshall W. Nirenberg Papers (1937–2003)
Marshall W. Nirenberg

National Library of Medicine, *Profiles in Science*: http://profiles.nlm.nih.gov/JJ/. Manuscript papers; 159 boxes and oversize materials; 72½ linear feet; photograph courtesy of *Nature* © 2011

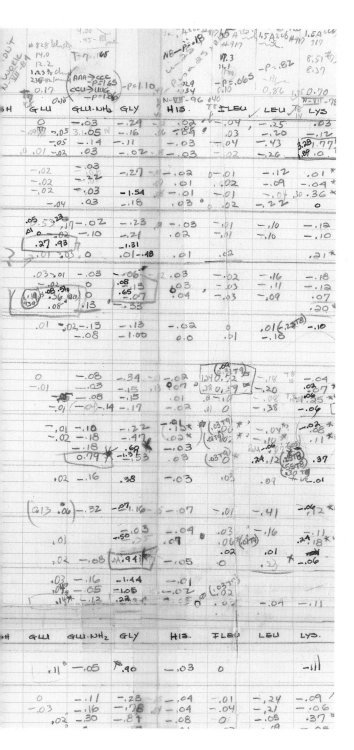

The photograph is dramatic, more dramatic in its own way than the famous one of James Watson and Francis Crick. Like that photograph, this one portrays two young scientists in the throes—the joys—of collaboration. The names are not as well known: the young men are Marshall Nirenberg (1927–2010) and Heinrich Matthaei (b. 1929). But their accomplishment was just as important. Watson and Crick worked on molecular reproduction—the DNA molecule formed of two entwined strands, each strand holding the information that guides life's unfolding, each strand crucial as cells divide. Nirenberg and Matthaei worked on molecular function. For the structure of DNA lent itself to thinking of a "code." With a pattern of nucleic acid base pairs, A, T, G, and C, laid out to form a strand of DNA, a key was needed to provide meaning—just as Morse code translates dots and dashes into letters and words. In this case the dots and dashes were nucleic acid bases, the letters were amino acids, and the words were proteins, the complex molecules that guide cellular actions such as "break down a sugar," or "create a cell wall," or even "make a new molecule of DNA." Nirenberg and Matthaei cracked that code.

Their approach was simplicity itself (which didn't make it easy). Make a synthetic nucleic acid, run it through a ribosome (which assembles proteins), and see what comes out. First, put in a strand of all U's (uracil, a stand-in for T, in this case). Out comes a synthetic molecule made solely of the amino acid phenylalanine, multiple copies joined head-to-tail like a protein. So UUU (the code was formed of three bases) means phenylalanine. Vary the amounts of the nucleic acid bases and see what amino acids join up and in what proportions. Keep it all straight with a chart made of graph paper taped together (dated January 18, 1965, 19½ x 19¹³⁄₁₆ in. [49.5 x 50.2 cm]; detail left) or, actually, many such charts, each a refinement of the last. Work so hard that in a scant four years (starting in 1961 and finishing in 1965) it's all straight—all the combinations of bases are matched with all twenty amino acids. Three years later, in 1968, pick up a Nobel Prize.

We don't mind the staginess of the 1962 eight-by-ten glossy. It flatters us. From our place "behind the blackboard" we see science being made, at least as we like to think it's made: two men, at the height of their powers, united in a common purpose, working successfully at one of the great challenges of modern biology. The vantage point the photographer provides is pure genius; a more realistic position would put their backs to us or have them looking away from their work. We're placed in the midst of their creation. We think: "Look, they're working it out for *us!*"

The photograph and chart come from the extensive collection of letters, photographs, and laboratory notebooks connected to Nirenberg's work on the genetic code; other papers deal with his ideas on how the brain works, his next research topic.

—Paul Theerman

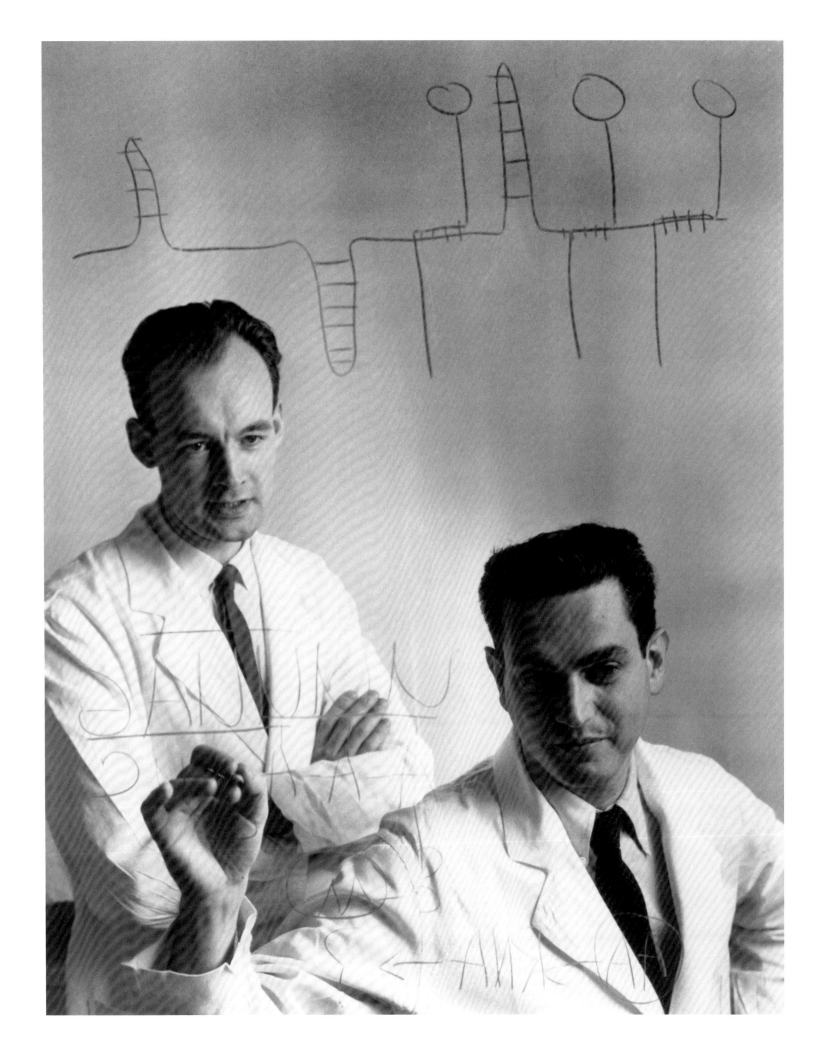

Mechanics of the Human Walking Apparatus (1836)
Wilhelm Eduard Weber and Eduard Weber

Mechanik der menschlichen Gehwerkzeuge. Göttingen, Germany. Printed book with atlas containing lithographs, 426 pp. + 10 pp.; text: 4¾ x 7⅞ in. (12 x 19.8 cm); atlas: 8 x 10 in. (20.5 x 25.4 cm)

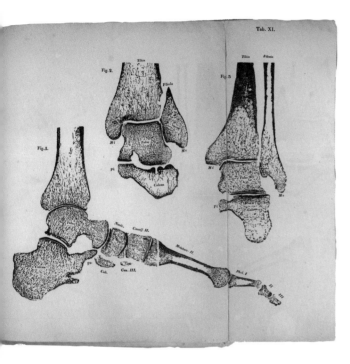

ABOVE: Imprints taken from cross sections of the skeletal foot demonstrate that the articular surfaces joining the lower leg and foot are round only in one direction, rotate almost entirely in one direction, and therefore can be considered hinges. *Mechanik* atlas, pl. 11

OPPOSITE: Two figures provide a model of how the motions of running and springing can be accurately drawn. *Mechanik* atlas, pl. 16

"Few movements in a living human depend so much on external forces, occur so evenly and are so little altered by the Will" as walking. So wrote Wilhelm Weber (1804–91) and Eduard Weber (1795–1881) in their treatise on the mechanics of human motion, a work that continued a line of inquiry that began in the seventeenth century. René Descartes's conception of the human as a machine animated by a soul and Giovanni Borelli's application of mechanics to anatomy in *On the Motions of Animals* (1680–81) had helped to initiate the long debate over mechanism versus the immaterial soul and materialism versus vitalism. The suggestion that mechanics—matter and motion defined by mathematically expressed laws—could explain perception, thought, will, and action was politically dangerous and morally suspect. To consider the human a mere "engine" bordered on atheism. Borelli prudently avowed that the principal cause of movement is the soul and the active instrument is the will.

At the beginning of the nineteenth century the Weber brothers also avowed that walking and running "depend on free will," but then methodically demonstrated that "such mechanical movements can be predicted by calculation," so that "a voluntary act of will is not needed to move the active instruments successively in the necessary order." That the legs can oscillate like a pendulum, for instance, is a property that makes possible the regularity of successive steps. "It appears," they determined, "that the constant period of the oscillations results from the force of gravity without requiring an act of will."

The Webers were the first investigators to systematically study the mechanics of human motion. To do that they needed to devise a way of capturing reliable data. Artists, they argued, had misrepresented the curvature of the spine and angle of the pelvis. The investigator seeking an accurate visualization of body mechanisms must instead use mechanical and mathematical approaches. The Webers employed the crosshairs of a telescope to measure pelvic tilt at different phases of movement, and then analyzed the phases using differential equations. To illustrate "the bases of the human walking machine" they encased bones in plaster blocks and sawed them into segments to make imprints on paper (left). This method, they claimed, "is so true that it replaces the actual specimen." A draftsman using their equations to determine the body's position at different phases of motion could illustrate running and springing figures as they might appear on a stroboscopic disk (opposite). Because the legs articulate "like hinges" set in a frame or the cogwheels of a watch, they obey strict rules. Such mathematically reconstructed figures can create an impression of movement "corresponding exactly to nature."

By using mechanical principles so rigorously, the Webers contributed to the ascendancy of a new materialist science of life. Increasingly, inventions such as pumps, telegraphs, combustion engines, and assembly lines would be made to serve as models of organisms and body parts—and would even eventually replace or augment them. Humans and machines seemed now disconcertingly equivalent: the mechanics of living bodies subverted the idea not only of spirit enlivening the human frame but also of free will and even God.

—ALLISON MURI

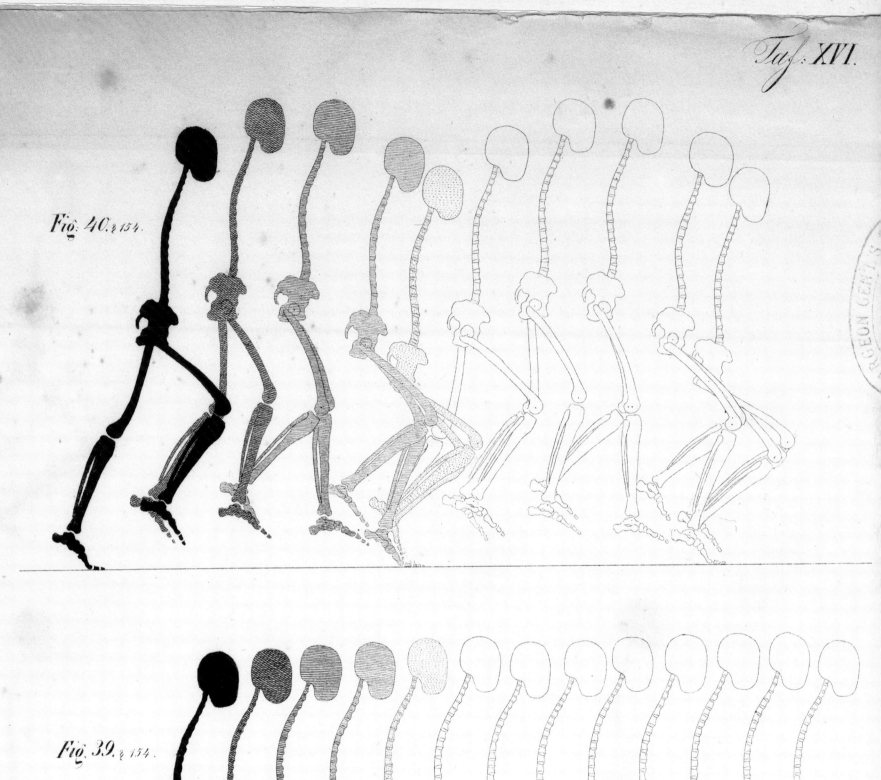

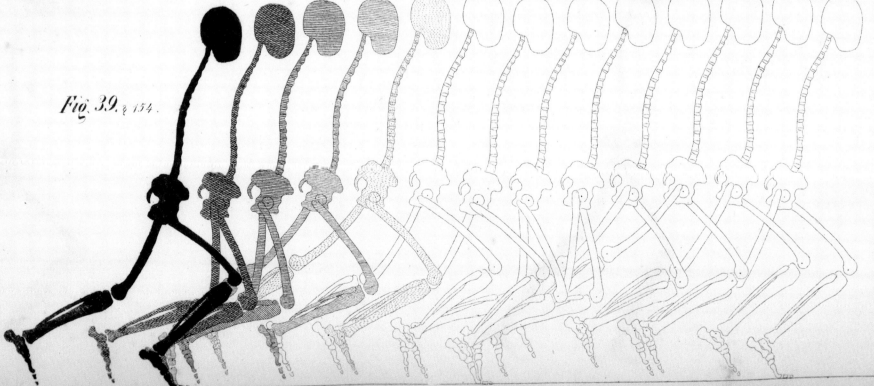

Fig. 40. z 154.

Fig. 39. z 154.

Man and Sunlight (1924)
Hans Surén with photographs by Gerhard Riebicke, C. J. Luther, J. Gross, and Paul Isenfels

Der Mensch und die Sonne. Stuttgart, Germany. Printed book, 224 pp.; 5⅛ x 7⅝ in. (13.1 x 19.7 cm)

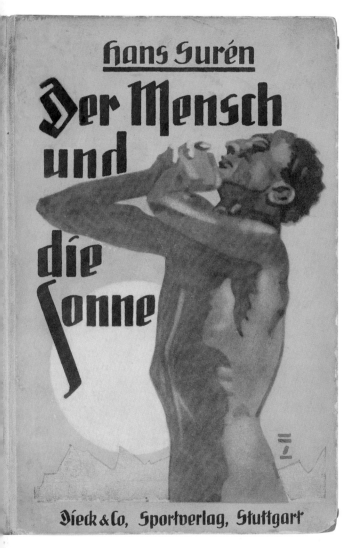

ABOVE: A man, probably Hans Surén, turns toward the sun. Cover art: Ludwig Hohlwein (1874–1949), a renowned poster artist who worked for the Nazis even before 1933 and helped to shape the visual image of Nazi Germany. *Der Mensch und die Sonne*, cover

OPPOSITE: Book pages (left) showing a female "water nude" in a pose that conceals her breasts and genitals and (right) Surén training a man in gymnastics. *Der Mensch und die Sonne*, pp. 14–15

Published in Germany in 1924 and translated into English in 1927, this little volume—an homage to sunlight and its revitalizing effects—was the best-selling "naturist" tract of its time. Its author, Hans Surén (1885–1972), a former army officer and fervent advocate of *Luft- und Sonnenbad* (air- and sunbathing), was nudism's foremost exponent.

Exposing the naked body to the sun may have seemed scandalous in Wilhelmine Germany, but nudism gained popularity with the craze for body culture in the postwar Weimar Republic. Nudism also had a politics. It was allied with eugenics, which aimed to strengthen the nation by strengthening the individual body: according to Surén, the "future of a *Volk*" depended on the "bodily and moral armaments" that nudism could provide.

Der Mensch und die Sonne advised readers on how to sunbathe for health: the largest possible part of the body's surface should be exposed to the sun's rays so that the skin could "breathe." It argued that nakedness was not immoral. After all, the ancient Greeks exercised in the open and without clothes. (The original meaning of gymnastics came from *gymnos*: "naked.") *Surén-Gymnastik*, practiced during "Surén weeks" (training camps for naturists), played a central role. Sunbathing had to be complemented by exercise, skin care, and oiling and shaving the body to harden and smooth its surface. The goal was to make the body resemble a Greek bronze. Whiteness as an ideal of beauty was replaced by a classical or even primitivist aesthetic. Surén boasted that his "healthy, natural brown skin color" could compete with "any Arab inhabitant of the middle of Africa." At the same time the metallic look of tanned, oiled skin over hardened muscles resonated with contemporary physiological models of the masculine body as an armored machine. In contrast Surén's women often had a marble-white complexion, denoting purity, and were posed in the postures of classical statues, although he could also show them as active and modern.

To attain the ideal body Surén relied on two visual instruments: the mirror and the photograph. Under surveillance in the mirror, the naked body could not hide "defects" and "abnormalities." In the early twentieth century the new technology of the halftone photograph was becoming a pervasive feature of mass culture. Naturist publications always featured photographs of beautiful naked people, presented as the "living truth" one should strive for. Such photographs functioned as the other side of the photographic archives of "abnormal" and "exotic" naked bodies shown in criminology, medicine, and anthropology texts. The photos in *Der Mensch und die Sonne* (mostly by Gerhard Riebicke [1878–1957], a newspaper photographer who specialized in shots of athletic bodies in motion) mobilized and controlled the eroticism—which partly accounted for the popularity of nudist publications. The "artistry" of the nudes (and Surén's insistence on their moral purpose) gave readers the license to take pleasure in viewing them.

Surén's popularity continued after the Nazis gained power. The 1936 edition, retitled *Man and Sunlight: The Aryan-Olympic Spirit*, replaced "naked truth" with "*völkisch* truth" and presented photographs of the nude "Aryan" body as the "realization of the racial ideal."

—MAREN MÖHRING

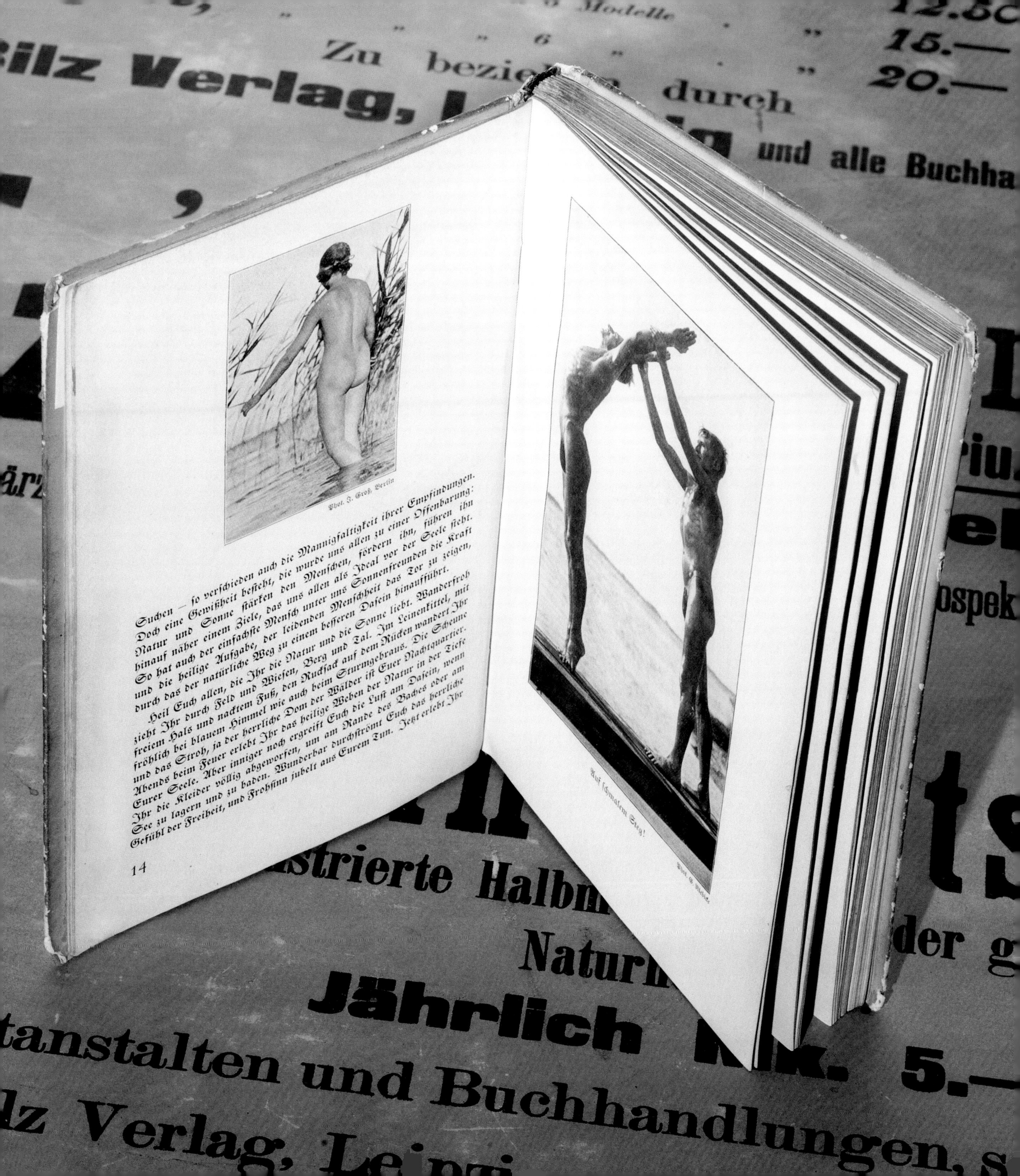

Phot. J. Groß, Berlin

Suchen — so verschieden auch die Mannigfaltigkeit ihrer Empfindungen. Doch eine Gewißheit besteht, die wurde uns allen zu einer Offenbarung: Natur und Sonne stärken den Menschen, fördern ihn, führen vor der Seele sieht. So hat auch der einfachste Mensch, das uns als Ideal hinauf näher einem Ziele, und die heilige Aufgabe, der leidenden Menschheit die Kraft durch das der natürliche Weg zu einem besseren Dasein hinaufführt.

Heil Euch allen, die Ihr die Natur und die Sonne liebt. Wanderfroh zieht Ihr durch Feld und Wiesen, Berg und Tal. Im Leinenkittel, mit freiem Hals und nacktem Fuß, den Rucksack auf dem Rücken wandert Ihr fröhlich bei blauem Himmel wie auch beim Sturmgebraus. Die Scheune und das Stroh, ja der herrliche Dom der Wälder ist Euer Nachtquartier. Abends beim Feuer erlebt Ihr das heilige Weben der Natur in der Tiefe Eurer Seele. Aber inniger noch ergreift Euch die Lust am Rande des Baches oder am See zu lagern und zu baden. Wunderbar durchströmt Euch das herrliche Ihr die Kleider völlig abgeworfen. Gefühl der Freiheit, und Frohsinn jubelt aus Eurem Tun. Jetzt erlebt Ihr

14

Auf schmalem Steg!

Phot. G. Riebicke

Rodney (1950)
Lucifer Guarnier (director), for the National Tuberculosis Association

New York. Motion picture, color, sound, animation, 16mm; 10:16

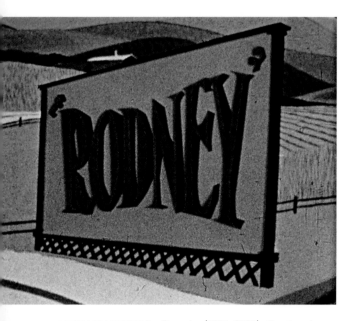

ABOVE AND OPPOSITE: Lu Guarnier (1914–2007), director of *Rodney*, was an exponent of the new modernist cartoon animation of the 1940s and early '50s. Cartoon modernism emphasized abstraction, bold lines, dynamic distortion, and the elimination of unnecessary detail. The new style was economical (it required fewer cells and less drawing per cell) and brought visual elements from cubism, surrealism, art deco, minimalism, even abstract expressionism to the mass movie and television audience. Stills from National Tuberculosis Association's *Rodney* reprinted with permission, © 2011 American Lung Association. www.Lung.org

It's 1950 and a fine upstanding teenager named Rodney is stricken with the deadly tuberculosis bacterium (*Mycobacterium tuberculosis*). But rest assured—and rest he will, in a tuberculosis hospital—science is on top of the disease.

The early 1950s was a time of high anxiety in American culture. The United States had won the world war, but after the Soviets exploded their atomic bomb in 1949, fears of nuclear war began to proliferate, along with some undefinable unease about the consequences of scientific progress. Yet the 1950s was also a time of optimism, when many believed that you could overcome anything by adopting a positive attitude and taking timely action.

And so this cartoon is both happy and haunted—by the threat of illness and attack. Stark posters of a dark profiled man and woman, with the legend "Have a Chest X-Ray," loom strategically in background storefront windows as Rodney happily strolls down the sidewalks of his town.

Because TB is an invader within. Like the great science fiction films of the 1950s—such as *The Man from Planet X, The Day the Earth Stood Still, Invasion of the Body Snatchers*—*Rodney* plays off cultural dread and suspicion of the Other.

That Other could also be people of a different social class or ethnicity. At one point Rodney (who lives in an all-American small town) says to his doctor that he thought only people who live in the slums get TB. The doctor counters, almost poignantly, "Germs don't know one person from another." Tuberculosis, it turns out, is a modern, democratic disease. Even white middle-class people get it, and it's nobody's fault. With the defeat of Nazism and its racial ideology, and in the aftermath of the genocide that killed six million Jews, there was a changed climate of opinion in America: discrimination is wrong.

Rodney's modernist cartoon animation renderings of cars, people, lungs, bacterial invasion, diagnostic technology, and treatment methods capture that moment in American life and medicine when everything felt modern. The main vector of modernity here is the X-ray. (The National Tuberculosis Association commissioned *Rodney* for a campaign to encourage X-ray screening.) A few years later the emphasis would shift to antibiotics, but *Rodney* takes place on the doorstep of the antibiotic revolution: drug treatment of tuberculosis had already been invented but became practicable only in 1952, when isoniazid, the first oral mycobactericidal drug, was created. *Rodney* makes no mention of antibiotics—and, surprisingly, only one fleeting mention of the tuberculin test.

There is another vector of modernity: the motion picture itself, made in a contemporary idiom that powerfully communicates to the public. And the messages are: See your doctor regularly (and get regular chest X-rays). If he says you have TB (which may not be evident), listen to your doctor and go to a "modern tuberculosis hospital," where you will rest and recover and be isolated until you no longer pose a danger to your family and community. If that doesn't do the trick, the fatherly doctor explains, surgery to collapse a lobe of the lung will give it even more rest. Happily that turns out to be unnecessary in Rodney's case.

—KATHY HIGH AND MICHAEL SAPPOL

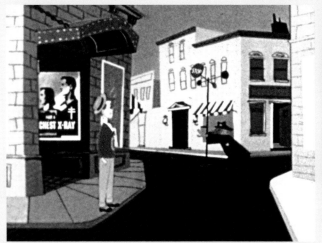
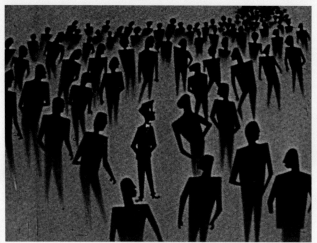
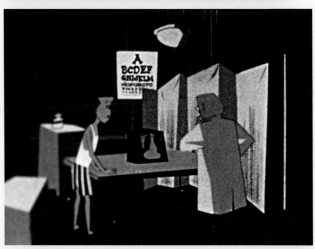
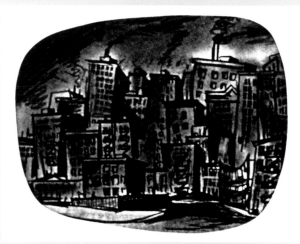
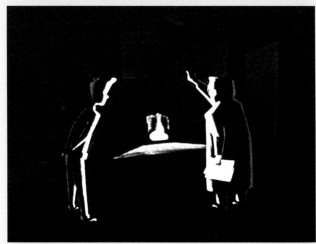
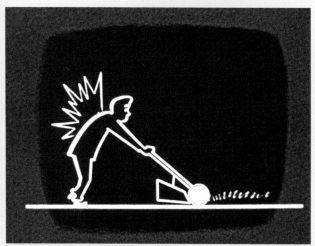
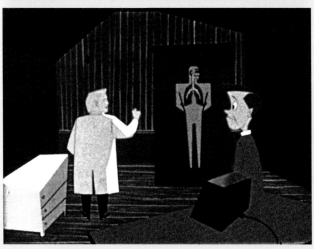
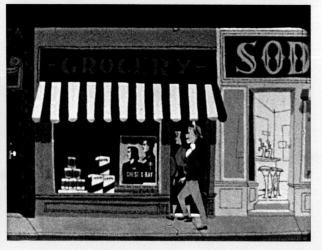

The Wonder in Us (1921)
Hanns Günther (Walter de Haas), ed.; cover design by W. Thamm

Wunder in uns: Ein Buch vom menschlichen Körper für Jedermann. Zürich–Leipzig, 2d ed. Printed book, 454 pp.; 5¾ x 8¾ in. (14.7 x 22.3 cm)

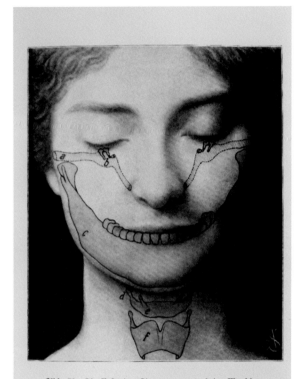

Abb. 73. Die Refte des Kiemenapparats beim Menfchen.

Es entftehen aus dem 1. Kiemengang der Ohr-Nafengang (a), aus dem 1. Kiemenbogen die Gehörknöchel (b) und das Knorpelgerüft des Unterkiefers (c), aus dem 2. Kiemenbogen die Fortfäße des Zungenbeins (d), aus dem 3. Kiemenbogen deffen Körper (e), aus dem 4. Kiemenbogen der Schildknorpel des Kehlkopfes (f).

ABOVE: "The vestiges of the branchial apparatus in humans." A photomontage superimposes an anatomical diagram over the photograph of a young woman—which is parallel to an evolutionary superimposition: our evolutionary past coexists in our body with the evolutionary present. The structures of the human eye, ear, nose, jaw, and throat shown here correspond to the gill structures of fish. *Wunder in Uns*, pl. 19

OPPOSITE: "An attempt to represent our brain's setup, shown graphically." The anatomy of the brain and nervous system is here reconfigured as linked rectilinear offices of functions—and covered over with printed tissue paper. *Wunder in Uns*, pl. 13

In the early decades of the twentieth century a modernizing imperative took hold. Suddenly it seemed that a new age was dawning—an era of new technologies, fashions, and political philosophies—modern times. In the aftermath of the Great War (1914–18), with the overthrow of the old European empires, it was all the rage to strip off the veneer of fussy decoration and unnecessary detail that choked the preceding era and to replace it with designs and inventions that emphasized machine power, strong lines, bold colors, and smooth surfaces of metal, glass, concrete, and rubber.

Wunder in Uns: Ein Buch vom Menschlichen Körper für Jedermann bears the marks of this moment. In 1921 Hanns Günther (the pseudonym of the German popular science writer Walter de Haas, 1886–1969) compiled twenty-eight essays on the human body into "a book for everyone." Furnished with a cover illustration showing a boldly minimalist outline of a human heart, *Wunder in Uns* presented illustrated lessons on "recent developments" in medicine and "modern physiology." Central Europe was then afflicted by postwar political and economic turmoil, but even in troubled times the book attracted a wide readership and quickly sold out its first edition.

Part of its appeal was its colored plates, which feature stylized cutaway diagrams of the interior of the human body. Although anatomical illustrations had long been a staple of popular medical books, they typically presented a static view of structures. In contrast, the most striking illustrations in *Wunder in Uns* deploy images of industrial production to visually explain the body's functions.

The head was the most modern part of the body. Plate 13 (opposite) represents the brain as bundles of wires connected to telecommunication offices staffed by little switchboard operators, file clerks, and messengers, who sort and redirect sensory electrical messages received from the eyes, nose, mouth, and lower body. In another plate, on digestion, foods tumble off a conveyor belt down the esophageal chute into the stomach and intestines, depicted as a sweaty mine or furnace room tended by manual laborers. The body then had a class system—the clean head office controlled the dirty body factory—which reflected the social organization of twentieth-century industry (with one glaring inaccuracy: the workers are represented as adult men, even though switchboard operators were usually women).

Both the form and content of *Wunder in Uns* signified modernity. Its admixture of text, drawings, and photographs was in the graphic style that had recently been developed in American newspapers and magazines. Each colored plate was preceded by a tissue-paper overlay printed with captions, a slick packaging concept.

America was another signifier. *Wunder in Uns* tried to do things the modern industrialized American way. Its illustrations of the industrial body were borrowed (then colorized) from an American encyclopedia, *Pictured Knowledge* (1919). Later in the 1920s, *Wunder in Uns* essayist Fritz Kahn (1888–1968) developed modernist medical illustration in a series of popular publications. In the 1940s, as a refugee from the Nazis, he returned the genre to America.

—Michael Sappol

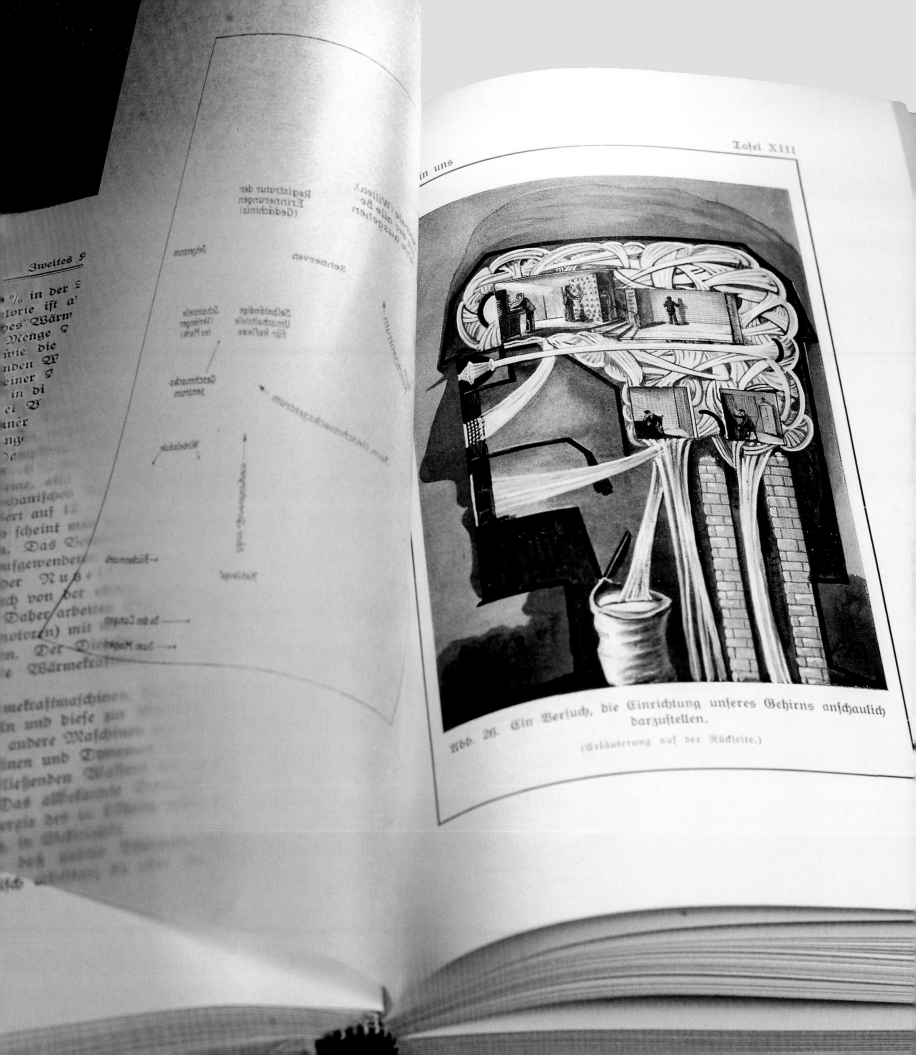

Abb. 26. Ein Versuch, die Einrichtung unseres Gehirns anschaulich darzustellen.

(Erläuterung auf der Rückseite.)

Health and Hygiene Puzzle Blocks (ca. 1960–66)
Number 10 Shanghai Toy Factory

Shanghai, China. Eight blocks; printed in four-color on six sides; 1⅜ x 1⅜ in. (3.5 x 3.5 cm)

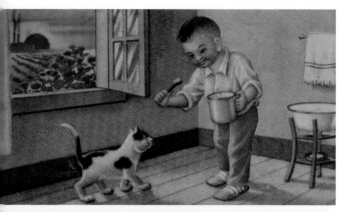

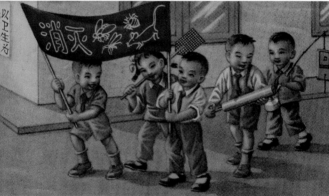

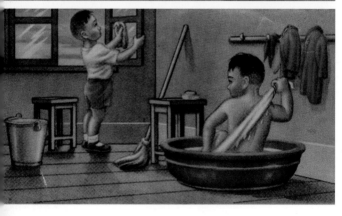

ABOVE: Selected scenes from the puzzle blocks

*I*n 2005 the National Library of Medicine acquired more than fifteen hundred Chinese public health posters plus an assortment of other materials, mainly from the Communist era (1949 to the present). Among these riches is a charming set of eight block puzzles. The pictures on the sides of each block, when put together, make six scenes aimed at fostering revolutionary consciousness and teaching hygienic behavior through the cycle of a day.

Scene one: As a cat looks up at him and the sun rises through an open window, a boy brushes his teeth (left, top). He will next use the basin and towel behind him to wash his face. The dawn is to the new day as the boy is to the new political order: optimistic, bright, and full of promise.

Scene two: The boy joins his sister and older brother, walking on a country road. They stretch out their arms to exercise before school begins.

Scene three: In class the boy reads while other boys rub their eyes, which are strained from reading. A wall poster urges, "Protect your eyes; rest at regular intervals." (The exhortatory poster campaign was a hallmark of the Communist regime.)

Scene four: The boy and his sister join a mass health campaign (left, center). He helps hold up a banner that says "Exterminate!" and shows drawings of a mosquito, fly, rat, and louse. His sister waves a flyswatter. One boy holds a pesticide sprayer; another carries a bamboo pole dangling a mousetrap. "Carry out sanitation to make things beautiful" reads a sign on a wall as they march past.

Scene five: Now home, the boy and his sister wash their hands and face. Their mother brings steaming dishes to the table as dusk falls outside the window. The boy looks to his mother, anticipating a tasty supper.

Scene six: Their blue jackets and red scarves hang on a rail, and it's time to get ready for bed (left, bottom). The boy's older brother bathes in a large red tub, and the ever diligent boy cleans the window as the sun sets. A green bucket and mop wait for cleaning up after bathing. Soon all the children will have a good night's sleep.

The Number 10 Shanghai Toy Factory probably produced these blocks between 1960 and 1966. Since no posters of Mao Zedong are seen on the home, school, or village walls, the blocks likely were issued before the Cultural Revolution (1966–76), when Mao's portrait became ubiquitous. The "Four Pests" banner suggests the years following the Great Leap Forward (1958–61): in May 1958 Mao ordered that "the whole people, including five-year-old children, must be mobilized to eliminate the four pests" (sparrows, rats, mosquitoes, flies). In March 1960 Mao replaced sparrows (targeted for eating too much grain) with lice.

The two-year campaign nearly exterminated sparrows in China. Without natural enemies to keep them in check, swarms of locusts proliferated, consuming large quantities of grain and contributing to a famine in which 35 to 50 million people died—among them children who participated in the earliest Four Pest extermination campaigns portrayed on these very blocks.

—Marta Hanson

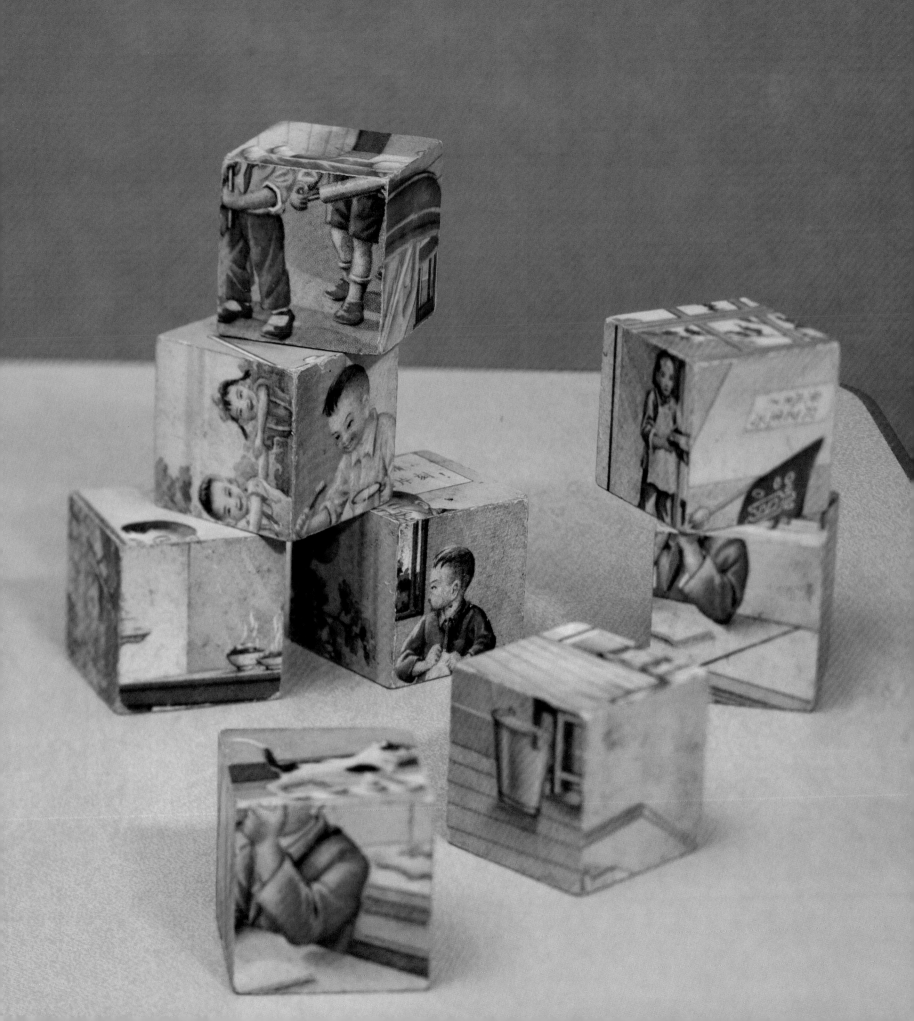

"There ain't no match for a mucous patch"

Huber the Tuber (1943) and *Corky the Killer* (1945)
Harry A. Wilmer

New York. Printed books with line drawings, *Huber*: 83 pp., 6¾ x 9⅞ in. (17 x 25.2 cm); *Corky*: 67 pp., 7 x 9⅞ in. (17.5 x 25.2 cm)

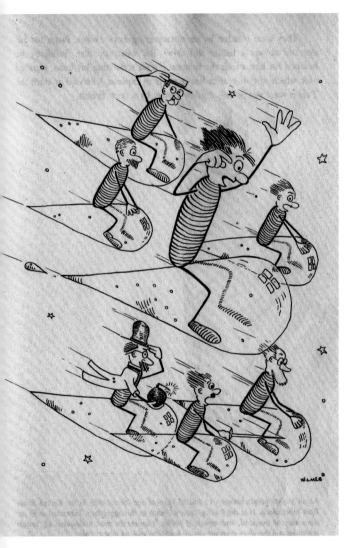

ABOVE: Huber the Tuber and his associates ride cough droplets to their next human victim. *Huber the Tuber*, p. 3

OPPOSITE: (Top row) Corky the Killer and friends contemplate locating a snug place in their victim's body where they will be secure from attack by the body's dog-faced defenders. *Corky the Killer*, pp. 31, 53. (Bottom row) Huber the Tuber and his associates find lodging in a victim's lungs. *Huber the Tuber*, pp. 35, 59. Excerpts from National Tuberculosis Association's *Huber the Tuber* reprinted with permission, © 2011 American Lung Association. www.Lung.org; *Corky the Killer* courtesy the National Social Hygiene Association © 2011

Tuberculosis attracted considerable attention from artists and writers. Along with syphilis and polio it was so rampant that cautionary visual messages appeared in myriad public places, from offices to restrooms. A wall in my third-grade classroom routinely displayed public health flyers, pamphlets, and posters—some benign, others nightmarishly frightening. They were specters of horror that left mental scars on an impressionable little me.

In the "Crusade Against TB," tuberculosis was often symbolized by hooded demons or skeletons. They were not pleasant to look at but did the job of raising awareness. Yet not every anti-TB product was scary. The logo for TB, the cross with the double horizontal crossbars, was a friendly brand. Even friendlier was *Huber the Tuber, a Story of Tuberculosis*, which was conceived, drawn, and written for the National Tuberculosis Association in 1943 by Dr. Harry Wilmer (1917–2005), who was then recovering from his own bout with tuberculosis. This entertaining little illustrated book stars Huber, an anthropomorphic tubercle (a lung nodule caused by the *Mycobacterium tuberculosis*), who goes on a series of adventures in "The Promised Land 'o' Lung." In the course of his escapades he gets caught up in a war that looks suspiciously like the one then raging in Europe and Asia and meets up with Nasty von Sputum, Rusty the Bloodyvitch, and Huey the Long Tuber (a reference to Senator Huey Long). And the reader gets otherwise serious lessons about the causes, diagnosis, pathology, and treatment of tuberculosis.

A few years later Wilmer created a companion volume, *Corky the Killer, a Story of Syphilis*, for the American Social Hygiene Association, an anti–venereal disease advocacy group. *Time* magazine described *Corky* as "a slightly bawdy blend of fact and fancy that seeks by cartoons and comic-strip dialogue to tell about the syphilis spirochete and how it works."

The villain is Corky, a nasty 1/3,000th of an inch tall, with a corkscrew body (characteristic of the spirochete), a nose like a golf tee, and spindly legs. He is the leader of a band of syphilitic saboteurs and the Mayor of Chancretown, whose anthem is "Down by the Old Blood Stream." Dodging anti-syphilitic "magic bullets" (the drug Salvarsan, developed by Paul Ehrlich), Corky makes a mad dash through "Man World" and latches on to the first blood cell that floats by. Soon he rejoins his fellow saboteurs, who love to cause nasty skin eruptions (chancres). Eventually caught, he is brought to trial and, after losing his case, sentenced to the Soap and Water Chamber of Torture, where he is scrubbed to death. The moral of the story: syphilis can be prevented or cured, if caught early and treated appropriately.

Wilmer, a passable pen-and-ink draftsman in *Huber*, greatly improved his craft in *Corky*. But somehow the drawings in *Huber*, which look like doodles, are more effective. Both books have a bit of magic in them: the health message is subordinated to the sheer joy of visual storytelling. Like the best illustrated children's books—and graphic novels and animated cartoons—each creates an imaginative universe that refers back to the real world with wit, humor, and insight.

—STEVEN HELLER

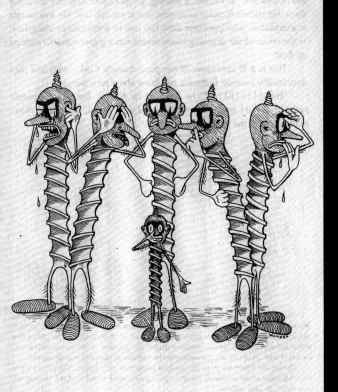

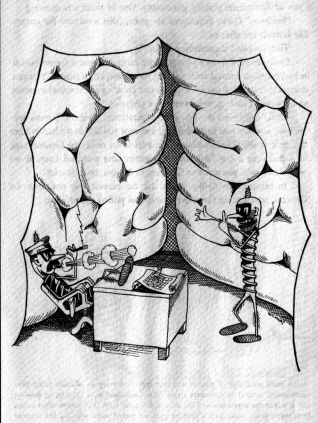

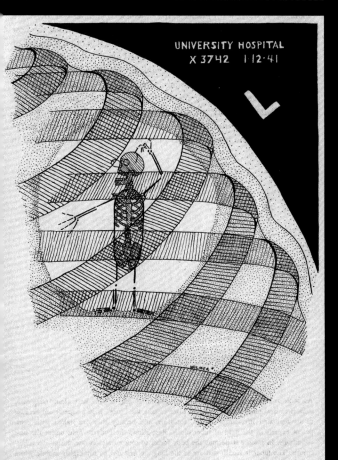

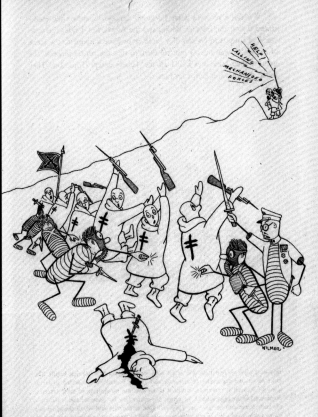

Chinese Anti-Tuberculosis Flyers (1940s)
National Anti-Tuberculosis Association of China

Shanghai, China. Printed flyers, 5⅛ x 7½ in. (13 x 19 cm)

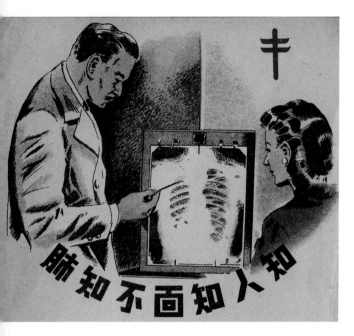

ABOVE AND OPPOSITE: Flyers from a larger series of anti-tuberculosis flyers (Shanghai, 1940s and '50s), Chinese Public Health Collection, National Library of Medicine

Tuberculosis carried a social stigma for both the individual and the nation in the early twentieth century, when China was depicted as the "Sick Man of East Asia."

The adoption of Western ideas, standards, and practices of health was taken to be a yardstick of progress, while traditional religious beliefs and health practices were disparaged as superstitious and backward. When the newly founded National Anti-Tuberculosis Association of China began conducting anti-tuberculosis campaigns in 1933 it used images, motifs, and visual styles influenced by, and sometimes directly borrowed from, European and American posters, flyers, and pamphlets. The anti-TB campaigns and the formation of an activist public health movement were tied to modernization efforts.

The Chinese anti-TB campaigners believed that visual images must play a vital role in health education and mobilization campaigns in a nation where many were poorly educated or illiterate. The flyers shown here are part of a series made in the 1940s under the anti-communist Kuomintang government. Branded with the double-barred Cross of Lorraine, the international anti-TB trademark, the flyers placed the fight against tuberculosis in a distinctively Chinese framework. In one flyer (opposite, bottom left) the domestic scene is completely Western, but in the far background next to the window can be seen a Chinese painting of winter-plum blossoms. Winter blossoms symbolize perseverance and vitality in a harsh environment, a common theme in traditional Chinese art and rhetoric. Next to the image of a mother kissing her baby the flyer says "love but don't harm your son." In keeping with contemporary Western campaigns it argues that kissing is bad because it transmits germs that cause TB.

Another flyer (opposite, top right) shows a man in traditional dress spitting a gob of sputum—which is revealed by a microscope to contain bacteria—in an alley where innocent children play. The text cautions that spitting is an "unforgivable mistake" because it spreads tuberculosis, and instructs readers to correct this bad habit. An old woman in another flyer kneels before an altar and prays for health, with a poster inset that advertises traditional nostrums and quack remedies (opposite, top left). The flyer featuring a seated man, with a question mark and whirls of confusion around his head (opposite, bottom right), urges people to see a doctor at the first sign of illness rather than engage in wishful thinking and passively hope that diseases will go away on their own.

In contrast, a detail from another flyer (left) shows a doctor explaining a lung X-ray to a young woman. The title, "Knowing people's faces but not their lungs," plays on the Chinese proverb "Knowing people but not their hearts." The accompanying text argues that to prevent and treat TB, people should seek the advice of doctors trained in scientific medicine (the germ theory, good hygiene, nutrition, physical fitness, and sanitary engineering), who are equipped with the latest technologies—the microscope, X-ray, tuberculin test, BCG vaccine, and mass media. The underlying premise is that in heeding the advice of health experts the Chinese people can modernize themselves and their nation.

—LIPING BU

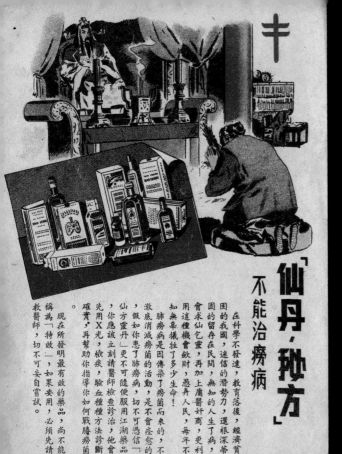

「仙丹、秘方」不能治療病

在科學不發達，教育落後，迷信的潛勢力，還根深蒂固的我國，經濟貧困的留存在民間，無知的老人生了病，會求仙乞靈，再加上庸醫奸商，更利用這種機會欽財，愚弄人民，每年不知有多少生命！

肺癆病是因傳染了癆菌而來的，不澈底消滅癆菌的活動，是不會癒的，假如你患了肺癆病，切不可愚信「仙方」「仙丹靈方」更不可隨便服用江湖藥品，你應該立刻請醫師檢查診治，他會用X光、驗痰、驗血種種方法診斷，確實，再幫助你指導你如何戰勝癆菌。

現在所發明最有效的藥品，尚不能稱為「特效」，如果要用，必須先請教醫師，切不可妄自嘗試。

Form 14 100M 5-38
中國防癆協會編印　　上海(16)楓林橋醫學院路一三八號

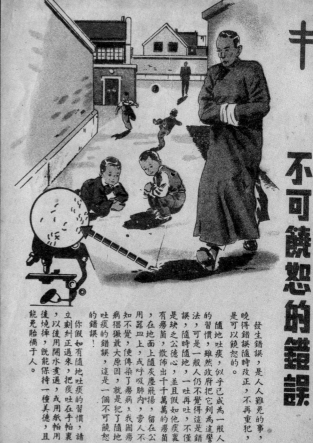

不可饒恕的錯誤

發生錯誤，是人人難免的事，曉得錯誤隨時改正，不再重犯，是可以饒恕的。

隨地吐痰，似乎已成為一般人的習慣，雖然政府把它列為違警法，可是一般人仍不覺得這是錯誤，隨時隨地，不覺再吐，是缺乏公德心，並且假如他吐痰有癆菌，留在地面上隨灰塵飛揚，旁人不知，就是犯了隨地吐痰撒散大原因，我國癆病猖獗戴的錯誤，這是一個不可饒恕的錯誤！

你假如有隨地吐痰的習慣，請立刻糾正過來，把痰吐在手帕裏，以後燒掉，或用開水燙過，或用廢紙包裹，既能保持一種美德，且能克胎禍于人。

Form 17 100M 5-38
中國防癆協會編印　　上海(16)楓林橋醫學院路一三八號

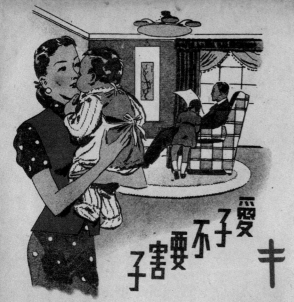

愛子不要害子

沒有一個做父母的不愛他子女，可是我要你們告訴我，假如你是患有肺癆病，也許因為你的親熱，會帶給他們終身或口腔食物最危險！

肺癆病在家庭裏最容易于女也最喜歡他子女，中國差不多有世世代代，都是患著癆病的傳染，這種病的來源，天性的傳染，並非遺傳來，他並且可愛于女的父母，是要設法防止自己的危險！

你為愛你的子女，要告訴你的父母，不能和子女太接近的你，也應該告訴子女的傳染機關去全受施行健康檢查，並告訴你如何保護你的子女不受癆菌的傳染，以用結核菌素的測驗來證明你的子女是否已受感染，可以接種B.C.G.苗，未受感染而有防癆的功效！

凡雇用乳娘或褓母時，必須先要用X光檢查肺部，如果患有肺病，萬不可用，以免傳染你的子女。

Form 15 100M 5-38
中國防癆協會編印　　上海(16)楓林橋醫學院路一三八號

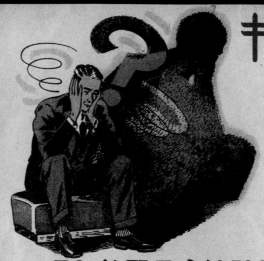

打破諱疾忌醫的心理

有許多人生了病，往往不願把去看醫生，起初自己還安慰自己，以為它會慢慢好起來的，住其拖延，直等到不堪收拾再去尋醫，往往已病入膏肓，雖名醫亦告束手，終于無辜犧牲了性命！

肺癆病初發作的時候，大都是感冒症，至夜晚盜汗，胃口不開，或身體重逐漸消瘦，一般人總認為是咳嗽，無現象，及至體重減輕，再經醫師診斷，已是已演成嚴重的肺癆病了，假如能及早就醫，就能節省時者錢，諱疾忌醫的心理，我們應該立刻打破。

你假如對你健康發生懷疑，請立刻到防癆機關或醫院去檢查，醫師會給你適當的指導，保障你身體的健康。

可以燎原，不要以星星之火，以至不可收拾地步，那纔悔之晚矣。

Form 16 100M 5-38
中國防癆協會編印　　上海(16)楓林橋醫學院路一三八號

Chinese Public Health Slides (1950s–70s)
Hangzhou and other cities, China

Painted and printed glass slides in cardboard and cloth-stitched frames, 4 x 3⅛ in. (10.2 x 7.9 cm)

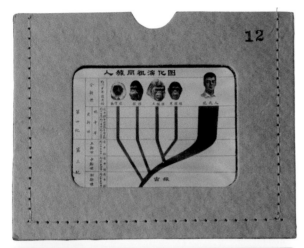

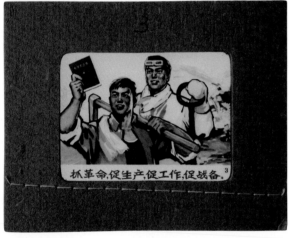

ABOVE, TOP: Slide 12 from a series on human evolution shows the relationship of humans with apes.

ABOVE: Slide 3 from the series "Love the Nation Hygienic Movement" features Mao's little red book held high.

OPPOSITE: Slides instruct parents on the need to protect their children against TB.

The National Library of Medicine owns perhaps the world's largest collection of materials relating to public health in China, dating from the 1800s into the Communist era (1949 to the present). In this treasure trove of posters, pamphlets, and ephemera is a unique collection of more than forty sets of slides designed for projection in classrooms and other spaces where audiences assembled. Most of them were made for health campaigns: tuberculosis vaccination; eradication of flies, rats, and mosquitoes; child hygiene; prevention of childhood diarrhea, pneumonia, and rickets; family planning; rural drinking water sanitation; coal-smoke and natural-gas poisoning; first aid; vomit and phlegm sanitation; processing human manure into fertilizer; prevention of dysentery, liver-fluke disease, hepatitis, diphtheria, tuberculosis, and meningitis; and methods to reduce intestinal disease, and so forth. The oldest sets, consisting of glass slides sewn into cloth frames, date to the 1950s–60s. The more recent ones, from the 1970s, are mostly film in cardboard frames, produced for the public health campaigns of the Cultural Revolution.

The glass slide set illustrated here (opposite) comes from a 1950s-era campaign for BCG (Bacillus Calmette-Guérin) vaccination to prevent tuberculosis. Made in Hangzhou, Zhejiang province, the slides are each stamped in blue, "It is the parents' responsibility to get their children the BCG vaccine." The first slide presents French scientists Albert Calmette and Camille Guérin, who developed the vaccine. The campaign's focus on children is signaled by scenes of children playing in the village and nursery. The second row of slides depicts the subcutaneous injection method, symptoms of tuberculosis, and three stages to expect after vaccination (redness, swelling, scarring). The third row presents a mother bringing her son to be checked by a doctor, a hospitalized child, and the four stages of child development. The show concludes with slides that tell parents how to get BCG vaccinations for their children (they can go to a clinic or wait until doctors come to their village). The final image, of a young girl next to an enlarged BCG vial, advises, "Children who want to prevent consumption quickly get vaccinated with BCG!"

Other sets range from nine to more than fifty slides. Ten slides on the "Love the Nation Hygienic Movement" document the peak of the Cultural Revolution with Chairman Mao quotations, his red book, revolutionary banners, and proletariat workers. More than fifty slides depict human evolution from apes and illustrate Engel's maxim that "Labor created humanity." Some sets still have booklets that give the lectures and sometimes the year of the campaign they were connected to (1972, family planning; 1974, intestinal disease prevention among soldiers).

Slide lectures were held in conjunction with postering, parades, publications, exhibitions, mass rallies, public address announcements, theatrical performances, and film—some of which can be seen in their projected images. Communist-era Chinese public health campaigns used a coordinated approach to media as a socialist technology of total mobilization for vaccination, sanitary engineering, personal hygiene, and revolutionary consciousness initiatives. These rare slides give viewers a glimpse of that lost world.

—MARTA HANSON

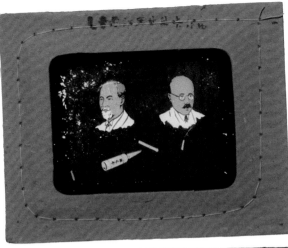
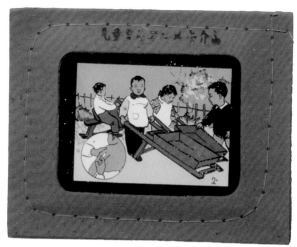
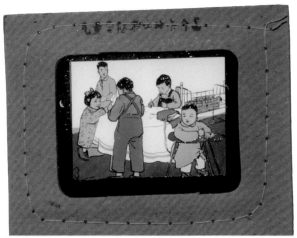
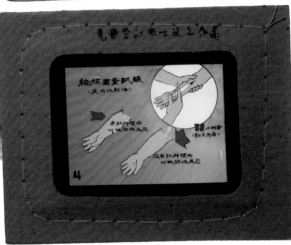
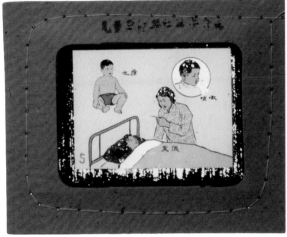
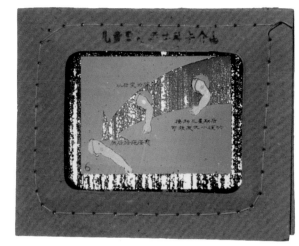
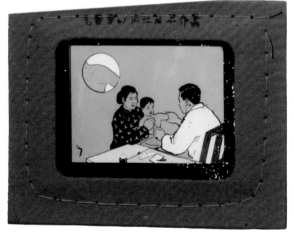
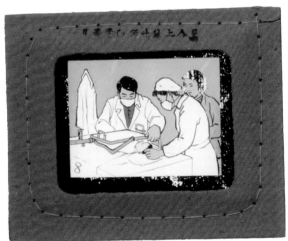
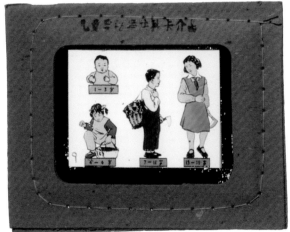
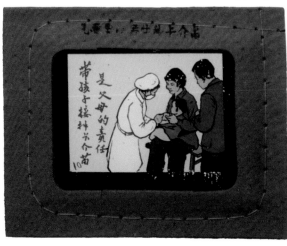
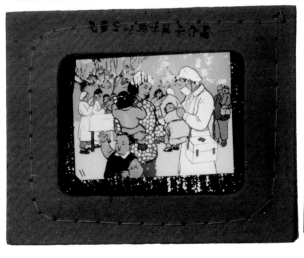
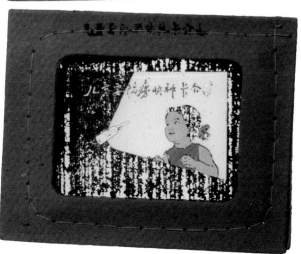

Elementary Hygiene for the Tropics (1902)
Azel Ames

Boston. Printed book, 180 pp.; illustrated; 5 x 7¼ in. (12.5 x 18.3 cm)

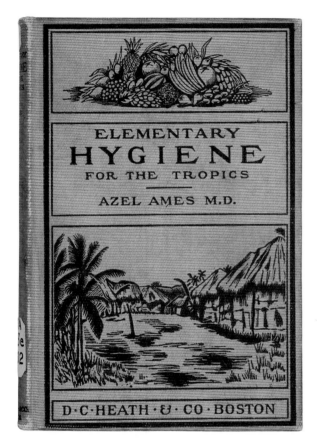

ABOVE: A native village street adorns the cover of this guide to living in the tropics.

This sometimes charming, sometimes dreadful little book offers a series of profusely illustrated lessons designed to teach "the young" how to stay healthy amid the many dangers in the tropics. Its intended readership is not native-born children but the offspring of white settlers—military officers, businessmen, colonial officials, and missionaries. Native people, we are told and shown, have a regrettable tendency to live in damp, overcrowded, and unsanitary dwellings in close quarters with domestic animals, rodents, and insects. Their customs and ways of doing things threaten their own health and the health of others. The book's author, Azel Ames (1845–1908), was well known for his writings on medicine and health. A major in the U.S. Army, he was a veteran of the Civil War and Spanish-American War and later represented the United States Public Health Service in the Philippines as military and civil sanitary inspector and in Puerto Rico as director of vaccination.

Ames begins his book by lecturing on the importance of being well. Sick people cannot work or find pleasure; if a man cannot earn anything for his family, he will be "poor, hungry and wretched." With good health, however, the same man is likely to be prosperous, contented, and happy. Ames lists the "musts"—the things we must know and must understand and laws we must obey lest we become ill, wretched, and dead.

After this rather terrifying introduction his advice is generally sound. We need to breathe clean air, eat nutritious food, rest and sleep well, and reduce wastes of every kind. At the end of each chapter he poses questions for the reader to answer. The question "What are the air cells in our lungs like?" has two possible right answers: masses of air cells are like "very great bunches of very small grapes"; single air cells, however, are like "small red toy balloons with very thin gutta-percha skins, blown up full of air."

He often uses colorful metaphors. The body, he says, like a well-kept horse, will repay us well for our good treatment. His advice on nutrition is a mix of the scientific knowledge of the time and a dose of common sense. Ames does not hesitate to disapprove of others' customs; he frowns on the French habit of having only coffee and bread for breakfast. In parts of the tropics, he says, people eat reptiles such as iguanas, but these are *not* fit food for decent people. As for clothing, Ames insists that children should wear flannel bands to keep their bowels warm. While native people laugh at the idea of wearing flannel bands around the body, he says, many of their children die.

Ames has a particular horror of "impurities" of every kind and sees their pernicious effects everywhere. These include foul air, vile odors, dirty water, rotting filth, decaying animals and plants, bodily wastes, and dangerous vapors from sewer pipes. These must be countered by the most scrupulous attention to cleanliness. He tries to be cheery and uplifting but mainly depicts the tropics as a disease-plagued environment that poses a grave risk to white children. I feel fortunate to have missed reading this little volume when growing up as a child in British Malaya.

—ELIZABETH FEE

OPPOSITE: A photograph shows tropical natives polluting their water supply. *Elementary Hygiene*, p. 89

Food mu...
be caref...
cleaned

are typhus, typhoid, and scarlet fevers, dysentery, cholera, and agues, besides which worms or t... often enter... in the wat...

To ... from thi... we must... of every... springs, ... wells from... draw it. Wi... care this can be...

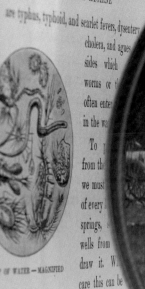

A DROP OF WATER — MAGNIFIED

How to keep water pure Cattle and hogs or other animals must not be allowed to wallow or wade, or women to wash clothes in, or people on the hillsides to throw their refuse into the streams from which people lower down take their water supply. Rotten vegetable and animal matter must not be thrown upon, or buried in, the ground near springs or water-courses for the next shower to wash into them. *Every one must be constantly careful* to keep all sources of water supply clean. Drinking-water must always be kept in clean vessels, which should be carefully covered. If not tightly covered, they should be protected with fine netting.

Food if
pleasan...
sight a...
smell d...
gests b...

The us...
cookin...

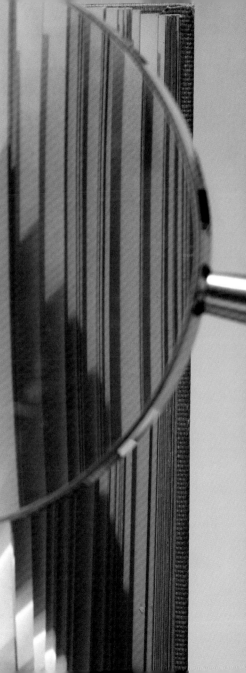

A USEFUL STREAM

...w ways these people are polluting the water

...or de... ficult to keep all impurities are to drink... sandy, we can filter it... means to remove How to purify water need to use it very soon, we can stir into it a little powdered alum, which will throw the mud to the bottom, and we can then pour or draw off the water, above the mud that has settled. This method has been used for many years by the people on the lower Mississippi River, and in the United States and the British armies.

Malaria Pinup Calendars (1945)
Frank Mack, for the U.S. Army

Washington, DC. Printed posters, color; 6⅜ x 7¼ in. (16.2 x 18.2 cm)

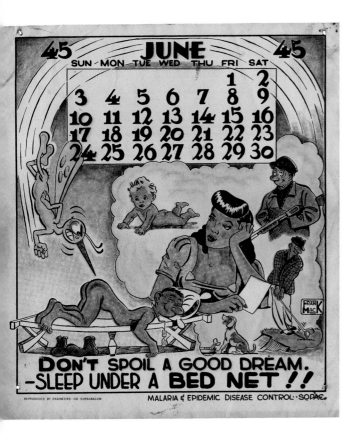

ABOVE: Sleepytime down SOPAC (South Pacific) way. If Moe is too recklessly macho to let fears of a wee mosquito bite prick his dream balloon of hetero homefront joys, maybe the threat of figurative (and literal!) buggery will drive the point home.

OPPOSITE: A swell pair of all-American gams serve as a risqué reminder to keep pulling for victory over both Japan and mosquitoes. These pinup calendars were part of a larger antimalaria campaign that emphasized the use of bed nets, mosquito repellent, Atabrine (an antimalarial pill), avoidance of places where mosquitoes swarm at night, and keeping skin covered.

To young American GIs waging World War II in the South Pacific malaria posed a threat as dire as that of the enemy's military forces. Tens of thousands of men died, due in part to shortages of quinine, then the only available treatment.

Early in the conflict the army's surgeon general established a malaria control office that provided ample supplies of the newly developed antimalarial agent Atabrine. Soldiers in the field, however, didn't view the threat seriously enough to swallow the bitter pill and risk its malaria-mimicking side effects: headaches, nausea, and vomiting. Consequently, only one-third of his troops were fit for combat at any given time, according to General Douglas MacArthur, the rest either afflicted by the disease or recovering.

In response, Armed Forces Radio began broadcasting so many malaria advisories that it became known as "the mosquito network" among the grunts, and "antimalaria squads" offered education and treatment in the field. But, as with the *Private Snafu* series of animated cartoons, GIs responded most avidly to information presented as entertainment. In 1944 an enlisted artist named Frank Mack was assigned the duty of designing pinup calendars to reach these homesick, bored, and horny soldiers, sailors, and marines.

If Mack, who went on after the war to work on the "Ripley's Believe It or Not" newspaper syndicated comics feature, lacked the artistic skill that peers such as Dr. Seuss brought to their own wartime posters, his rambunctious style, well showcased in the "Malaria Moe" comic strips he drew for the *Stars and Stripes* military newspaper, was an ideal choice for the task at hand.

The two months featured here are charming examples of Mack's work. In the pinup for May 1945 a comely redhead in a see-through nightie poses à la Rita Hayworth alongside a photo of her soldier boy, promising hubba-hubba-and-how, if only he'll thwart the insect foe and return, hale and hearty, to her yearning arms. Mack draws her with the kind of clunky eroticism GIs already enjoyed in novelty postcards, aircraft nose art, Tijuana bibles, and tattoos.

More homespun desires, with a note of slapstick ribaldry, turn up in June's pinup. Here, Malaria Moe himself, buck naked and barracks-bound, dreams of the pleasures waiting back home, blissfully unaware that the gum-bubble sheen of his upturned buttocks provides an irresistible target for an especially ornery and enormous specimen of, perhaps, *Anopheles flavirostris*, dubbed "Skeeter" in Mack's *Stars and Stripes* comics.

These rare pinup calendars are fascinating not only as images but as objects—souvenirs of military life as lived. The tack holes in their corners testify to active duty decades ago, perhaps hanging on a medic's office wall to attract the eye of some green, buck-naked private. There, vulnerable as Frank Mack's hapless Moe, he might find distraction from "bend over and cough" indignity by counting the remaining calendar days until—thanks to his bug net, his M1, and a bit of luck—he'd come marching home, ready to lay that pistol down and commence the postwar mission of producing bouncing baby boomers.

—SPORT MURPHY

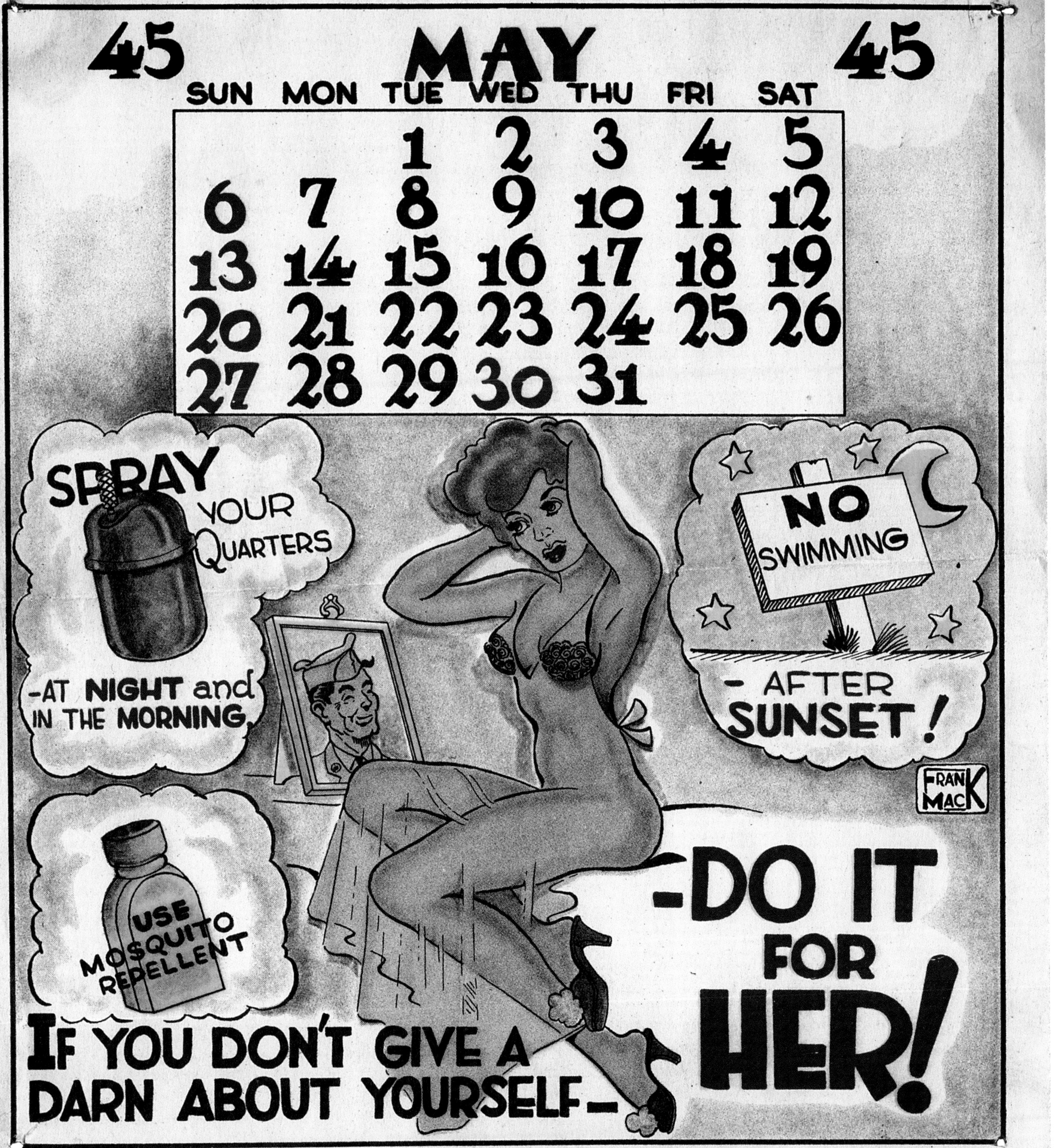

REPRODUCED BY ENGINEERS · HQ · SOPACBACOM

MALARIA & EPIDEMIC DISEASE CONTROL · SOPAC

Commandments for Health (1945)
Hugh Harman Productions, for the U.S. Navy

Washington, DC. Motion pictures, black-and-white, sound, animation, 16mm: *Personal Cleanliness* (5:00);
Cleaning Mess Gear (5:00); *Drinking Water* (6:00); *Use Your Head* (5:00); *Native Food* (6:00)

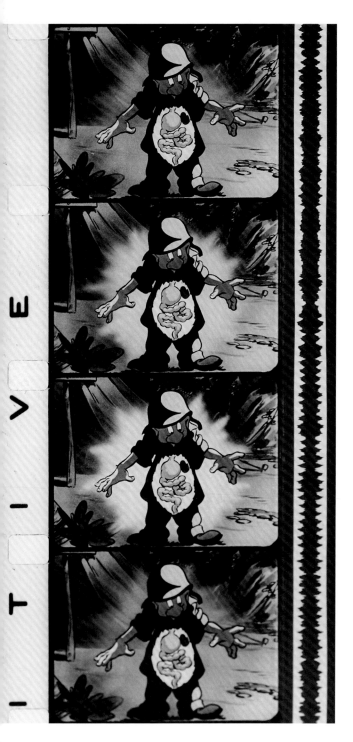

*I*nspired by the U.S. Army's popular *Private Snafu* animated cartoon series, late in World War II the navy hired Hugh Harman (1908–82) to do a similar series, focused on health. His *Commandments for Health* may have consisted of ten short black-and-white cartoons (mirroring the Ten Commandments) but was not widely distributed or shown. Today it is extremely rare. The National Library of Medicine holds five titles; only two others are known to exist.

Harman began his career in the 1920s with Walt Disney and Warner Bros. in the 1930s. For the navy's film series he hired top talent Mel Blanc (the voice of Bugs Bunny) to voice the dim-witted McGillicuddy and the smart regular-guy narrator. But unlike the *Snafu* series, the animation is jerky and backgrounds are static, sure signs that the cartoons were made quickly and cheaply. (Animation in the 1940s was labor intensive: the more drawings, the smoother the action.) Each film follows the same formula: the main character, the hapless U.S. Marine private McGillicuddy (a Snafu clone), violates a health commandment, endangering himself (and sometimes also his fellow soldiers). In *Drinking Water*, "Mac" ignores the third commandment: "Thou shall not drink water from any source other than that designated." Instead, after using up his water and baking under a scorching sun (drawn as a caricature of Japan's prime minister Tojo), the parched Mac jumps into a stream contaminated with a gorilla, "dead Japs," and a native village's latrine. (McGillicuddy cartoons contain a dose of anti-Japanese propaganda that goes over the edge into racism.) In the end Mac has to make so many urgent trips to the "head" (a toilet) that his feet dig a trench.

Personal Cleanliness also has a third commandment—another sign that the cartoons were rushed through production—"Thou shall keep thy personal habits clean." Mac, predictably, refuses to bathe. His socks walk off by themselves, his skin itches, and slant-eyed athlete's-foot "germs" attack his toes with saws and jackhammers (opposite, middle right). The film concludes with more racial stereotyping: natives who appear to be cannibals and speak in minstrel-show dialect pick him up and dump him into a kettle, but only to give him a bath.

Cleaning Mess Gear's fifth commandment is "Thou shalt faithfully wash thy mess gear...for verily if thou become negligent in this habit thy guts shall be like knots in a wet rope." Once again, Mac doesn't comply. He licks his plate clean instead of sterilizing it in scalding water. Later, an X-ray view shows his intestines literally tied in knots (left; the line running down the right is the sound track). In the next scene, sadistic doctors subject him to a stomach pump, a huge dose of castor oil, and a 50-gallon enema. In *Use Your Head* the seventh commandment is "Thou shalt not use any spots except chosen ones for the deposition of your excrement." But Mac makes his own private toilet, attracting a swarm of Japanese-featured flies (opposite, top center) that gives the whole camp dysentery. When a Japanese radio announcer thanks Mac by name (opposite, top left), the marines use a steam shovel to dump him and his latrine into a pit.

—MICHAEL RHODE

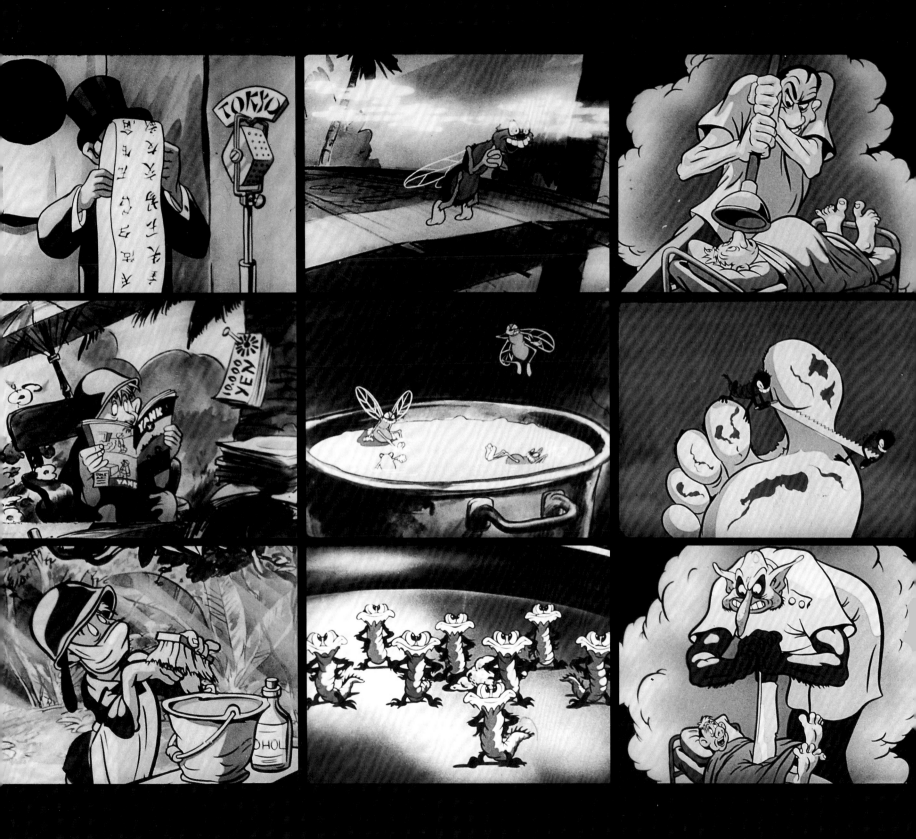

St. Elizabeths Magic Lantern Slide Collection (1855–1890s)
American Stereoscopic Company (Philadelphia); T. M. McAllister (New York); James W. Queen & Co. (Philadelphia); and unknown manufacturers

Glass slides in wooden frames; photoprinted and handpainted

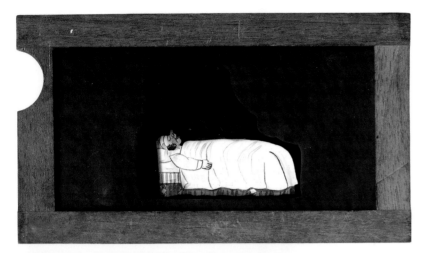
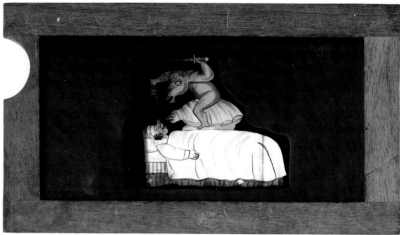

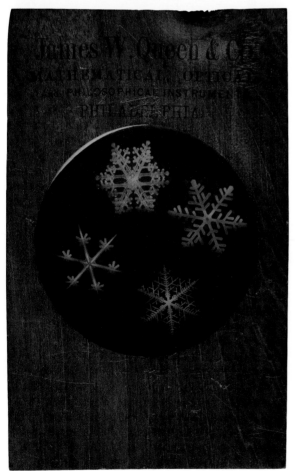

*P*icture the scene. Seated in a lecture hall, several hundred well-dressed mental patients—watched carefully by attendants—await the entrance of the medical director of their hospital. Gaslight dims and the doctor emerges, striding toward a lectern. "Today's topic," he announces, "is the symmetry of natural forms." An attendant at the back hunches over an elaborate contraption that burns streams of hydrogen and oxygen over a cylinder of calcium oxide. The resulting beam of intense white light—limelight—is focused on a glass plate coated with tiny particles of silver salt affixed to the glass with albumen. Cast across the auditorium onto a screen is the perfect image of microscopically observed snow-flakes, ten feet in diameter.

According to the art historian Emily Godbey and the psychiatrist George S. Layne, such magic lantern displays were more than a pastime to amuse nineteenth-century patients. Originated in the early 1850s by Dr. Thomas Kirkbride (1809–83) of the Pennsylvania Hospital for the Insane, in collaboration with German émigré photographers William Langenheim (1807–74) and Frederick Langenheim (1809–79), they were an important part of the "moral treatment" of patients. Subscribing to John Locke's "impression" theory of mental process, early American asylum superintendents believed that rational, orderly imagery could be "impressed upon the mind," thus—according to Kirkbride—effacing "delusions and morbid feelings, at least for a transitory period." Many of the images (some mechanically reproduced, others hand-painted), accordingly, were manifestly instructive: several illustrate the perils of drink and tobacco; others depict order and beauty drawn from nature and travel. Some of the images even moved. Using "slip slides"—a pair of sequenced images slipped into and out of a wooden frame—operators created the first form of animation, preceding flip books by several decades.

The therapeutic use of magic lantern slides spread well beyond Philadelphia. The images gathered here are from St. Elizabeths Hospital—originally the Government Hospital for the Insane—a federally funded institution built in 1855. All of them were produced by

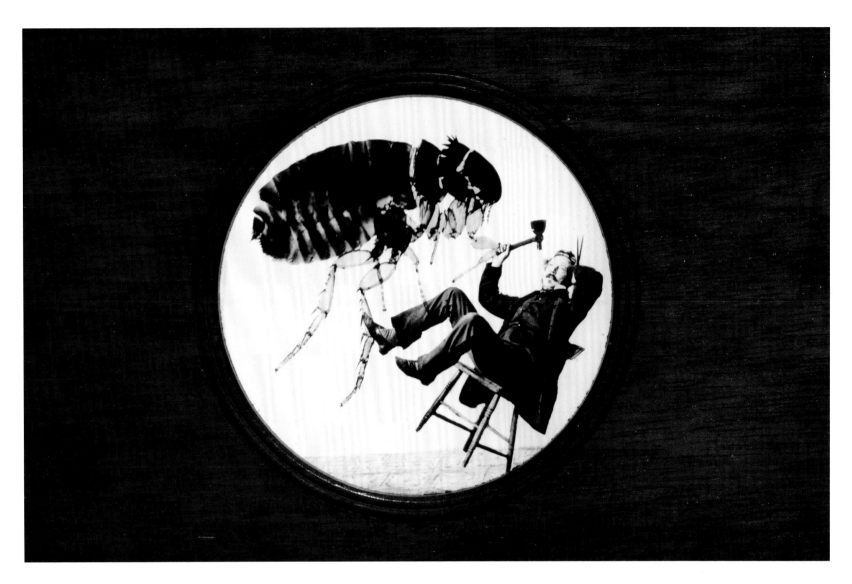

ABOVE: "The Attack of the Monster (Pulex Irritans)." Lantern Slide 136

OPPOSITE, TOP: Slip slides, with two glass cells in the same frame, were manipulated to create the illusion of motion. Lantern Slide 80

OPPOSITE, BOTTOM: Snowflake. Lantern Slide 47, James W. Queen & Co.

commercial companies, for the general public, and many were designed purely for entertainment purposes. The most famous is the Langenheim Brothers' "The Attack of the Monster (Pulex Irritans)," a surreal and somewhat horrifying double exposure in which a magnified flea menaces an ax- and shears-wielding man—actually one of the brothers. Other images in the St. Elizabeths collection similarly highlight the ludicrous and the bizarre: a man trying to chop off his own foot; a pair of eyeglasses becoming two people; a sleeping man having a nightmare featuring a blue mare astride a giant turtle brandishing a sword and lobster; a cook bearing a human-headed dish of pudding; a bather jumping into a huge fish's mouth.

Given that many patients were delusional and/or medicated with dream-inducing opiates, one wonders about the wisdom of serving up these ready-made hallucinations, magnified to terrifying proportions. But theory trumped such considerations. According to a leading practitioner of moral treatment, Dr. John Minson Galt, asylum amusements should feature techniques of "revulsion"—that is, psychological interventions that would cause patients to recoil from their delusions by externalizing them and subjecting them to the ridicule of others. In particular, "hilarity" would help "supplant the place of delusive ideas and feelings.... If you can get [the insane] to laugh natural, it is quite apt to explode the whole affair."

—Benjamin Reiss

Disease Warning Sign Collection (ca. 1890–1960)
Various public health departments

United States. Cards printed on colored stock

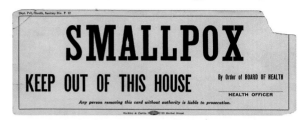

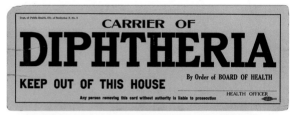

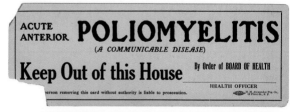

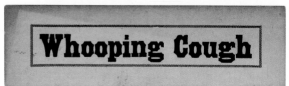

ABOVE: Examples of public health warning cards in the National Library of Medicine's collection, probably late nineteenth century. The smallpox and poliomyelitis cards were printed in San Francisco, the others in unidentified locales.

OPPOSITE: Salk polio vaccination campaign sign, ca. 1955.

*T*he history of public health cannot be understood without artifacts such as those pictured here—the handbills, forms, public notices, signs, educational circulars, and pamphlets that document and in part constitute the street-level history of public health. They are relics of the infectious-disease prevention campaigns of late-nineteenth- and twentieth-century state and local public health agencies as they sought to isolate the sick, encourage physicians to report cases, and educate ordinary men and women. Such humble pieces of disposable paper and cardboard document vital links between the worlds of law and medicine, the laboratory and the bedside, public policy and the political and professional stakeholders who created and enforced those policies.

Disposable printed items, called "ephemera" in the book and printing trades, until recently had only a small place in our most prominent libraries. The shelves of our established medical libraries are laden with words written to be preserved: theses, medical journals, monographs, and textbooks. Learned books and articles *were* the history of medicine for generations of its chroniclers. This cumulative record of intellectual achievement excluded by definition the ephemeral—print with an instrumental, transactional, or commercial purpose, to be used and discarded. But in recent years a new historical sensibility has made such ephemera indispensable, as we seek to link high culture with low, theory with practice, medical institutions with everyday life. Only the more prescient libraries, such as the National Library of Medicine, have purposefully collected such undignified materials.

These objects reflect a changing consensus of epidemiological and laboratory knowledge. They also illuminate the not always direct relationship between that knowledge and public health practice. Smallpox, for example, had been known to be transmitted from person to person since at least the eighteenth century, yet late-nineteenth-century outbreaks of the disease, which gave rise to an aggressive policy of isolation and official encouragement of vaccination, had to struggle against resentment of compulsory measures and in some instances the organized opposition of anti-vaccinationists. Newer immunizations for scarlet fever, diphtheria, and whooping cough, which joined the list of reportable ills in the late nineteenth and early twentieth centuries, similarly required the education and mobilization of an often wary public. And thus ongoing campaigns for childhood immunizations remain a reality in the twenty-first century—just as they were a half century earlier in the era of Jonas Salk's novel polio vaccine.

Each threatened epidemic has provided a new focus for debate and discussion. Today fears of emerging diseases, and the needs and anxieties of a global health community, underscore the continued importance of outreach and implementation as well as research. The past half century has witnessed a revolution in mass media, and the need to deploy old and new modes of communication remains as central to the tasks of medicine and public health today as when these health signs were printed many decades ago.

—CHARLES ROSENBERG

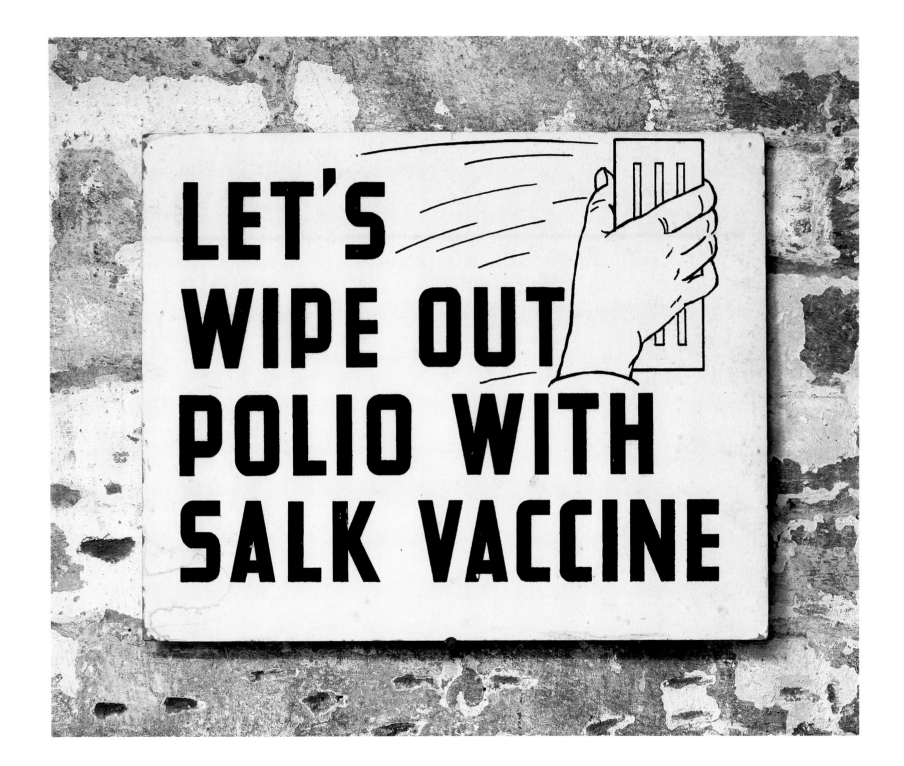

Easy to Get (1947)
Army Pictorial Service, Signal Corps (Official Training Film T.F.8 1423)

Washington, DC. Motion picture, black-and-white, sound, 16 mm; 22:00

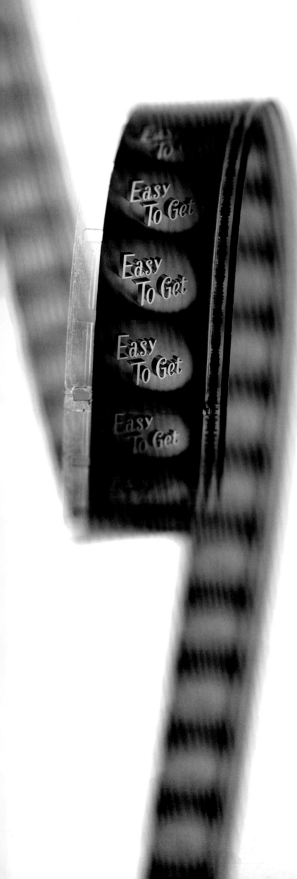

*T*his curious little nightmare movie is addressed to black soldiers. It depicts black men as overgrown, impulsive, hypersexualized children who are unable to contain their primordial desires. The film's title refers to venereal disease but could equally refer to women, who in this bleak tale of misogyny are invariably represented as sexually promiscuous and solely to blame for passing along the pox. The title is perhaps also self-referential—its message is "easy to get." It was produced as part of a larger wartime "Easy to Get" multimedia anti-VD campaign (aimed at all male soldiers, not just black men). There were "Easy to Get" comic books, animated cartoons, posters, pamphlets, radio skits, even matchbooks—which tried to recruit the attention of their target audience by showing views of provocatively sexy women alongside queasy glimpses of festering genitals, oozing sores, and congenital deformities. An unbeatable combination.

The film's daytime segments—its ego, if you will—take place in the office of a white doctor, played with dripping condescension by Wendell Corey. The first of two representative black GIs, Corporal Baker, normally "one happy mister," visits the doc to find the source of a baffling infection. Believe it or not, says the doc, the shy, "clean-looking" gal Baker met in the drugstore at home—the girl with the soft voice, the one whose parents are "good people"—turns out, like every other woman in the film, to be "filthy and diseased." Why, implies the doc, would anybody ever take such a foolish risk?

We soon see why. A series of evocative, artful noirish sequences form the film's id, from which the daytime scenes seem impossibly distant. At night the film's second representative black GI, Private Anderson, "something of a playboy," picks up a smoldering bad girl in a wild jitterbug joint. "Sure, he knew she was a whore, so what?" Even worse, instead of jumping up afterward to chummily soap down his cock with other soldiers in the "pro [prophylactic] station," Anderson languidly lights a cigarette, lays back, and figures he can afford a second helping.

The horror show that follows—the film's superego—displays the consequences of such undisciplined behavior. One soldier, a former athlete, now has knees like basketballs; another collapses and dies suddenly at a luncheonette counter; a third can't remember three words in a row because "the syphilis germs got into his brain." In close-up we see the swollen, oozing genitals of a guy who "rubbed whiskey on his rod after a pickup." Nastiest of all, one man passes the disease to his wife, who gives birth to a monster spawned from undisciplined desire—a cretinous gargoyle with a misshapen skull, half a nose, and eyes rolling back in its head.

This ghastly sight is juxtaposed with images of black heroes, men who have sublimated their lusts so as to better serve their race and their nation: heavyweight boxing champion Joe Louis and Olympic track stars Jesse Owens and Ralph Metcalfe. As a grand finale, speaking magisterially from behind an imposing desk, Paul Robeson bellows a final exhortation. Grow up, boys, and leave women alone!

—MIKITA BROTTMAN

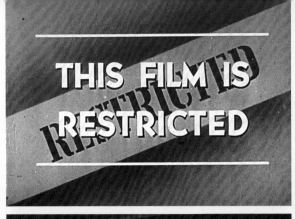

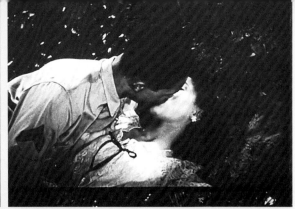

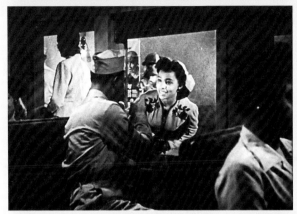

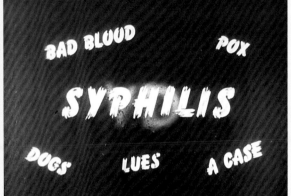

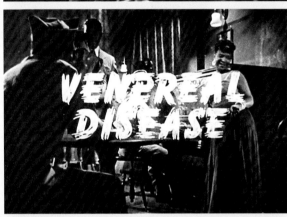

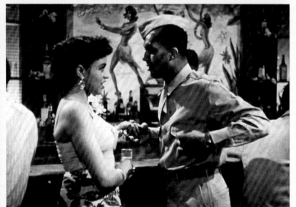

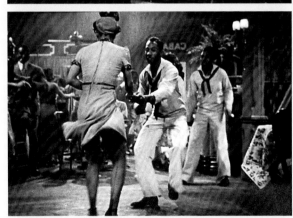

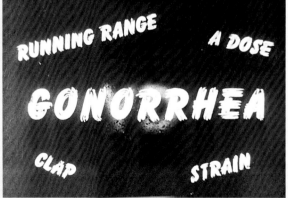

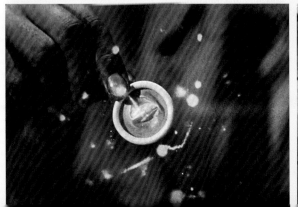

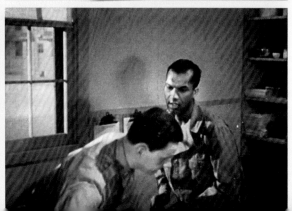

Civil War Surgical Card Collection (1860s)
Army Medical Museum and the Surgeon General's Office

Washington, DC. 146 numbered cards, with tipped-in photographs and case histories; 9⅞ x 11⅞ in. (25 x 30 cm)

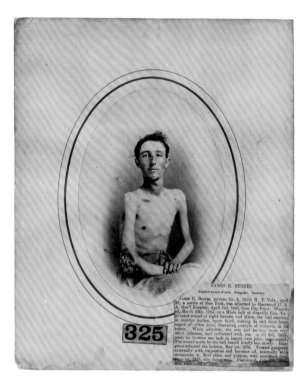

ABOVE AND OPPOSITE: The Army Medical Museum's staff mined incoming reports for "interesting" cases—such as a gunshot wound of the "left side of scalp, denuding skull" or "gunshot wound, right elbow with gangrene supervening"—and cases that demonstrated the use of difficult surgical techniques, such as an amputation by circular incision or resection of the "head of humerus and three inches of the left clavicle."

On May 21, 1862, Surgeon General William Hammond (1828–1900) issued two "circular" letters to the officers of the Army Medical Corps. Circular No. 2 directed officers to submit medical and surgical specimens to the newly formed Army Medical Museum. Circular No. 5 asked them to submit "details of cases…and the results of investigations" for publication in a *Medical and Surgical History of the War of the Rebellion*. Contributing to the museum and book served to affirm and reshape the professional identity of Union army surgeons and physicians. It articulated a new epistemological foundation for American medicine, based on the experience of dealing with thousands of wounded and sick patients, the critical comparison of cases, and a commitment to learning and developing new theories and techniques. And it prompted the officers to make photographs of unique and interesting cases.

Those photographs were mounted on cards, along with a short printed text detailing the subject's case history: where he was wounded, course of treatment, results, and attending physician's name. The cards became medical records, used to determine the amount of pension that the wounded men would receive. They also became teaching and research aids with visual and verbal documentation of wounds inflicted by minié ball, cannonballs, and accidents; camp and hospital diseases; gangrene, ulcers, and surgical techniques. Soldiers are posed and identified by name, rank, company, regiment, and state in many of the photographs, but the disease or wound or amputation is meant to be the focus of the picture.

Some photographs were made by officers at the Army Medical Museum, but most were made by Lieutenant Colonel and Surgeon Reed Brockway Bontecou (1824–1907) while in charge of Harewood General Hospital, a three-thousand-bed facility in Washington, where he was posted from October 1863 to May 1866. The images show a wide array of war diseases and injuries—gunshot wounds of the legs, arms, head, face, eyes, chest, abdomen; resections, amputations; cases of acute erysipelas (bacterial skin infection), sloughing and spreading gangrenous ulcers, and prosthetic limbs. Taken together, they provide an extraordinary document of the damage the war wrought and the challenges facing Civil War medical practice.

Bontecou's cards are in a number of repositories, but the National Library of Medicine's set is unique. Many of its cards are marked with hand-drawn arrows in red ink, showing the entry and exit of the bullet. Lesions or gangrenous ulcers are circled and colored red. Some cards also have pencil or pen notations. Bontecou and his colleagues prided themselves on their modern, scientific approach to medicine and surgery and they regarded the photographs as a kind of two-dimensional clinic. A set of cards was exhibited at the Philadelphia Centennial Exposition of 1876.

These images of patients set squarely before the camera are touching and disquieting, a powerful display of suffering. Many of the soldiers willingly offered themselves up as photographic subjects, proud to record the terrible marks of their service to the nation—and proud to contribute to the advancement of medical knowledge.

—SHAUNA DEVINE

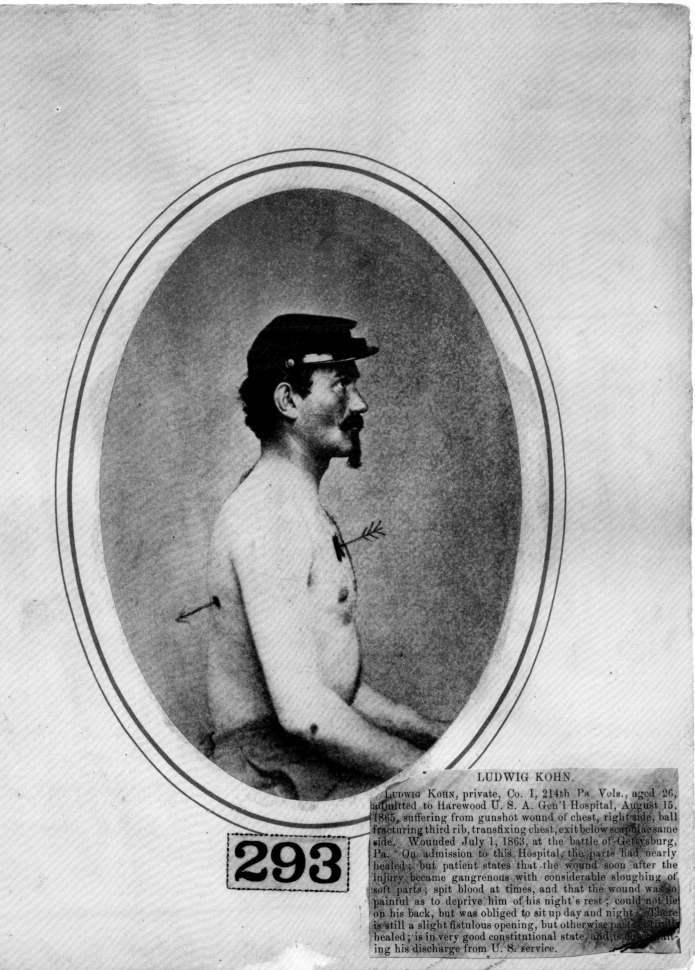

293

LUDWIG KOHN.

LUDWIG KOHN, private, Co. I, 214th Pa Vols., aged 26, admitted to Harewood U. S. A. Gen'l Hospital, August 15, 1865, suffering from gunshot wound of chest, right side, ball fracturing third rib, transfixing chest, exit below scapulae same side. Wounded July 1, 1863, at the battle of Gettysburg, Pa. On admission to this Hospital, the parts had nearly healed; but patient states that the wound soon after the injury became gangrenous with considerable sloughing of soft parts; spit blood at times, and that the wound was so painful as to deprive him of his night's rest; could not lie on his back, but was obliged to sit up day and night. There is still a slight fistulous opening, but otherwise parts entirely healed; is in very good constitutional state, and is await- ing his discharge from U. S. service.

Nightingale Collection (1845–1939)
Florence Nightingale

London and other locations. Books, pamphlets, letters, photographs, engravings, lithographs, sound recordings

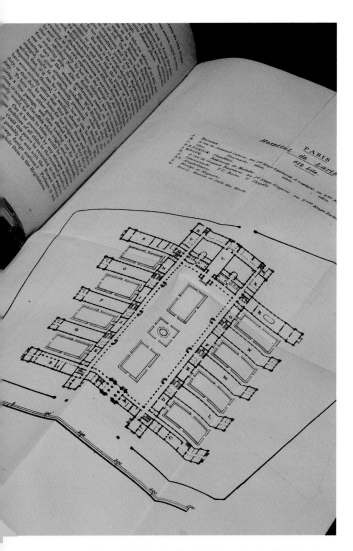

ABOVE: Plan of the Hospital Lariboisiere, Paris. Nightingale approved of the hospital's pavilion design but criticized some features (e.g., privies in the middle). Nightingale, *Subsidiary Notes as to the Introduction of Female Nursing into Military Hospitals in Peace and War* (London, 1858)

OPPOSITE: "Diagram of the Causes of Mortality in the Army in the East," in *A Contribution to the Sanitary History of the British Army during the Late War with Russia* (London, 1859). Anonymously published, *Contribution* was a brief but powerful indictment of unnecessary, because preventable, deaths among British soldiers in the Crimea. Nightingale's bold use of color in the summary chart was far ahead of its time.

There are few figures in medicine who are also iconic figures in world history. Florence Nightingale (1820–1910) is one such individual—the mythic lady with the lamp, founder of professional nursing, savior of the British soldier in the Crimea and India, and decisive advocate for clean and orderly hospitals. It is all true if oversimplified, yet her heroic personal narrative obscures one key aspect of her success.

That is her skill in communication, her ability to deploy an array of words and images as rhetorical tools in convincing her readers that the current state of health and disease is intolerable, and that both logic and morality dictate a new institutional order. She used not only figures of speech, but figures—numbers, in the form of statistics and raw data, as well as plans, tables, and charts that dramatized instructive differences in morbidity and mortality. Words and images allowed her to reach out from her invalid's rooms in London to influence a generation of reformers throughout the world. Nightingale's simple arithmetic demonstrating the—culpable—difference in death rates between hospitals constituted in itself a powerful argument for reform. That difference was both diagnostic and motivating. If death rates could be lower, then they should be. Nightingale was a master of the Is and Ought.

And she was a pioneer in using the power of graphic representation to show how the Ought could become the Is. Her *Notes on Hospitals* (in its third enlarged and revised edition by 1863) was filled with floor plans indicating the placement of beds and windows to allow a health-preserving circulation of air in one-story pavilion-style wings or freestanding buildings. That same influential book also provides model forms for tabulating, managing, and reporting every aspect of a hospital's cumulative experience. Nightingale's summary indictment of the British army medical staff and its hospitals in the Crimean War (published in 1859) used a then novel color-coded chart to show month by month the proportion of preventable deaths to those from wounds and other causes. It was a grim and damning reality that could be changed for the better by the nursing and hospital reforms she orchestrated.

Knowledge demanded responsibility, and responsibility action. The three things that destroyed so many soldiers in the Crimean War, Nightingale contended, were ignorance, incapacity, and "useless regulation." "Health is known to depend on the observance of certain laws," she argued. "Surely, before a picked body of men in the prime of life could have been cut off by a mortality greater perhaps than that of any pestilence on record, there must have been some very glaring disobedience to these laws." Cleanliness, order, ventilation, and sound diet ensured health—disorder, filth, and poor diet brought an inevitable punishment in the form of cholera, scurvy, dysentery, and fevers. In the Crimea, Nightingale was an activist on the ground, but for the remainder of her long life she was a publicist for reform—a powerful rhetorician who used words and images to invoke a health-sustaining world of predictable order. She was more modern than she knew.

—CHARLES ROSENBERG

DIAGRAM OF THE CAUSES OF MORTALITY
IN THE ARMY IN THE EAST.

2.
APRIL 1855 TO MARCH 1856.

1.
APRIL 1854 TO MARCH 1855.

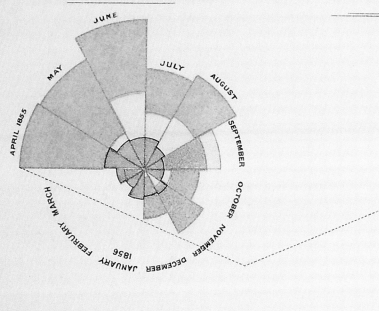

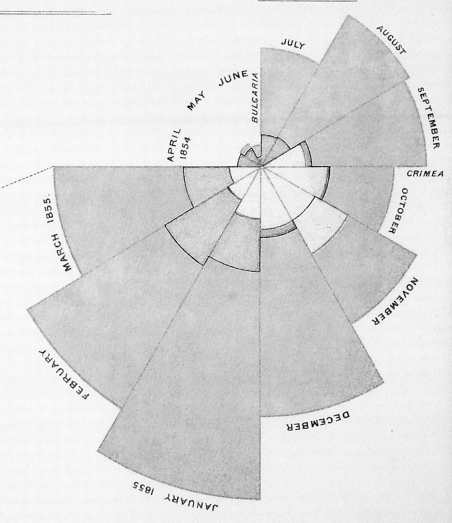

The Areas of the blue, red, & black wedges are each measured from
the centre as the common vertex.

The blue wedges measured from the centre of the circle represent area
for area the deaths from Preventible or Mitigable Zymotic diseases, the
red wedges measured from the centre the deaths from wounds, & the
black wedges measured from the centre the deaths from all other causes.

The black line across the red triangle in Nov.ʳ 1854 marks the boundary
of the deaths from all other causes during the month.

In October 1854, & April 1855, the black area coincides with the red,
in January & February 1856, the blue coincides with the black.

The entire areas may be compared by following the blue, the red, & the
black lines enclosing them.

First Aid on the Battlefield (1869)
Johann Friedrich August von Esmarch

Der erste Verband auf dem Schlachtfelde. Kiel, Germany.
Printed book with illustrations, 23 pp., 3¾ x 6¾ in. (9.5 x 17.2 cm); with printed bandage, 36 x 36 x 51½ in. (91.4 x 91.4 x 130.8 cm)

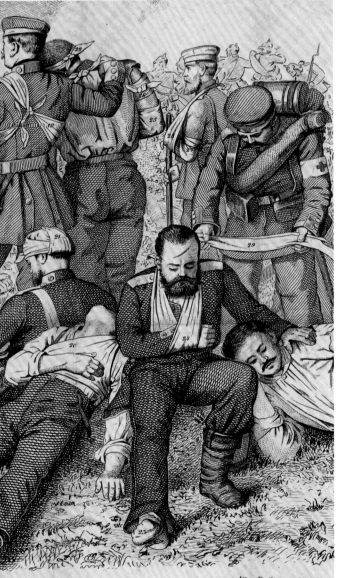

ABOVE AND OPPOSITE: Esmarch's triangular bandage for a battlefield first-aid kit. The realistic, crowded battlefield scene was later considered to be demoralizing and too visually complex. It was dropped in subsequent editions and replaced with a simpler diagram of six men (against no background at all), illustrating how the bandage should be tied around different limbs.

In 1870–71 the Prussian war machine tore through France with ruthless efficiency, eliciting fear and admiration in equal measure. What impressed international observers was not only the power and precision of the Prussian army but also the arrangements it had made for the prevention of disease and the evacuation and treatment of casualties. Whereas the French army suffered more than 200,000 cases of smallpox, the Prussians had fewer than 5,000, and whereas the French wounded often went untended, the Prussians made extensive use of railways to evacuate casualties and dealt with them far more effectively on or near the battlefield.

These vaunted achievements were the fruit of bitter experience. Those who planned the medical evacuations during the Franco-Prussian War included many veterans of earlier conflicts, beginning with the First Schleswig War of 1848–51, when Germans in that duchy attempted to secede from Denmark. The secession, at first crushed by the Danish army, was achieved by force with the support of Prussia and Austria in 1864. Two years later the battle-hardened Prusso-German army went on to defeat Austria, signaling the reemergence of Prussia as a major military power. In these earlier conflicts, German forces had failed to plan effectively for the treatment of their war wounded.

At the heart of this turmoil was Friedrich von Esmarch (1823–1908), who was to become one of the most famous surgeons of his day. Born on the west coast of Schleswig-Holstein, Esmarch was a German patriot who strove for independence from Denmark. He obtained his medical degree from Kiel University in 1848 and shortly afterward enlisted as a surgeon in the army of the Schleswig Germans. His experience as a frontline surgeon led him in 1851 to write a treatise on bullet wounds in which he showed that injured limbs could sometimes be saved, avoiding amputation. When war broke out again in 1864, Esmarch served in the field hospitals of Flensburg, Sundewitt, and Kiel. After war was declared against Austria he was called to Berlin in 1866 to become a member of the hospital commission and to oversee surgery in military hospitals there. This accumulated experience formed the basis of his best-known work, *First Aid on the Battlefield*.

The pamphlet had enormous influence on first aid in both military and civilian life. It endeavored to make first aid comprehensible to laymen and was included in a kit to be carried by soldiers. This kit famously contained a triangular cloth bandage (pictured here) printed with instructional illustrations for securing injured limbs and reducing bleeding on different parts of the body.

Esmarch went on to make other important innovations in surgery and first aid, including a rubber tourniquet bandage that enabled what he referred to as "bloodless surgery." His works on surgery and first aid were translated into other languages and went through many editions. As someone who was revolted by what he termed "the terror of war," Esmarch through his life and work exemplified the complexities of an age in which barbarism and humanitarianism marched hand in hand.

—Mark Harrison

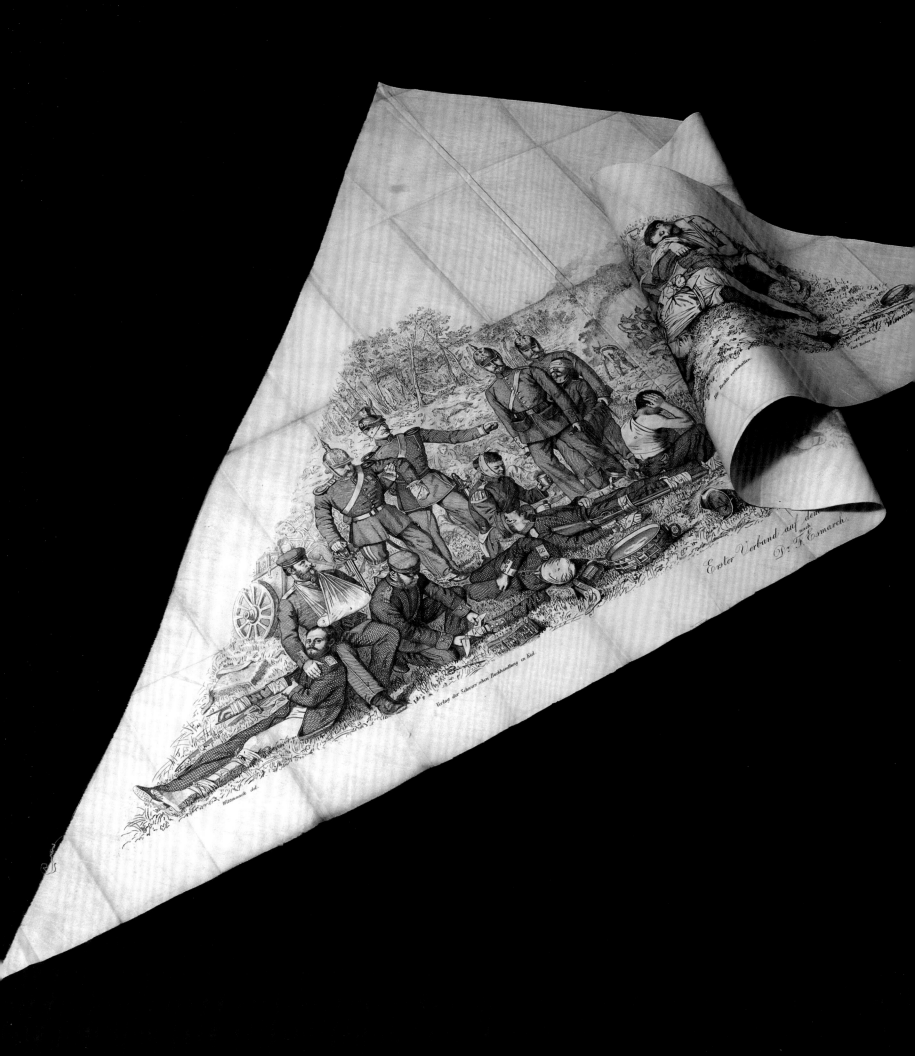

Erster Verband auf dem nach Dr. F. Esmarch.

Plastic Reconstruction of the Face (1918)
Filmmaker unknown

Paris. Motion picture fragment, black-and-white, silent, no intertitles, 16mm; 6:00

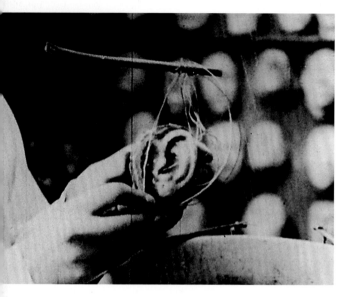

A woman dips a sculpted ear into a chemical solution and adjusts the current. The ear, plated with copper, will then be attached to a soldier. To make the attachment, a cast was made of his disfigured features (after his wounds had healed), a suffocating ordeal. The sculptor used the cast to re-create the man's missing parts and prewar appearance. Details such as eyebrows or mustaches were made from real hair or slivers of tinfoil and glued on. It was difficult to paint masks to convincingly resemble flesh, despite the skill that went into their creation. Children were known to flee in terror at the sight of a masked veteran.

A tiny, black-robed woman scurries down a deserted street and ducks into an alley overgrown with ivy. The black-and-white film flickers, as though what is left of the emulsion might crumble away at any moment. The alleyway dissolves; we find ourselves in an artist's studio. The walls are lined with plaster heads. Are these death masks, works of art, or a gallery of lost souls? Abruptly a young soldier standing in the foreground removes his chin to reveal a scarred hollow where his jaw once was. He reattaches the chin. A woman in military uniform appraises the fit. She is Anna Coleman Ladd (1878–1939), an American sculptor and former socialite. This is the Studio for Portrait Masks, where, as the soldiers put it, you come to get a "tin face."

A bearded sculptor holds up the cast of a head. As he turns it, the profile switches from classical elegance to terrible deformity. He is Francis Derwent Wood (1871–1926), an artist who pioneered the use of masks to hide the destroyed faces of the men who fought in World War I. Soldiers are routinely maimed in war, but trench warfare dramatically increased facial injury. These galvanized copper masks offered a way to "face" the world.

The psychological toll was enormous. Some men went on to become cinema projectionists, hiding from the world in the darkness of the projection booth. It would surely have been disturbing for them to view again and again films of profound paranoia, centered on the face and shifting identities, in contemporary films such as Louis Feuillade's *Fantômas* (1913–14), in which Paris is terrorized by a criminal mastermind who with the help of fake beards or facial prosthesis could become any- and everyone, or Fritz Lang's *Dr. Mabuse* (1922), another master of disguise.

Plastic Reconstruction inverts the ideals of Western art. The plaster casts of classical Greek sculpture that adorned the nineteenth-century sculptor's studio are replaced by casts that denote the wreckage of those ideals of beauty and symmetry. We see a young woman painting the tip of a soldier's nose. She appears to be flirting with the handsome mustachioed officer, shown in profile (opposite, fig. 9). The image recalls *The Corinthian Maid* (1782–84), a painting by Joseph Wright of Derby, based on a story by Pliny, in which a Grecian girl traces the silhouette of her departing lover on the wall, substituting an image for the man she is about to lose. *Plastic Reconstruction*, in contrast, looks to a mythic future where man is no longer quite human. Beyond L. Frank Baum's Tin Man, these soldiers of flesh and metal, hidden behind reproductions of themselves, anticipate the androids and cyborgs that would populate science fiction yet to come.

After the war people stopped paying attention. The war wounded became just another part of the human landscape. The last image in *Plastic Reconstruction* is of a soldier who literally takes off his face (opposite, fig. 12). He turns directly to the camera, fixes us with his one good eye, and the film abruptly ends. We are left with an indelible afterimage: a "faceless" man.

—Zoe Beloff

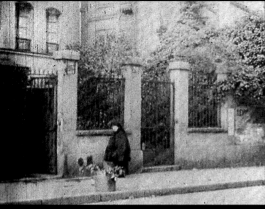

1. Paris, the Latin Quarter. The entrance to the Studio for Portrait Masks.

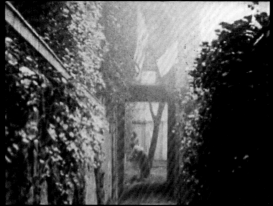

2. An alleyway leads to a courtyard populated with statues.

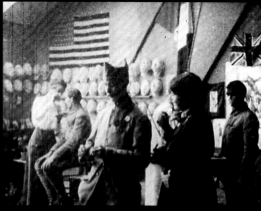

3. Lining the walls of the studio, filled with flowers and draped with flags, are masks in progress.

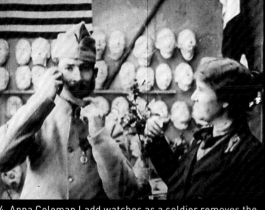

4. Anna Coleman Ladd watches as a soldier removes the mask that covers his missing chin.

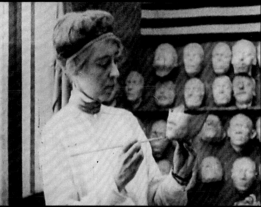

5. Painting a copper facial mask. Between 1918 and 1919 220 masks were made here.

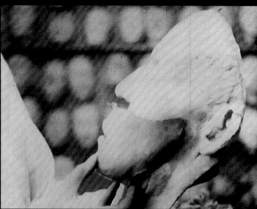

6. Fitting the mask over a plaster cast of the soldier's face.

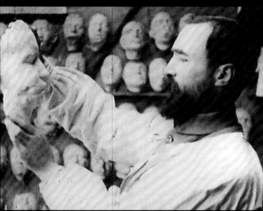

7. Francis Derwent Wood studies the life cast .

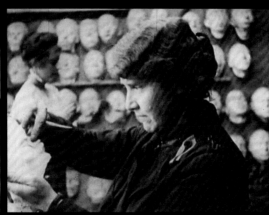

8. Ladd creating a nose.

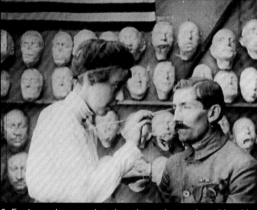

9. Each mask was painted on the patient to best blend in with his complexion.

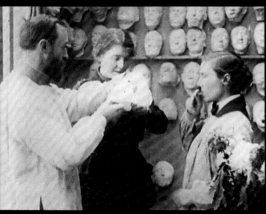

10. An assistant smokes anxiously as Wood appraises a cast.

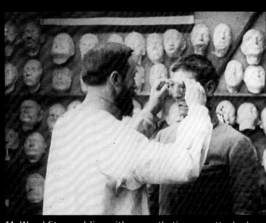

11. Wood fits a soldier with a prosthetic nose attached to glasses.

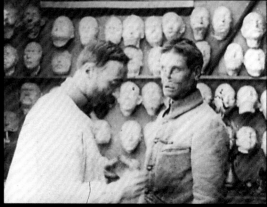

12. The final shot. A "faceless" man.

The Mess Kit and *The Silver Chev'* (1919)
Various U.S. military hospitals

Camp Grant, Illinois; Camp Merritt, New Jersey. U.S. military hospital magazines, color lithographic and halftone covers;
Mess Kit: 8¾ x 13 in. (22 x 33 cm); *Chev'*: 8¼ x 11 in. (21 x 28 cm)

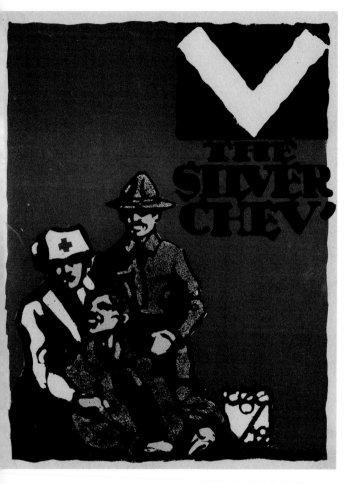

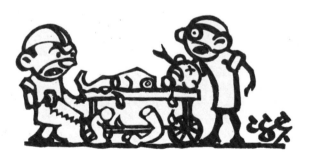

Cartoon detail from *Silver Chev'*, June 1, 1919, p. 7; drawing probably by Sgt. Christian G. Christensen.

Between 1918 and 1919, across twenty-one states and the District of Columbia, at least fifty military hospitals produced official in-house magazines—"house organs." Endorsed by the Surgeon General's Office, magazines such as *The Mess Kit* of Camp Merritt Base Hospital, New Jersey, *The Silver Chev'* of Camp Grant Base Hospital, Illinois, and *The Come-Back* of Walter Reed General Hospital, Washington, DC, were brought to life by wounded soldiers and military staff who contributed articles, jokes, poems, illustrations, and other material. Magazine work served to distract from bullet, shell, and bayonet wounds, influenza and other infectious diseases, gas exposure, gangrene, and shell shock. Like counterpart publications produced in British hospitals, these magazines served as "safety valves" to help relieve the stress experienced by frontline soldiers and their caregivers. And, like their British counterparts, American house organs took up the latest developments in the print culture of their time: editors playfully interwove a variety show of cartoons, embellishments, photographs, and texts.

One editor, Corporal Sydney Flower, conveyed the spirit of the publications. "*Mess-Kit*," he wrote, is "written by the enlisted man for the enlisted man…. *The Mess-Kit* is…his *voice*." Corporal Flower continued: "This magazine, belongs first to the Khaki [Army] and the Serge [Navy]; afterwards to humanity generally, and particularly to patriotic humanity. Its field is very wide; its contents are varied; its uses many. In this number…you will find Cup, Plate, Knife, Fork, Spoon, and a good meal, for the small sum of One Dime, served with some little attention to the picturesque. You have only to draw up your chair. You are welcome."

Readers of such magazines likely did feel welcome. Columns such as "Ward Gossip," "Funny-isms," "Nurses Department," and "Recreation News" informed and entertained readers and encouraged them to participate in the social life and programs of the hospital camp. Profiles of charitable organizations such as the Jewish Welfare Board, Knights of Columbus, Salvation Army, and YMCA described how recreational activities were as integral to hospital life as medicine and surgery. Advertisements from local businesses showed the support that army hospitals received from surrounding communities and offer us glimpses of the commercial and civic life of the towns where soldier-patients spent time while on leave from their institutional confines. The purchase of magazines by readers also helped to support hospital activities: in many instances a portion of publication revenues funded recreation programs for soldier-patients and staff.

There is perhaps no better assessment of the value of military hospital magazines than that offered by Martha Alberta Montgomery, an aide who taught wounded soldiers writing, drawing, and painting as occupational therapy. As "strict products of soldier talent," Montgomery observed, hospital magazines "furnished meaningful occupation" and "afforded diversion from affliction…instilled into all a pride in their organization." They also "aroused local interest in…uplift work," "drew the public into sympathy with Army life and plans…for soldier care, comfort, and amusement," and "served as a medium for reaching men for re-enlistment in the various branches of the service."

—JEFFREY S. REZNICK

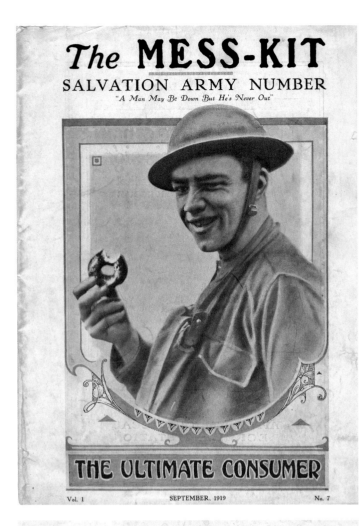

The MESS-KIT
SALVATION ARMY NUMBER
"A Man May Be Down But He's Never Out"

THE ULTIMATE CONSUMER

Vol. 1   SEPTEMBER, 1919   No. 7

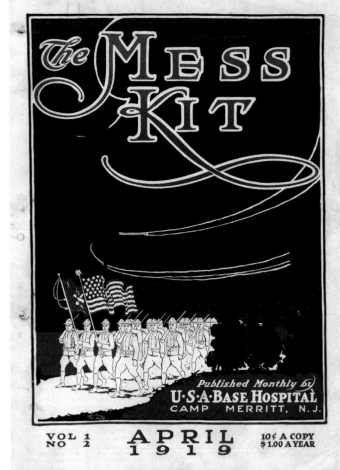

The MESS KIT

Published Monthly by
U·S·A·BASE HOSPITAL
CAMP MERRITT, N.J.

VOL 1   **APRIL**   10¢ A COPY
NO 2   **1919** $1.00 A YEAR

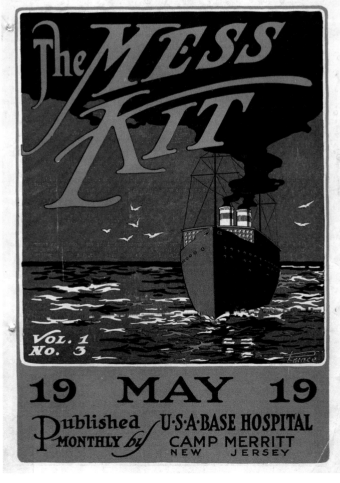

The MESS KIT

19 MAY 19

Published   U·S·A·BASE HOSPITAL
MONTHLY by   CAMP MERRITT
NEW JERSEY

Vol. 1
No. 3

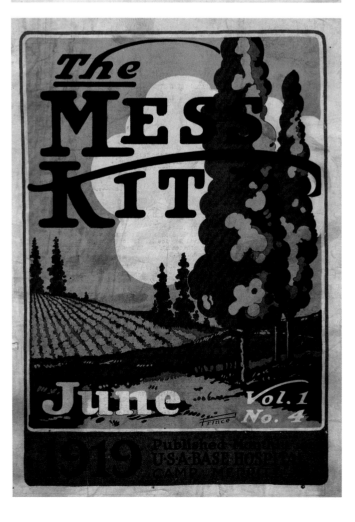

The MESS KIT

June

Vol. 1
No. 4

1919

Published Monthly
U·S·A·BASE HOSPITAL
CAMP MERRITT

Russo-Japanese War Photo Album (ca. 1905)
Compiler unknown

Japan. Album of 50 original gelatin silver photographs; handwritten captions in Japanese; 8¼ x 5⅞ in. (21 x 15.2 cm)

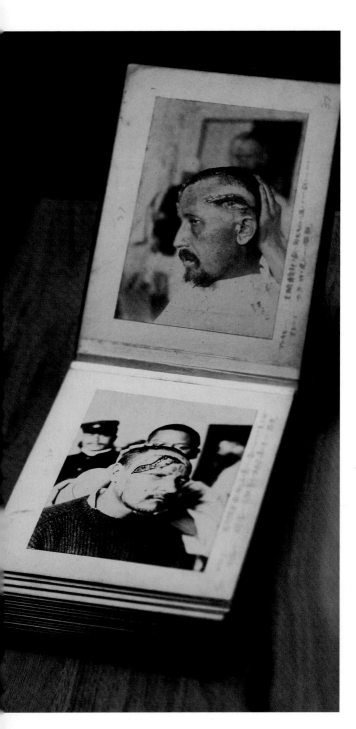

*D*uring the Russo-Japanese War (1904–05) Japanese forces lost 85,600 men, while the Russian army incurred from 40,000 to 70,000 deaths. At least 20,000 Chinese civilians died as well. The Japanese army suffered from supply shortages that limited the use of heavy artillery and forced General Maresuke Nogi to take the fortified positions outside of Port Arthur through three bloody assaults. The army sustained more than 56,000 casualties in the battle of Port Arthur. (Nogi atoned by ritually disemboweling himself after the Meiji emperor died in 1912.)

This collection of photos from the war centers on Port Arthur (modern-day Lüshunkou), the Russian Hospital located there, and the care of Russian soldiers by Japanese medical personnel. Many of the pictures reveal the gruesome realities of fighting in Manchuria across the winter months of 1904 and 1905, including frostbitten limbs that required amputation (opposite). Western audiences, through the reports of foreign observers, received a glowing picture of how the Japanese army treated friend and foe alike. The American doctor Louis L. Seaman, touring hospital facilities in Japan and Manchuria during the war, marveled at how well trained, staffed, and supplied the medical corps were. According to Seaman, Japan had the most sophisticated military triage system and field hospitals in the world. Doctors and stretcher bearers took the wounded from the front to dressing stations, where they received superficial treatment before being conveyed to a field hospital. After surgery the wounded were carried to the nearest railroad station and sent on to the main hospital base in Dairen (modern-day Dalian). Once rested, the wounded traveled to hospitals in Japan.

Reports of men treated at field hospitals in Manchuria, however, tell a very different story. Lieutenant Tadayoshi Sakurai, who lost his right arm during the siege of Port Arthur, left a bleak account of life inside field hospitals. In his memoir *Nikudan* (*Human Bullets*), Sakurai wrote, "Large armies of flies attacked the wretched patients, worms would grow in the mouth or nose, and some of them could not drive the vermin away because their arms were useless…. Those in charge of the surgical work…had to crowd more than a thousand patients into a field hospital provided for two hundred [so] they were powerless to give any better care to the sufferers."

Seaman, no doubt, was shown only what his hosts wanted him to see: the best hospitals in Port Arthur and Liaoyang. In the same vein, these photographs were designed to depict the civilized approach of the Japanese army to the treatment of the war wounded and the advanced state of Japanese military medical services.

We don't know how this collection came to the National Library of Medicine. The photographs, furnished with captions that offer detailed analysis of battlefield wounds, are aimed at a Japanese-speaking medical audience. They do, however, fit the pattern of wartime reporting—newspapers, photojournalism, and woodblock prints—which was designed to bolster domestic morale and international support by portraying Japanese soldiers in acts of bravery or compassion and stoic Russian soldiers suffering defeat with dignity.

—Alexander Bay

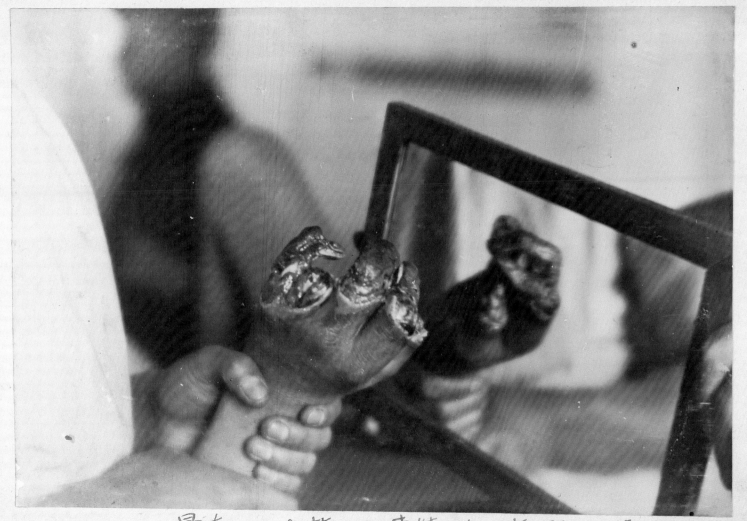

門脈平吉　最左ノ〻ハ小指ニシテ凍傷ノ為〻壊疽ヨリ萎縮ス　壊
指ハ銃創ニヨリ挫折セラル各指ノ背面ニアル白線ハ分界線

Hitler as Seen by His Doctors (1945–46)
Military Intelligence Service Center, United States Army, European Theater

Frankfurt-am-Main, Germany. Bound photocopy of typescript, 2 vols., with photographs and charts; 7 x 11½ in. (17.7 x 28.2 cm)

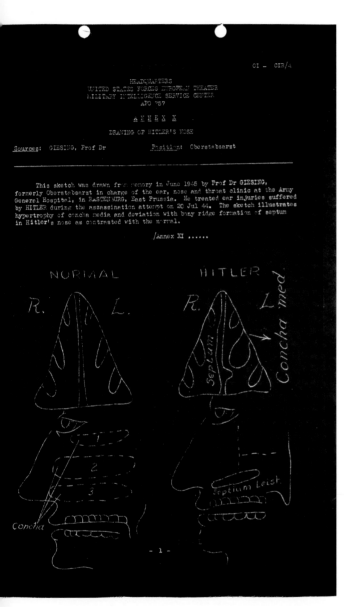

ABOVE AND OPPOSITE: Sketches and X-ray of Hitler's nasal passages and teeth. *Hitler as Seen by His Doctors*, annex X and unnumbered prints of X-ray photographs between annexes I and III

Compiled by American military intelligence in the months after the German surrender, this report contains all of Adolf Hitler's available medical records plus interrogations of several physicians who cared for Hitler. Whether the confidential document was shared with America's wartime allies is unclear, but by 1958 it had been declassified.

Everyone connected with the report had an agenda: the doctors who defended their medical care of Hitler while downplaying their Nazi allegiances, and the intelligence officers, who wanted to debunk myths about Hitler, guard against future Hitler impostors, and provide "research material for the historian, the doctor and the scientists interested in Hitler." The authors almost certainly had another, unstated, goal: to see if there was a medical explanation for the brutal behavior of the world's most infamous mass murderer.

The report is revealing. Hitler was a victim of "VIP Syndrome": his medical care was compromised because of his fame. His primary physician from 1937 to 1945 was Theodor Morell (1886–1948), a "shrewd, money-crazed quack," who dosed his hypochondriacal patient with twenty-eight different "medications"—including vitamins, stimulants, hormones, and pills containing dangerous amounts of atropine and strychnine. (Morell had a proprietary interest in his nostrums, which Hitler ordered German hospitals to buy.) Hitler was Morell's guinea pig; Morell was Hitler's enabler. Like other famous patients, the Führer worsened his problems by self-medicating. Hitler's other doctors, more competent and conventional, resented Morell's primacy. Three were fired after openly criticizing their unorthodox colleague.

In a sense, the report is all that remains of the Führer's corporeal remains. Hitler and Eva Braun killed themselves in April 1945 as Soviet troops swept into Berlin. Their bodies were burned (but it is rumored that his skull was taken to the Soviet Union). *Hitler as Seen by His Doctors* contains evaluations of Hitler's body systems, tests such as electrocardiograms and blood counts, diagrams of his teeth and nose, as well as five X-rays of his head. The photographic and motion picture documentation of Hitler is vast, but here is a record of his insides.

Which leads one to wonder: If medical records might be considered "windows to the soul," what can we learn about Hitler from his charts? Could some underlying condition explain his mad quest for world domination and the evil he perpetrated? Could some explanation be found in his doctors' examination of his body and psyche?

Although one summary statement noted that Hitler's facial expressions "had an intense quality that subdued and captivated most individuals," this was more opinion than scientific fact. When it came to exceptional medical findings, there were disappointingly few. Morell found Hitler to be emotionally labile but without hallucinations, illusions, or paranoia. Karl Brandt termed Hitler a "psychopathic personality," and Hans Karl von Hasselbach termed his persistent expectations of victory a delusion, but both, along with Erwin Giesing, agreed there were no phobias or obsessions. At least in the areas they tested, Hitler's judgment was good.

The U.S. Army interrogators had learned what they could from the doctors: Hitler remained an enigma.

—Barron H. Lerner

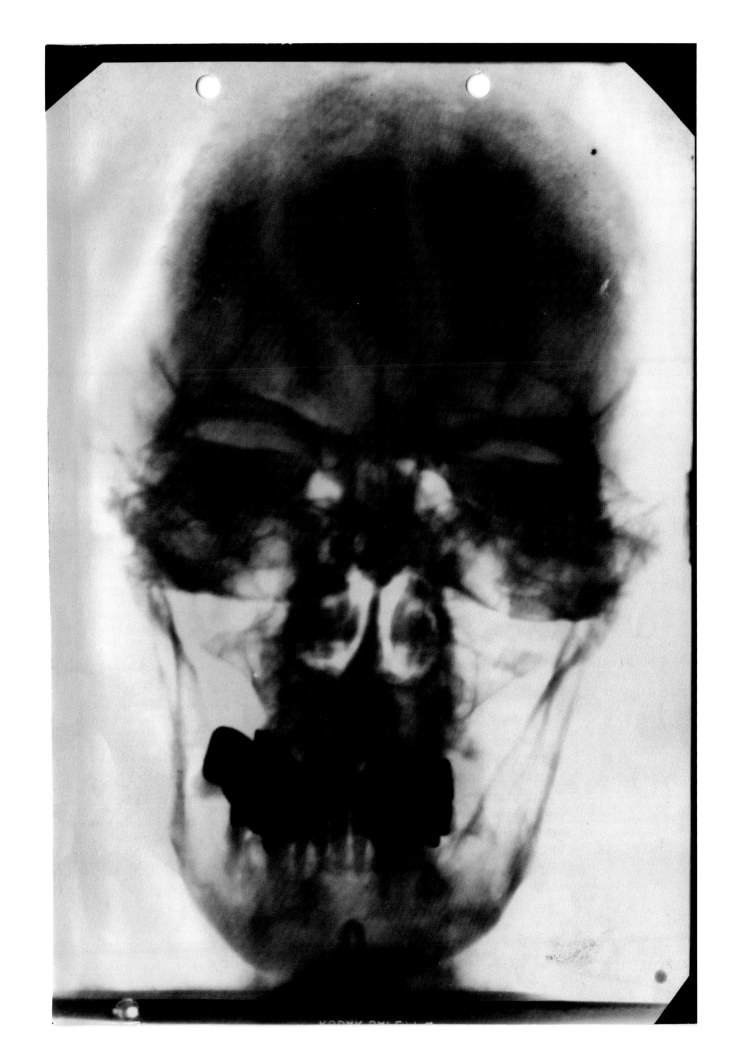

Medical Report of the Atomic Bombing in Hiroshima (1945)
Imperial Army Medical College and First Tokyo Military Hospital

Tokyo. Bound mimeographs with insert charts, diagrams, and photographs; 10¼ x 14½ in. (26 x 37 cm)

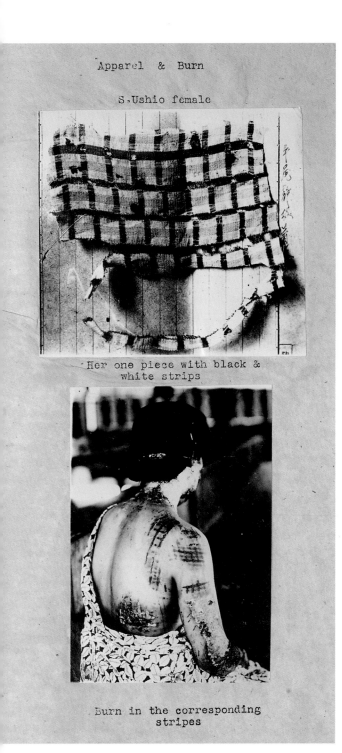

Apparel & Burn

S. Ushio female

Her one piece with black & white strips

Burn in the corresponding stripes

The atomic bomb exploded over Hiroshima on August 6, 1945. Some seventy thousand people died that day—upwards of a quarter of the city's population. Another seventy thousand were injured. Many would die from wounds, burns, and radiation poisoning over the next few weeks. The city was devastated, its doctors and nurses scattered or killed, its hospitals and clinics destroyed. Two days later, the Imperial Army Medical College and the First Tokyo Military Hospital sent doctors into the chaos of destruction. Over the next months these men were the mainstays of care—and data gathering and analysis.

Though the American medical investigation of the atomic bombing is well known, Japanese doctors provided the earliest and most detailed studies. Americans did not enter Hiroshima in any numbers until mid-October, forestalled by a hurricane and the formal commencement of Occupation. At that point, three separate American investigations (from the Army Medical Corps, Manhattan Project, and the navy) sprang up. Coordination was needed and, on October 12, the supreme commander for the Allied Powers, General Douglas MacArthur, set up the four-party "Joint Commission for the Investigation of the Effects of the Atomic Bomb on Japan" (the Japanese were the fourth party). The commission's work was completed by mid-1946 and the supporting materials shipped stateside. To continue the research, President Truman established the Atomic Bomb Casualty Commission. It remained in existence until 1975.

This report—entirely a Japanese production—preceded almost all of that work. Issued in November 1945, when the Joint Commission had only just begun, the mimeographed typescript of several hundred pages has a hand-lettered title page and glued-in tables. Its roughness evokes the dire circumstances of its production. Amid the catastrophe the Japanese army doctors labored to describe what they had seen and done, diagrammatically, quantitatively, professionally, and objectively. In charts, tables, and case histories, they laid out the symptoms of radiation sickness and patterns and circumstances of death. They prepared a hand-colored map of Hiroshima, distinguishing completely destroyed areas from those partially destroyed; drew the smoke cloud that the A-bomb left over the city; made diagrams of shock-wave patterns; described the treatments they administered; and inserted photographs of wrecked buildings and people, most famously a photo showing the pattern of a print dress rendered in flesh. And they provided case histories, such as the example of K. Ishida, a twenty-five-year-old officer.

> On the very day of bombing appeared vomiting.... Felt sore throat.... Was admitted to the...hospital. The tongue was coated brownly & had tendency of bleeding. Both tonsils were swelled. Scalp-hair were sparsely. Small petechias [red spots] were generalized on the whole body surface. On 29/VIII appeared bloody stool & epistaxis [nose bleeding], which was difficult to stop. On 1/IX appeared disturbance on consciousness.... Died on 2/IX.

Tellingly the Japanese medical officers wrote their report in English. They were already cooperating with the American military but perhaps had a larger goal: to bear witness to the scope of death and devastation in a form that could be circulated to the wider world.

—PAUL THEERMAN

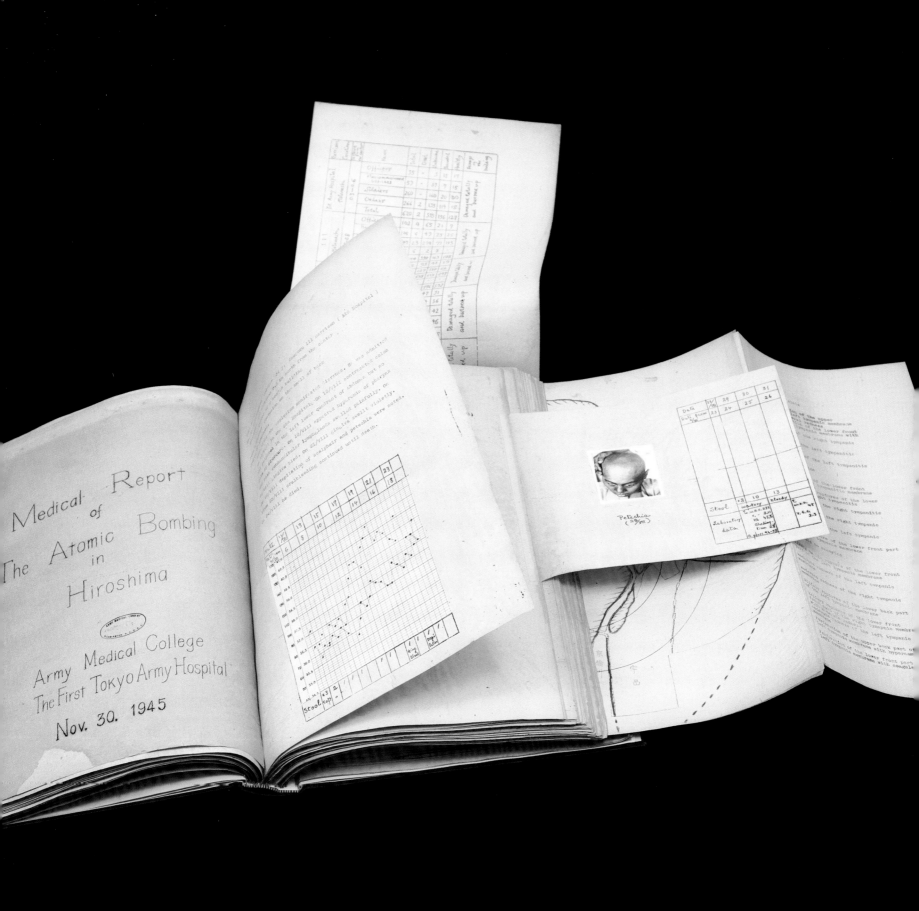

Anti–Germ Warfare Campaign Posters (ca. 1952)
Second People's Cultural Institute

Fuping County, Shaanxi Province, China. Hand-inked and painted posters on paper; 14¼ x 15 in. (36.2 x 38.3 cm)

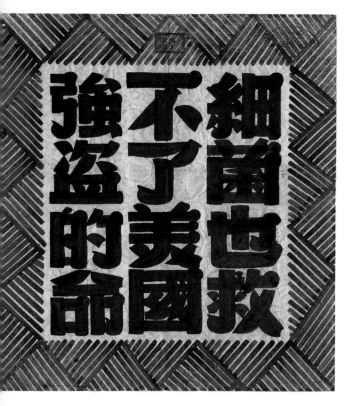

ABOVE AND OPPOSITE: Hand-drawn Korean War propaganda posters, from two incomplete sequences in the collection of Chinese medical and health materials acquired by the National Library of Medicine.

In spring 1952, in the depths of the Korean War, Chinese newspapers reported that American forces were conducting germ warfare against Chinese and North Korean forces and civilians. According to reports, vigilant citizens had spotted large quantities of fleas, flies, mosquitoes, and rats in unexpected places in Manchuria and the coastal city of Qingdao. Premier Zhou Enlai called upon the nations of the world to condemn "U.S. imperialists' war crime of germ warfare." Zhou's charges tied the health of the Chinese people to the war effort in Korea. A Patriotic Health Movement was launched throughout China: the Communist Party mobilized the masses to eliminate pests to prevent disease and contribute to the war effort. Trained and untrained artists threw themselves into the creation of health posters to support the anti–germ warfare campaign.

The posters shown here, selected from two series, are the handiwork of unidentified artists from the Chinese interior, far from the theater of war. A title poster (left), in bold red ink and framed with a deep blue pattern, proclaims "Even Germs Cannot Save the Fate of the American Bandits." Another poster (opposite, top left), "Flies Spread Diseases," shows flies dropping American cholera bombs. Under them, at the bottom of the image, are the roofs of houses. The caption reads: "Flies like to live in cesspools and like to sing in front of people too; they carry countless germs and throw germ bombs everywhere."

From the same series, another poster (opposite, top right) presents a domestic scene. A mother boils infected clothes and burns infected material. Her son kills a fly with a flyswatter. Her husband cleans the top part of the house. The caption reads: "Germs rely on pests as a way to spread diseases. To eradicate pests is to defeat the American imperialists."

A poster from another series (opposite, lower left) shows a fleeing, wounded American who spits out rats and carries them by the tail. A rat clinging to his back wears a hat with a swastika, another wears a Japanese army hat, signifying that the American enemy is morally equivalent to the now-defeated Nazis and Japanese imperialists. Disease-bearing insects swarm beneath and behind the "rat-man." The caption reads: "The American bandits, paying no attention to the just sanctions of humanity, openly dropped loads of germs on Korea, our country's northeast, and Qingdao city."

The next poster in the sequence (opposite, lower right) shows how to destroy the enemy. A soldier, doctor, and worker attack the rat-man with the weapons of their trade—gun, fumigation sprayer, and shovel. The caption reads: "Under the attack of the Chinese and Koreans, as well as peace-loving people all over the world, the heinous crimes of the Americans cannot save them from their inevitable defeat."

The poster images are predominantly blue and black, colors that in Chinese art usually signify fearful things. The limited palette may also be evidence of a shortage of colored paint. The posters must have been frequently displayed: the paper is worn, wrinkled, and stained, and there are many tiny thumbtack holes in the four corners.

—LIPING BU

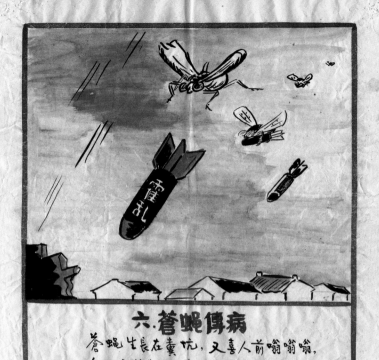

六.蒼蠅傳病

蒼蠅生長在糞坑，又喜人前嗡嗡嗡，
身帶病菌數不清，病菌炸彈到處扔。

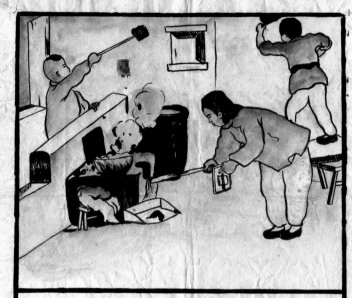

二.人人動手打老鼠，跳蚤虱子臭虫要消滅，
蒼蠅蚊子趕快撲殺淨，預防霍亂鼠疫傳染病，細
菌就靠害虫當媒介，消滅害虫就是打美帝。

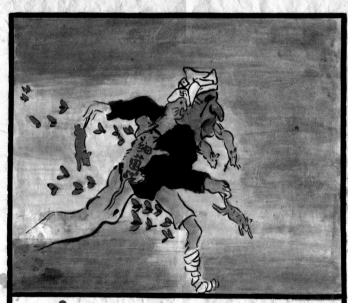

6.美國強盜竟然不顧人類正義的制
裁，公然在朝鮮和我國的東北和青島市大量撒佈細菌。

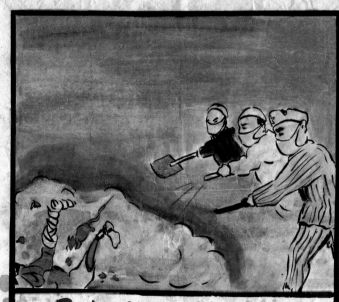

7.它的這種滔天罪行，在我中朝人民
及世界愛好和平人民的打擊下，終究也是
挽救不了它的命運的。

Selected Dictation of Curious Records (1818)
Ken Matsuzawa

Bunsen Kiroku. Japan. Bound manuscript with illustrations, 128 pp.; 6⅜ x 9⅛ in. (16.3 x 23.2 cm)

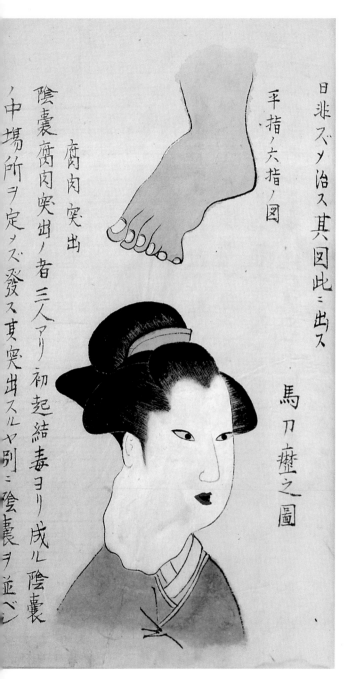

ABOVE AND OPPOSITE: Hand-drawn illustrations of tumors to be excised with general anesthesia. *Bunsen Kiroku*, pp. 46 and 67

This manuscript contains early records of the first surgeries ever done with general anesthesia. The Japanese surgeon Seishu Hanaoka (1760–1835) in 1804 used an anesthetic while performing a successful operation to excise a tumor of the breast. The records in this book date from around 1808. At the time Japan was closed to the outside world, except for limited contact with the Netherlands and China. Hanaoka, born into a family of doctors, studied Dutch surgery and Chinese medicine and was fascinated by the possibility of combining the two. He succeeded by re-creating the lost Chinese anesthetic *Mafeisan* for use in Western-style surgery. The development of *Mafeisan* was not easy. The main ingredients, datura and wolfsbane, can be lethal. The members of Hanaoka's family who volunteered as test subjects suffered terribly: his mother died; his wife lost her eyesight. The eventual success of the method, however, brought him wide recognition and many patients. He was awarded the rank of sword-wielding samurai. Students sought Hanaoka from all over the country, and he gladly took them into his school, *Shun-Rin-Ken* ("House of Spring Woods"), which trained more than a thousand doctors. Despite Hanaoka's large following, he left no records of his procedures, and information is scarce on his methods, including the exact recipe for *Mafeisan*. He used the traditional pedagogical method of hands-on apprenticeship to teach the secrets of the trade to his students, but he was so unusually secretive that he required his apprentices to submit a nondisclosure agreement signed in blood. Fortunately, Gencho Honma (1804–72) and other students wrote medical texts that provide information on the Hanaoka method. Accused of revealing his master's secrets, Honma was expelled from the school.

Other information comes from the notes of the apprentices. The National Library of Medicine's copy of notes by Hanaoka's disciple Ken Matsuzawa is a later recollection rather than a real-time record but appears to be stunningly accurate. The opening text reads: "Observing my Master Hanaoka's operations over the years, while it is clearly beyond the feat of this average person, I will record it in drawings for future generations." Good thing he did.

The manuscript is not a structured textbook. There are lists of unrelated medicines and accounts of successful surgical operations to excise tumors, but also of cases where Hanaoka refuses to treat a patient or where a patient is afraid to have her breast cut open and refuses treatment. Many of the cases deal with sexually transmitted diseases, the dark side of the often glamorized brothel culture of the period.

Hanaoka's pioneering work with general anesthesia never left Japan and was unknown in the West (where anesthesia was independently invented forty-two years later). He was both a traditionalist and an innovator. You can see Western scalpels in the drawings but his theory of medicine was mainly Chinese—he believed that dark/negative *chi* caused tumors—and he employed traditional folk remedies to increase breast milk and treat snakebite. The text recommends the application of earthworm guts for toothaches. Any volunteers?

—Hiroo Yamagata

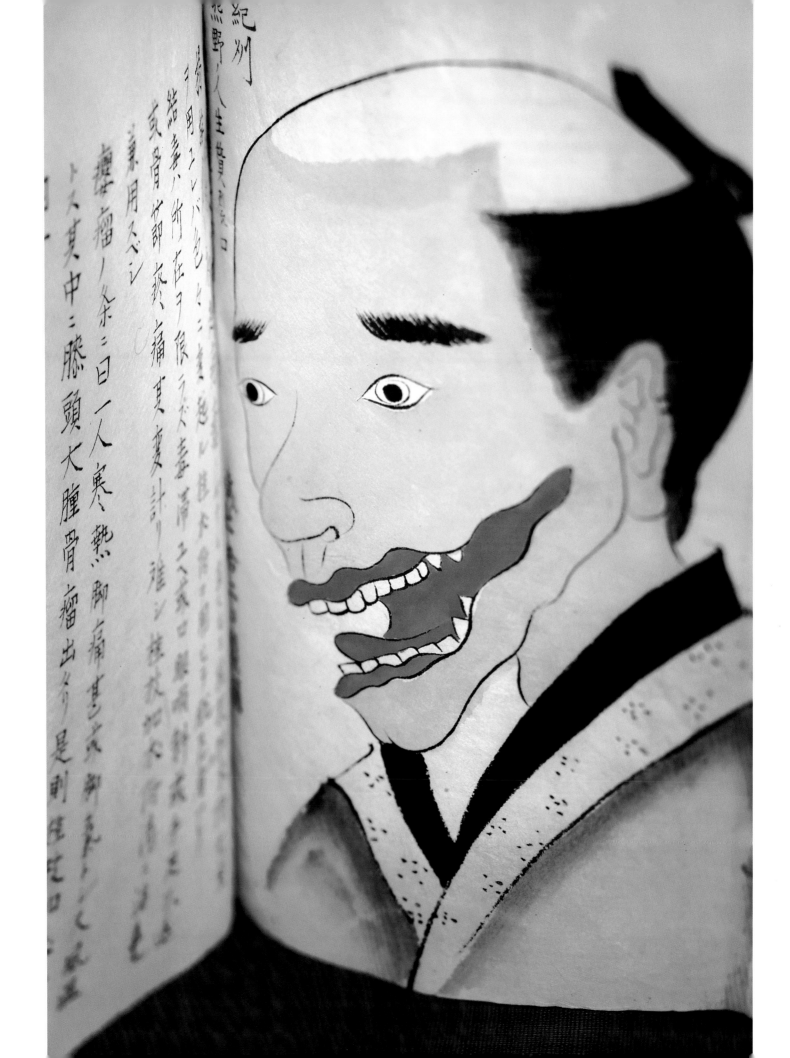

Catalogue of Educational Material (1941–44?)
American Society for the Control of Cancer

New York. Album with pasted-in pamphlets, flyers, and handbills, unpaginated; bound volume: 8⅜ x 10¾ in. (21.3 x 27.3 cm)
Detectives Wanted!: 5½ x 7¼ in. (14 x 18.4 cm)

.61-04 - "DETECTIVES WANTED" & SHIPPING

PRICE: $10.00 per 1,000
        $ 1.75 per 1,000 for imprint
                on last page.

ABOVE: This pamphlet was designed to recruit young fans of detective and gangster stories to the fictional Family Bureau of Investigation (FBI) to track down "Cancer the Gangster." *Detectives Wanted!* (1940; Westchester Cancer Committee, Bronxville, New York, 1942)

OPPOSITE: "Only X-ray, radium, surgery, ever cured cancer," illustration by Dorothy Darling Fellnagel (United States Public Health Service, 1941). Thomas Parran (1892–1968), a visionary surgeon general and modernizer, hoped to remake the U.S. Public Health Service into something like a European ministry of health. Under his direction the agency commissioned and produced posters, often featuring modernist designs, for many health campaigns.

found this odd little book by chance while browsing the dimly lit stacks of the National Library of Medicine. The catalogue record gave few hints as to its riches, but beneath its grubby, faded blue front cover is a treasure trove of material from the 1930s and 1940s—badges, buttons, posters, labels, string tags, transparencies, motion pictures, filmstrips, statistical charts, exhibition materials, window stickers, car cards, counter cards, booklets of sticky labels, and a wide selection of pamphlets.

The American Society for the Control of Cancer (ASCC) first released this catalogue sometime in the early 1940s, possibly December 1941, the date printed on the index page. The NLM's copy has a library binding dated July 23, 1946, but originally it came in a loose-leaf binder from which pages could be removed and others substituted or added. Most pages are individually dated to distinguish originals from replacements, and the NLM's copy includes pages labeled from December 1941 to December 1943. This catalogue offers for sale material on cancer prevention and treatment put out or distributed by the ASCC shortly before it became the American Cancer Society in 1944, when a new leadership of business people and advertisers transformed its educational programs.

At first glance the "X-ray-radium-surgery" image reproduced here would not seem to be a *hidden* treasure. It was designed by Dorothy Darling Fellnagel (1913–2006), a brilliant though not very well known graphic artist, who did her best work for the United States Public Health Service (which often collaborated with the ASCC). Digital copies can be found online at NLM and National Archives websites. But look at the mimeographed typescript beneath the image. Unlike the original posters and digital reproductions, this image comes with details of pricing and purchasing, as does the *Detectives Wanted!* (1942) pamphlet that encouraged children to remind family members to watch for the warning signs of the disease. The catalogue was made for those who wanted health education materials for display or distribution.

Here is all the information a school administrator, county public health official, local ASCC organizer, or community activist might need: shipping costs, product dimensions, special offers, service charges, "close out" supplies, "out of stock" materials, and instructions on how to order and sometimes how to display or use. Samples of some of the smaller materials are glued or taped onto the pages. (Some, such as *Detectives Wanted!*, have come loose because the adhesive has dried.) Larger materials, like the Fellnagel poster, are printed directly onto the page in reduced size (and somewhat altered color). Other pages include photographs of large artifacts such as exhibit displays. Some materials have no images or artifacts, just a short printed description as an aid to ordering (e.g., the movies, filmstrips, and *The Doctor Speaks on Cancer*—ten talks supplied to physicians for public lectures). This catalogue is a window into the material, visual, and literary culture of health mobilization in the early 1940s. It is also a glimpse of cancer from the order clerk's perspective.

—DAVID CANTOR

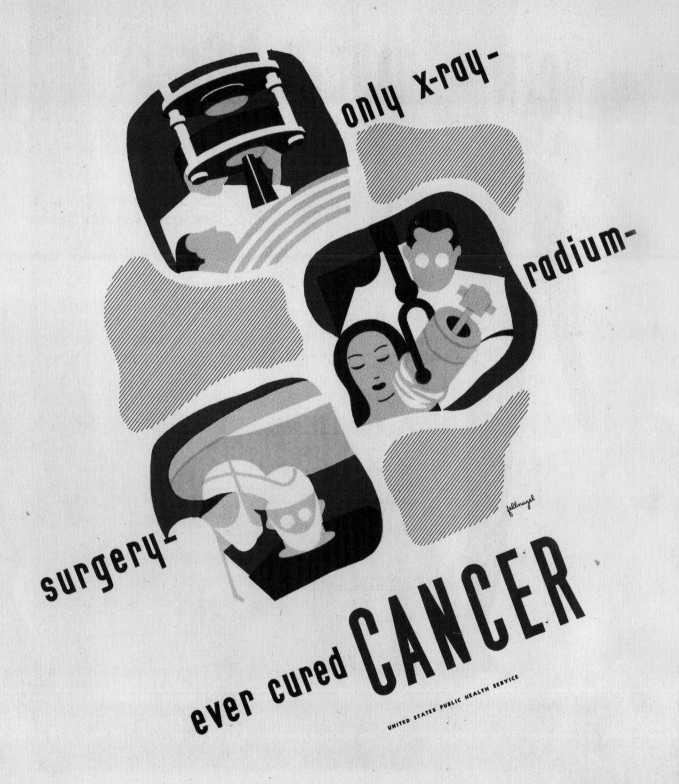

only x-ray—

radium—

surgery—

ever cured **CANCER**

UNITED STATES PUBLIC HEALTH SERVICE

PRICE: $0.05 each, $3.75 per 100
        Purchase orders should be placed with
        Superintendent of Documents,
        Government Printing Office,
        Washington, D. C.

A Materia Medica Animalia (1853)
Peter P. Good

Cambridge, Massachusetts. Printed book with chromolithographs, 272 pp. + plates; 5½ x 9⅛ in. (14 x 23.1 cm)

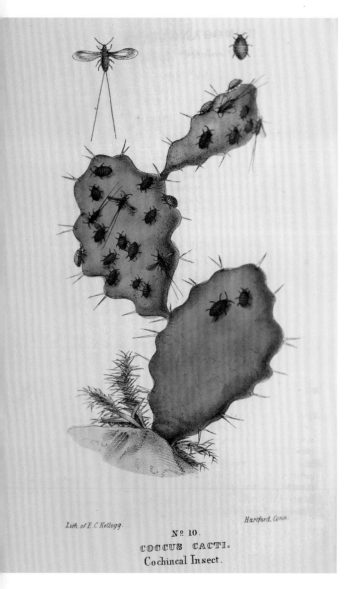

Lith. of E.C. Kellogg.

Hartford. Conn.

Nº 10.

COCCUS CACTI.
Cochineal Insect.

ABOVE: Cochineal insects swarm on a cactus. *Materia Medica Animalia*, pl. 10

OPPOSITE: A cuttlefish, valued for its "bone," which could be ground up to make a tooth powder, rests on a beach. *Materia Medica Animalia*, pl. 18

This is a rare book in several senses. Not only are surviving copies scarce but there is nothing much like it. Although a search of any serious library will reveal dozens—even hundreds—of books with "materia medica" in the title, they will likely focus on substances derived from plants. Peter Peyto Good (1789?–1875) did not set himself to swim completely against this tide: before he turned his attention to the animal kingdom, he had edited *The Family Flora and Materia Medica Botanica* (1845).

His animal material medica, "Containing the Scientific Analysis, Natural History and Chemical and Medical Properties and Uses of the Substances That Are the Products of Beasts, Birds, Fishes or Insects," is a kind of hybrid. It combines elements from traditional natural history compendia, including the bestiaries of the medieval period, with elements that reflect the zoology of his time. The introduction offers a brief outline of formal scientific taxonomy and locates each of the twenty-four creatures to be discussed within this system, but that is not the order in which they appear (at least if buyers followed Good's instructions about how to bind the installments—since each animal appeared in a separate installment, idiosyncratic orderings were theoretically possible). Instead, the table of contents suggests a view of the world as composed of randomly related phenomena: thus the sheep is followed by the oyster and the stag is followed by the blood-sucking leech.

The entries all ostensibly follow the same general structure. Headed by the Latinate and vernacular names of the creature, they first specify the nature and uses of the medicinal substance it produces, then proceed through sections on scientific analysis, natural history, and chemical and medical properties and uses. Sometimes Good offers surprising information. For example, he lists rattlesnake venom as a treatment for alcoholism, mercury poisoning, erysipelas (an acute bacterial infection associated with skin rash), fainting fits, and hydrophobia (rabies).

Despite their shared design the entries vary greatly in length and in the kind of material they contain; up-to-date zoology rubs elbows with folk wisdom and anecdote. Nor did Good always apply the same standard of relevance. To return to the rattlesnake, most of the long discussion of its "medical properties and uses" details treatments for snakebite; relatively little concerns the palliative qualities of venom. When Good considers farmyard species, most of which find a place in his catalogue, he tends to include digressions about the history and merits of their constituent breeds. The entry on the cochineal insect, on the other hand, fulfills its initial promise completely and efficiently, explaining how the creatures are collected, ground into powder, and then used to cure neuralgia and to color tinctures and ointments.

Even the illustrations reflect the miscellaneous traditions from which Good drew. (By the 1840s lithographs could be inexpensively reproduced, and brightly colored illustrations were available in books for popular audiences.) Some of the images, like that of the cochineal insect, recall an older botanical convention of disaggregation and separation, but most, like that of the cuttlefish, enjoy the richly delineated settings that came to characterize nineteenth-century natural history publishing.

—HARRIET RITVO

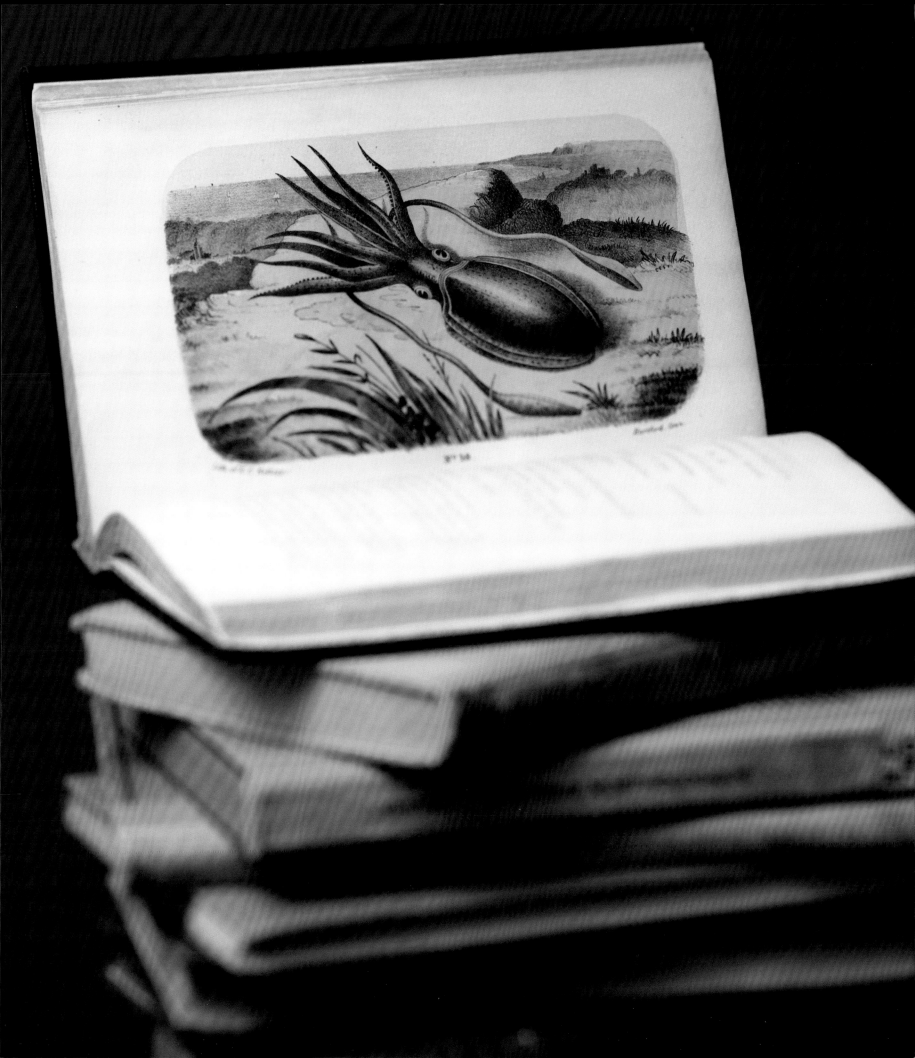

A Book of Receipts of All Sorts (1693–1730s)
Elizabeth Strachey

Somerset, England. Bound manuscript; 83 leaves and 14 loose scraps with recipes; 5½ x 7½ in. (14 x 19 cm)

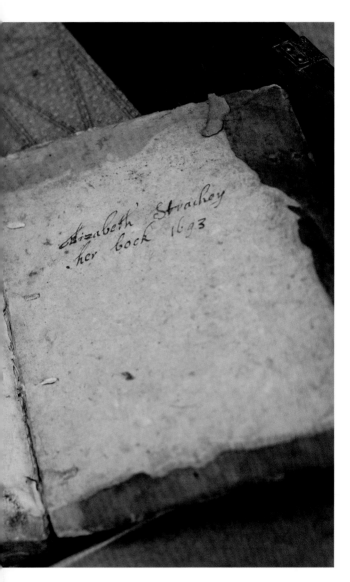

ABOVE: The inside cover of Elizabeth Strachey's recipe book bears her signature and a date.

OPPOSITE: A typical page of the diary features recipes to treat "A bluddy flux" and deafness.

In 1693 Elizabeth Strachey (ca. 1670–1722) wrote her name on the inside cover of a notebook. Over the next three decades she filled the book with recipes for remedies. While hundreds of such recipe books survive, many lack an attribution, making it difficult to understand the larger context in which they were made and used. But here we know that in 1692 Elizabeth Elletson married a gentleman, John Strachey (1671–1743), who inherited the family home at Sutton Court in Somerset. He was also a Fellow of the Royal Society who worked on geography and geology. She began keeping her recipe book the following year.

The book was a collaborative production; almost fifty people are credited with recipes. Some are family members, such as "Cousin Cross" or "Aunt Clarke." Others may have been friends with a shared interest in medicine. "Mrs. Newark," for example, is credited with a dozen recipes. The book was built up incrementally, over many years; recipes were added over time without any apparent larger structure. Mrs. Newark's recipes are in clumps of three or four, suggesting a visit or a letter prompted their inclusion. Strachey also drew upon the expertise of doctors. She mentions Drs. Hill, Butler, Chambers, and Griffiths, and she took advice from the philosopher John Locke, a family friend and a physician by training.

The book is not solely hers. Strachey died in 1722, but entries continue for about a decade afterward. Her successor (perhaps one of her daughters?) drew upon written sources, other manuscript recipe books, and printed works such as William Salmon's *Practical Physick* (1692). Elizabeth had drawn mainly upon her large network of friends and acquaintances.

The recipes deal with a wide array of conditions, including gout, fevers, webs in the eye, and scurvy—typical of the period. But you would never know from this volume that Strachey gave birth to nine sons and nine daughters: there are few recipes for reproductive problems and disorders. The recipes are not complex, relying upon local herbs and on measures like "as much as will lie on a penny." There's a powder to kill rats and mice, cunningly compounded of oatmeal, bacon fat, and lime. But Strachey was a sophisticated consumer and producer of medical knowledge. She recorded Richard Mead's remedy for the bite of a mad dog. She mastered the art of distilling. Many of the recipes reveal a careful accounting of efficacy: they are "approved," tested by trial and error, in much the same way her husband and his Royal Society colleagues assessed the results of their trial-and-error experiments.

Other recipes hint at a tenuous boundary between magic and natural knowledge. Strachey recommends a lodestone (a magnet) to draw away pain. On a corner of the page the word "abracadabra" is written as an acrostic. This age-old charm could have been written on a piece of paper that was worn next to the skin or chewed and swallowed. We cannot tell if it was merely a curiosity or a bit of insurance against the tide of ill health that any mother of eighteen confronted day in and day out.

—MARY E. FISSELL

for A bluddy fluxe

take franconsence. and put it in A chafin
of coals: put it in A close stool & sit o
it bare

for deafnes

take the Juice of ye Buds. Leaues, Inner
or yong branches of Elder: Luke warm
it into the yeares: It will breake the
Impostume within 4 or 5 days: And cure
the deafness

A nother

take the Juice of betony: And Juice o
Unnions: of each 6 ounces: A hanful of
Rosemary Leaues stamped: 3
ounces of bitter Almons: one white eele gro
choped: mix them altogether. And distill
them: then drop 2 or 3 drops in ye yea
2 or three nights together

A nother

take A stick of green Elme: or Ash
on ye fire: receive the water
ends of it: And th

Medical Trade Card Collection (ca. 1820–1940s)
Various manufacturers and retailers

France, Great Britain, Mexico, United States, and other countries. Donor: William Helfand

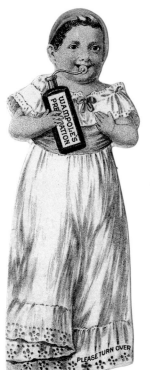 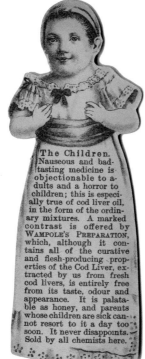

The Children.
Nauseous and bad-tasting medicine is objectionable to adults and a horror to children; this is especially true of cod liver oil, in the form of the ordinary mixtures. A marked contrast is offered by WAMPOLE'S PREPARATION, which, although it contains all of the curative and flesh-producing properties of the Cod Liver, extracted by us from fresh cod livers, is entirely free from its taste, odour and appearance. It is palatable as honey, and parents whose children are sick cannot resort to it a day too soon. It never disappoints. Sold by all chemists here.

PLEASE TURN OVER

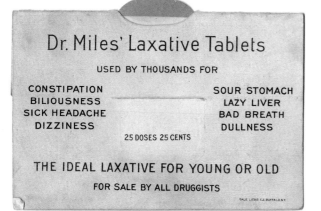

Dr. Miles' Laxative Tablets

USED BY THOUSANDS FOR

CONSTIPATION	SOUR STOMACH
BILIOUSNESS	LAZY LIVER
SICK HEADACHE	BAD BREATH
DIZZINESS	DULLNESS

25 DOSES 25 CENTS

THE IDEAL LAXATIVE FOR YOUNG OR OLD

FOR SALE BY ALL DRUGGISTS

SALE LITHO. CO. BUFFALO. N.Y.

ABOVE, TOP: Wampole's Preparation die-cut advertising card (Philadelphia, ca. 1895). The text on the reverse side, directed to parents, praises Wampole's chemists for their ability to disguise the taste, odor, and appearance of the product's basic ingredient, cod liver oil.

ABOVE AND OPPOSITE: Dr. Miles' Laxative Tablets movable, die-cut advertising novelty card (Elkhart, Indiana, ca. 1910). Above, reverse side of the card; opposite, the front of the card, lowered and raised

*T*he earliest medical cards, dating to the seventeenth century, were engraved advertising announcements used by physicians, apothecaries, pharmacists, and dentists, often featuring images relevant to their trade: mortar and pestle, distillation apparatus, drug jars, bandages, artificial teeth, or a portrait.

In the nineteenth century, as the speed and quality of printing techniques improved—especially lithography, which enabled printers to print bright colors cheaply in large quantities—medical cards became ubiquitous. Retailers and marketers of patent medicines increasingly used cards to advertise their products and services. The cards came in a variety of shapes and sizes, with attention-getting, colorful images on one side and hard sells on the reverse. Certain manufacturers—Ayer's, Hoods, Lydia Pinkham, Liebig, Wampole's Preparation, and the marketers of Holloway's Pills and Mrs. Winslow's Soothing Syrup—used cards as a primary vehicle of promotion to create brand names. There were also "stock" cards, for all types of product, that enabled the smallest pharmacists and producers to advertise, by having a printer add their name in a space left blank for that purpose. Printers such as Currier & Ives and Louis Prang made such cards available in small quantities. Postcards, embossed cards, die-cut cards, and, later, matchbook covers became advertising vehicles, incorporating public health warnings, information, and educational literature too. Although the pictures were sometimes the work of known artists, most were made by anonymous employees of commercial printers.

Like baseball cards, many medical cards showed heroes, men and women who had made great contributions to the healing arts and sciences. Cards for collectors came in the form of cigarette cards, biographical cards, and sets of playing cards that presented portraits of well-known physicians and scientists, alongside brief biographies of their productive lives. Vesalius, Galen, Hippocrates, Edward Jenner, Louis Pasteur, Claude Bernard (the French physiologist who was an exponent of laboratory experimentation), William Harvey, Florence Nightingale, and Paul Ehrlich are frequent figures in these series, as well as later figures like Ernst Chain (the biochemist who helped to develop penicillin) and Jonas Salk. Cards also featured mythical figures such as Asclepius and Hygeia and religious figures who were said to have performed healing miracles. Patent medicine manufacturers sometimes tried to make it seem as though the scientists and physicians portrayed on their cards had supplied testimonials. But sometimes the testimonials were authentic, and some cards bore testimonials from nonmedical figures, a king or celebrity, or made reference to some nonmedical historical event or fact. Cards could also be designed to be appealing playthings for children.

They remained popular until daily newspapers and monthly magazines proved more effective as advertising media. In their heyday, medical cards were frequently collected and pasted into albums and scrapbooks, an activity providing relaxation and entertainment prior to the advent of radio and television. The cards were intended to be ephemeral, but thankfully many have survived and serve as relics of past medical practices and remedies and of the innovative marketing practices of patent medicine manufacturers and distributors.

—WILLIAM H. HELFAND

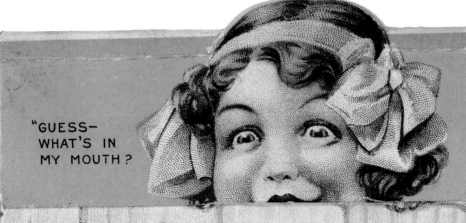

CHILDREN COAX FOR

Dr. Miles'
Laxative Tablets

BECAUSE THEY TASTE LIKE CANDY

PAT. NOV. 22, 1910.

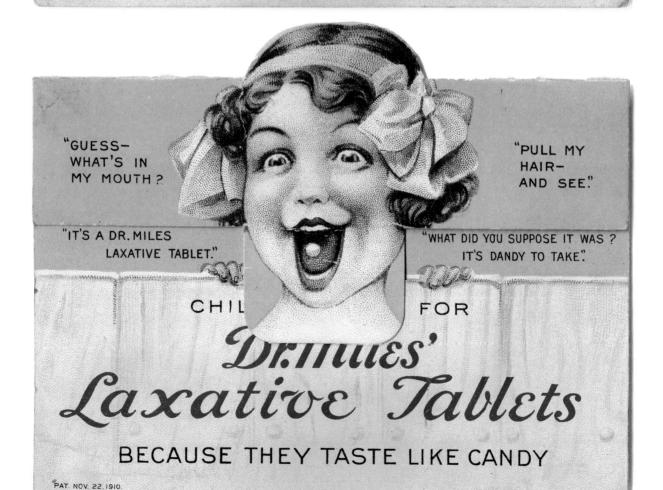

Scope Magazine (1941–57)
Will Burtin and Lester Beall (designers), for Upjohn Co.

Kalamazoo, Michigan. Printed magazines, color, 5 vols.; 8½ x 11 in. (21.5 x 27.8 cm)

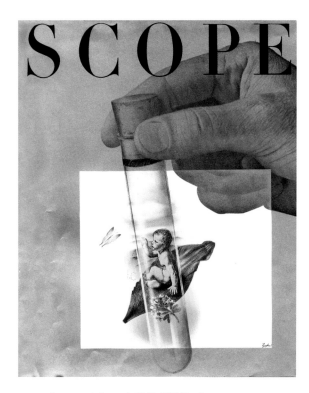

ABOVE: *Scope*, vol. 1, no. 1, 1941: Will Burtin

OPPOSITE (top row, left to right): *Scope*, vol. 1, no. 8, 1944 (Beall); vol. 1, no. 2, 1942 (Beall); vol. 1, no. 7, 1944 (Beall); vol. 1, no. 7, 1944 (Beall); (center row, left to right) *Scope*, vol. 2, no. 2, 1942 (unknown); vol. 1, no. 2, 1942 (Beall); vol. 1, no. 7, 1944 (Beall); vol. 1, no. 6, 1944 (Beall); (bottom row, left to right) *Scope*, vol. 1, no. 7, 1944 (Beall); vol. 1, no. 6, 1944 (Beall); vol. 1, no. 5, 1943 (unknown); vol. 1, no. 10, 1945 (Beall)

PAGE 212, CLOCKWISE FROM TOP LEFT: *Scope*, vol. 4, no. 3, 1954 (Burtin); vol. 1, no. 3, 1943 (Burtin); vol. 1, no. 7, 1944 (Beall); vol. 1, no. 3, 1942 (Unknown)

PAGE 213, CLOCKWISE FROM TOP LEFT: *Scope*, vol. 1, no. 5, 1943 (unknown); vol. 1, no. 6, 1944 (unknown); vol. 1, no. 6, 1944 (unknown); vol. 1, no. 5, 1943 (unknown)

*T*argeted at doctors, pharmacists, and other health professionals, *Scope* was a monthly magazine published by Upjohn Pharmaceuticals between 1941 and 1957. Its mission was to explain the latest medical research, to report on advances in diagnoses and treatment, and to advertise Upjohn's prescription drugs.

Uniquely among specialized magazines of its time and type, *Scope* richly featured technical content, presented in innovative ways. Two pioneering American graphic designers were hired during different periods to create colorful covers, pages, and spreads with visual impact. *Scope*'s first issue was designed by Will Burtin (1908–82) in 1941. On a field of metallic silver, it featured a dramatic image of a baby behind a test tube. Symbolizing the progressive nature of *Scope*, the cover of this first issue imagined a "test tube baby," some thirty-seven years before *in vitro* fertilization was invented.

The German-born Burtin, who came to the United States in 1938 after fleeing the Nazis, was a visionary, one of the first graphic designers to understand the importance of transforming highly scientific verbal content into coherent and clear visual form, using typography, diagrams, symbols, color, and photography that matched the special requirements of the subject matter. According to Burtin: "The extra-sensatory reality of science provides man with new dimensions. It allows him to see the workings of nature, makes transparent the solid and gives substance to the invisible…. The designer stands between these concepts, at the center, because of his unique role as communicator, link, interpreter and inspirer…. Through unceasing comparison and interrelation of factors, he gains an understanding and exciting insight into their nature and value, enabling him to depict even that which had been invisible. Thus he creates."

After that first issue Lester Beall (1903–69), Burtin's colleague, designed *Scope* for seven years in the 1940s, until Burtin returned as art director in 1948. The match between Beall's creative style and the progressive management at Upjohn led to magazine layouts that were unparalleled in the history of publication design. Beall's standing with the company was so high that he was given permission to design a cover, spread, or advertisement and send the original graphics directly to the printer without having to get a final approval from Upjohn. This uniquely open process enabled Beall to experiment visually and stimulated his creativity. Beall looked back on his years of designing *Scope* as "very exciting from so many different angles: the design and layout, the typography and the opportunity of interpreting in terms of photographs, drawings or paintings." His designs demonstrated what was possible when a brilliant designer was given freedom of expression. An aggressive self-promoter, Beall received accolades from the prestigious European design journal *Graphis* for many of his *Scope* pages.

The work of Burtin and Beall at *Scope* helped to spark the development of a larger theory and method of "visual reasoning," which sought to simplify complicated topics, banish complexity, and create in its place "a certain beauty of clear statement." *Scope* set the highest standard for the effective and beautiful blending of form and content, which still inspires designers today.

—R. ROGER REMINGTON

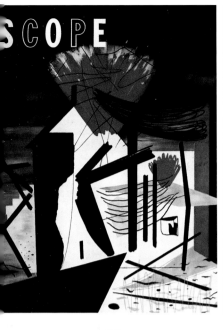

SCOPE

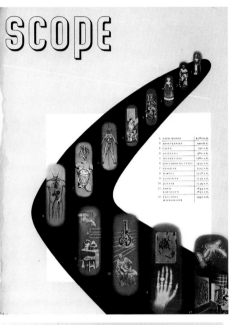

SCOPE

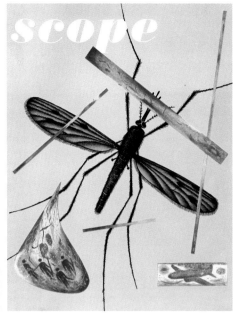

scope

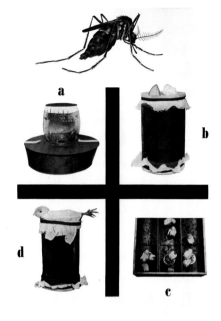

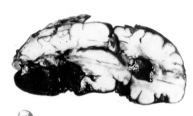

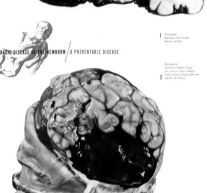

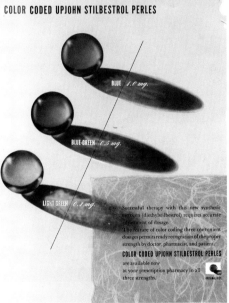

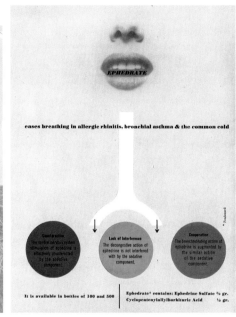

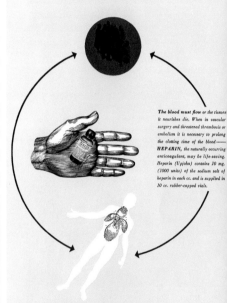

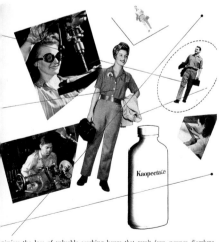

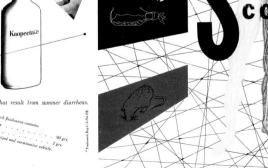

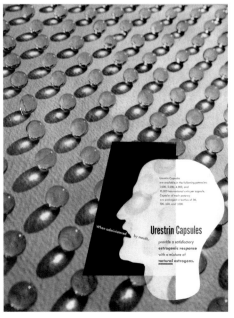

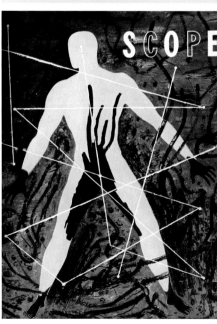

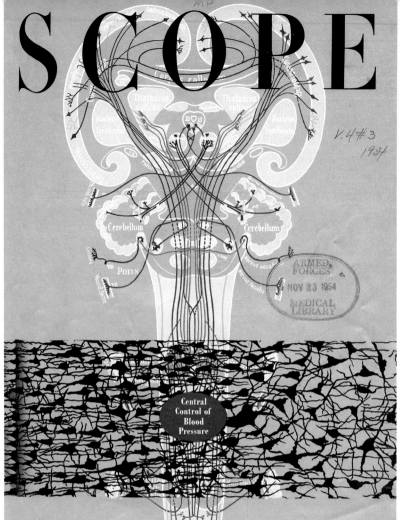

V.4 #3
1954

SCOPE

Central Control of Blood Pressure

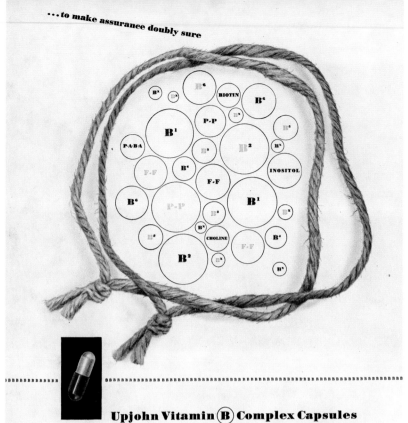

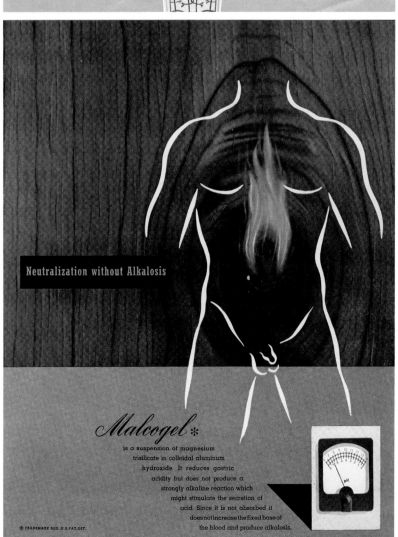

Neutralization without Alkalosis

Malcogel *

is a suspension of magnesium trisilicate in colloidal aluminum hydroxide It reduces gastric acidity but does not produce a strongly alkaline reaction which might stimulate the secretion of acid. Since it is not absorbed it does not increase the fixed base of the blood and produce alkalosis.

❋ TRADEMARK REG. U.S. PAT. OFF.

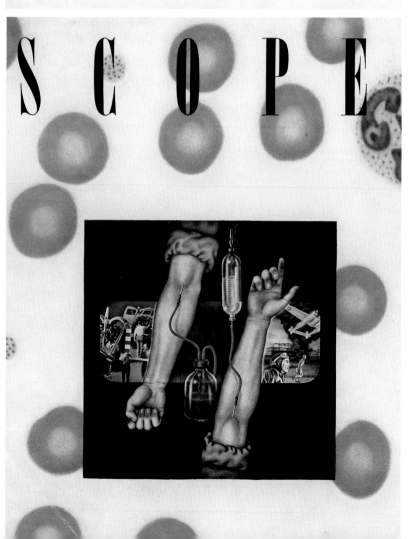

SCOPE

scope

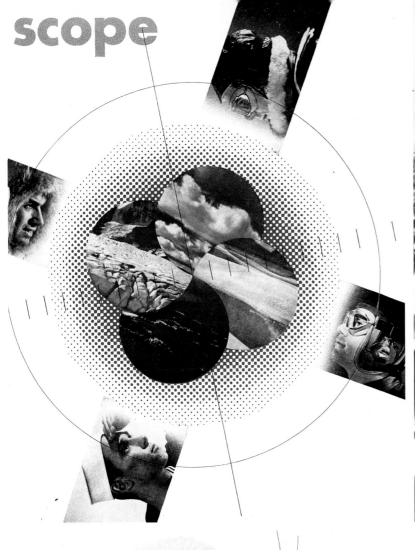

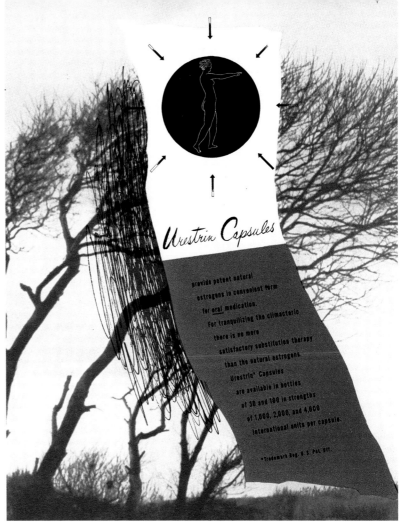

Urestrin Capsules

provide potent natural
estrogens in convenient form
for oral medication.
For tranquilizing the climacteric
there is no more
satisfactory substitution therapy
than the natural estrogens.
Urestrin* Capsules
are available in bottles
of 30 and 100 in strengths
of 1,000, 2,000, and 4,000
international units per capsule.

*Trademark Reg. U.S. Pat. Off.

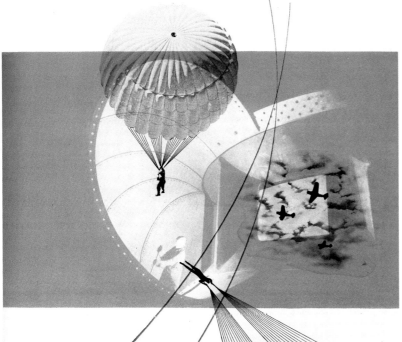

full capacity for men and machine

noted, sometimes with chills. There have also been
instances of urticaria of a transient nature, local
tenderness following intravenous injections, head-
ache, flushing of the face, and muscular pains. All
these phenomena are transient and of relatively little
significance. Quite probably even these mild reac-
tions will become less frequent as the preparations of
the drug become better. In some patients it seems
to have a tendency to produce thrombosis of the
vein at the site of the injection if concentrated solutions are used. There seems to be great individual
variation in susceptibility to this complication.
Penicillin as it exists today is one of the most powerful therapeutic agents thus far discovered, but perhaps of greater significance even than the immediate
value of the drug in the treatment of patients is the
fact that it opens up a new field of therapeutics into

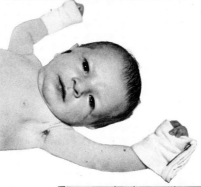

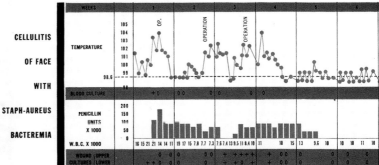

which Dubos' discovery of gramicidin gave us the
first glimpse. Undoubtedly the study of penicillin
will lead to the discovery of many other antibacterial
agents.

11. Chart showing the course of a patient with cellulitis of the
face treated with penicillin. This patient would undoubtedly have died were he not given penicillin.
(Courtesy of Dr. Chester Keefer, Boston)
12. (a) A newborn infant with a Staphylococcus pyoderma
(Ritter's disease?) shortly after the administration of penicillin. There are deep ulcerations of the cheek and axillae
and a perforation of the palate. Prior to the administration
of penicillin, sulfonamide drugs were used with doubtful
effect.
(b) Same patient about four weeks later. Superficial lesions
are nearly healed and the perforation of the soft palate has
closed spontaneously. The baby has remained well.
(Courtesy of Dr. R. J. Armstrong, Kalamazoo)

12

Studies in the Anatomy of the Nervous System and Connective Tissue (1875–76)

Axel Key and Gustaf Retzius

Studien in der Anatomie des Nervensystems und des Bindegewebes. Stockholm. Printed book, with color and black-and-white lithographs, 2 vols., 220 pp. + plates, 228 pp. + plates; 12 x 16 in. (30.4 x 40.6 cm)

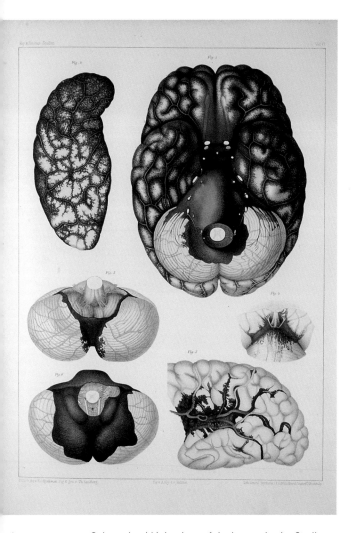

ABOVE: Subarachnoid injections of the human brain. *Studien*, vol. 1, pl. 6, figs. 1–6

OPPOSITE: Injections of the subarachnoid spaces and ventricles of the human brain. *Studien*, vol. 1, pl. 7, figs. 1–4

*J*t was owned by Charles Darwin, Jean-Martin Charcot, Hermann von Helmholtz, and other illustrious scientists. It was displayed as a triumph of Swedish science at the Centennial Exposition in Philadelphia in 1876, along with other Swedish exhibits (such as the model schoolhouse now known as the Swedish Cottage in New York's Central Park). Written in German, the most important scientific language of the day, the massive two-volume *Studies in the Anatomy of the Nervous System and Connective Tissue* deals with the brain and spinal cord (particularly the covering membranes and communicative passages between the brain's ventricles, serous spaces, and lymphatic vessels) and the nerves (their structure, sheaths, and endings).

Four men worked together closely for seven years to produce it: Key (1832–1901), Retzius (1842–1919), and the artists Nils Otto Björkman (1833–1900) and Theodor Lundberg (1852–1926). Key was professor of pathological anatomy at the Karolinska Institute in Stockholm and later its director. A liberal public intellectual, he had studied with Rudolph Virchow in Berlin and, like other Swedish scientists, was well connected to European scientific networks. Retzius, son of the prominent comparative anatomist Anders Retzius, was beginning a productive career that would range over histology (mainly of the nervous system and sense organs), comparative anatomy, physical anthropology, popular medicine, conservative politics, and even newspaper production. Björkman was an expert scientific draftsman, known for graceful renderings of the minute details of microscopic specimens and also for ethnographic travels to Lapland, where he made drawings and collected Sámi artifacts. The young and talented Lundberg would later become a celebrated sculptor and director of the Royal Academy of Art in Stockholm.

Their project of mapping the brain was a visual exploration. First, they acquired their numerous specimens of brains and spines, most likely from the autopsied bodies of people who died in public hospitals, jails, and workhouses. Then the anatomists adapted and developed histological techniques to make the specimens reveal the desired features. They injected them with colored substances and also dipped them in acidic salt solutions of gold, silver, and osmium (the same method Camillo Golgi later used when he discovered the nerve cell). Handling the specimens required expertise and first-rate equipment: the sharpest scalpels and microtomes for slicing the brains, the finest microscopes for examining them. The Karolinska Institute had extensive collections, and some of the specimens likely ended up there, among thousands of other microscopic slides. The artists drew the selected specimens with meticulous attention to detail, form, color, and depth. The printers then used the colored drawings to produce superb chromolithographic plates to go with the text. It was a costly book to print, in large format with superior binding and high-quality ink on fine paper, and could be completed only with support from a benefactor who donated 20,000 kronor—roughly $140,000 in today's money. (After marrying the wealthy philanthropist Anna Hierta in 1876, Retzius never again had to depend on donations to realize his projects.) In this and other works, Retzius collaborated

Tab. VII.

Tafel VII.

...dalräume und der Ventrikel des Gehirns.

...st eine Injection von einer durch lösliches Berlinerblau gefärbten Leimlösung in gewisse...

...spatium des Rückenmarks injicirt wurde. Die Leiche wurde nachher zum Frieren ge...

...durchgesägt. Die Zeichnung wurde nach dem gefrornen Präparate unter genauer Mass...

...Präparat in Alkohol eingelegt, und nach der Erhärtung wurde die Zeichnung in ihren...

...ärl Grösse. Die Figur dürfte in ihren Einzelheiten für Alle, welche Kenntniss von den...

...ndlich sein. Es ist hauptsächlich die Absicht gewesen, durch dieselbe die relative Lage...

...Subarachnoidalräumen und Ventrikeln zu zeigen. Man sieht, wie aufrecht in der That...

...i, und wie weit der letztere mit seiner vorderen Fläche, besonders nach oben, von der...

...ossen Cisternen (an der Figur die Cisterna media pontis) getrennt. Am oberen Rande des...

...rerurales (superficialis und profunda) sich einsenken; (die Scheidewand zwischen diesen...

...ach am Präparate bei der erwähnten Behandlung sehr undeutlich oder gar nicht hervor...

...se sieht man die Injectionsmasse durch die Dura fortgehen, um an der Oberfläche der...

...dieser und der, die Sella turcica überbrückenden Arachnoidea sich auszubreiten. An der...

...den hier befindlichen venösen Sinus. Nach vorn von der Lamina cinerea terminalis sieht...

...fläche des Corpus callosum (im Spatium subarachnoidale corporis callosi) war die Masse...

...Hinten und unten an der Figur sieht man, wie das hintere Subarachnoidalspatium des...

...llo medullaris übergeht. Der Durchschnitt geht hier gerade durch die Vallecula, und...

...hier, entsprechend der Incisura marginalis posterior, in die Cisterne hineinschiebt. Von...

...etzt sich die Injectionsmasse direct durch das Foramen Magendii oder Apertura inferi...

...t. Wenn man diese Figur mit der Figur 8 der Tafel III vergleicht, wird man es leicht...

...solchen Füllung und an einem Schnitt, welcher gerade durch das foramen Magendii geht...

...en Ventrikels bemerkt. Am Schädelgewölbe sieht man den durchgesägten Sinus longitu...

...cerebri entfernt. Nach hinten findet man bei Torcular Herophili die Mündung des Sinus...

...berhalb des Cerebellum gehenden, durch seine ganze Länge geöffneten Sinus tentorii, von...

...i die Vena magna Galeni abgeht. Man sieht weiter, wie tief das Subarachnoidalspatium...

...oder der hintere mittlere Theil der Cisterna ambiens) zwischen der Eintrittstelle der ge...

...st, und wie die Injectionsmasse hier theils nach hinten zwischen dem Cerebellum und der...

...terius, theils nach vorn in der Tasche zwischen dem Conarium mit seinem dünnen Mark...

...einerseits und der Lamina corporum quadrigem, andererseits fortgeht. Im dritten Ventrikel...

...rium an seiner ganzen oberen Fläche bis zur Spitze in dem Recessus supra conarium. Re...

...der Mitte des dritten Ventrikels findet man die quer durchgeschnittene, weiss gerichtete...

...l war, so weit wir finden konnten, keine Masse hineingedrungen, und er ist deswegen auch...

...ait dem betreffenden Schädel, ebenso behandelt wie der in der vorigen Figur abgebildete. Na...

...s sphenoideum an dem hintern Theil der Sella turcica, dicht in der Nähe und nach hinten...

...Man sieht u. A. die gefüllten Seitenventrikel, wie es scheint, in ziemlich natürlicher Au...

...e feinen, blauen Linien, welche von dem letzteren unterhalb des Fornix zu den Seitenven...

...zu sehen, wie sie abgebildet sind, und hängen davon ab, dass das Velum triangulare vo...

...eiche Fig. 4 Tafel IV). An der durchgeschnittenen Glandula pituitaria oder Hypophyse...

...ihr und die Sella turcica überbrückenden Dura, die Injectionsmasse in den hier befind...

...eingedrungen. An der unteren Fläche der Hypophyse findet man den durchgeschnittenen...

...die ganze Fläche sich ausbreitend. Seitlich am Os sphenoideum sieht man den Nervus trigeminus mit...

...von der Injectionsmasse umgebenen Nervus abducens, wie auch den Nervus trigeminus mit...

...ng, als zwischen ihren einzelnen Bündeln. Oben an der Figur bemerkt man die injicirten...

...t. hineindringend, theils in den venösen Seitenlacunen steckend (Vergl. Fig. 4 Tafel XXIX)...

...Leimlösung injicirten Präparate in natürl. Grösse gezeichnet. Die erstarrende Injection...

...angt. dagegen war sie von der Cisterna ambiens oder, wenn man so will und wie die Su...

...quadrigeminorum in das Velum triangulare hineingedrungen und hatte vollständig die Su...

...Vene in dem injicirten Subarachnoidalgewebe aufgehängt; die Injectionsmasse ist aus den...

...ur ihre Wände sind noch davon blau gefärbt. Gez. bei Harta. Obj. 4 und Ocul. 3

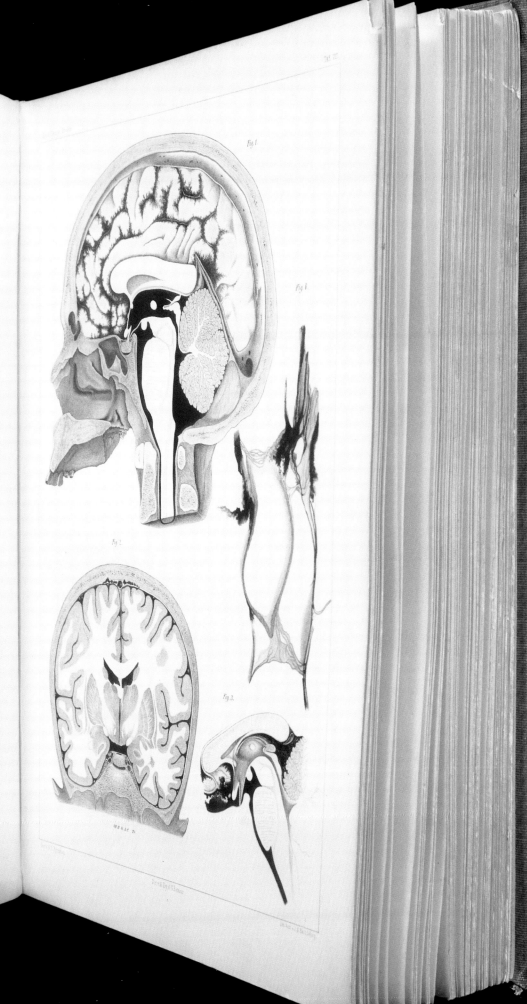

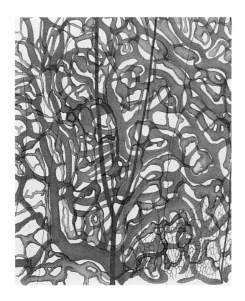

with the finest Swedish and German artists, photographers, and printers, although the collaborations were not always easy. Retzius eventually broke with Björkman, a superb draftsman, over stylistic matters. The artist, he believed, sacrificed accuracy in favor of aesthetics. Retzius thereafter chose to make his own drawings.

The images in these volumes are not mere illustrations of scientific findings—they *are* the findings. Without the image there is no scientific result. But scientific illustrations also do other work. Illustrated monographs and articles help to build personal and institutional reputations and to attract funding and students. Today's neuroscience is just as dependent on technologies of visualization, but with computed tomography, positron emission tomography (PET), and magnetic resonance imaging (MRI) scientists can look into the brains of living people—something that would have been inconceivable to Key and Retzius. However, the beauty of their lithographic brain images has never been surpassed.

—Eva Åhrén

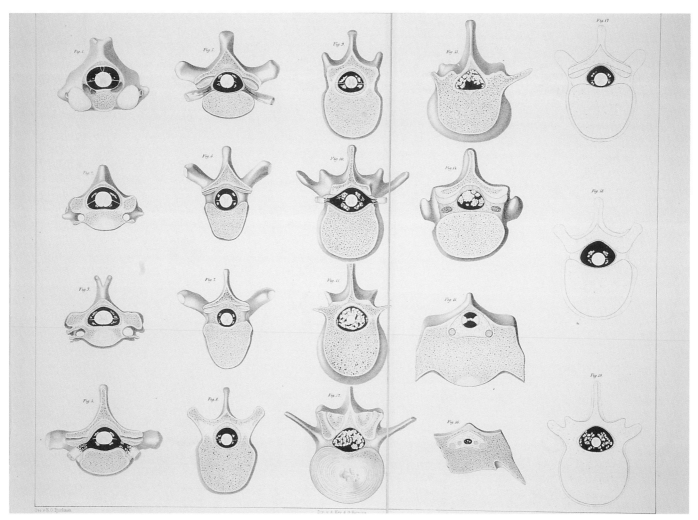

ABOVE, TOP: Section through the olfactory tissue of a rabbit, with blood vessels in red, lymph ducts in blue. *Studien*, vol. 1, pl. 37, fig. 3

ABOVE: Transverse sections of the human spinal column. *Studien*, vol. 1, pl. 2, figs. 1–19

OPPOSITE: Arachnoid villi, or pacchionian bodies, of the human brain. *Studien*, vol. 1, pl. 30, figs. 1–5

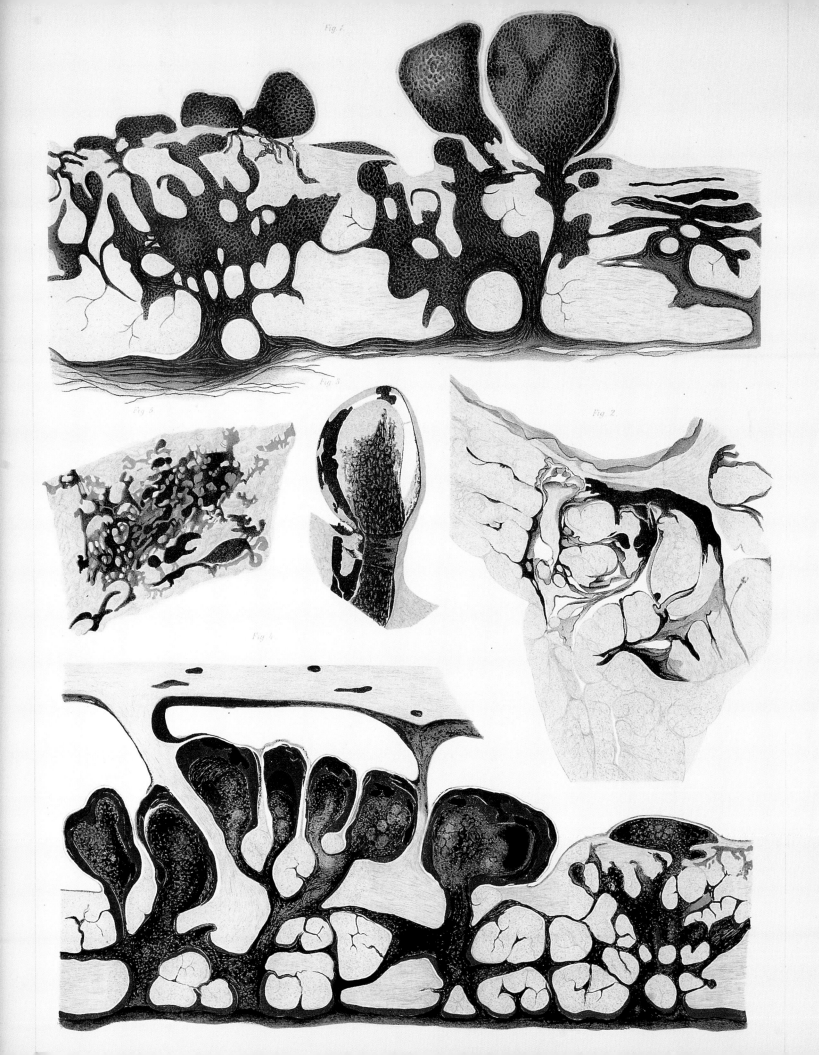

Fig. 1.

Fig. 3.

Fig. 5.

Fig. 4.

Fig. 2.

"Molecular Structure of Nucleic Acids: A Structure for Deoxyribose Nucleic Acid" (1953)

James D. Watson and Francis H. C. Crick

London. *Nature* 171.25 (April 1953): pp. 737–38. Printed journal, with line drawing; height 9⅞ in. (25.1 cm). Double helix DNA model. Plastic, stainless steel tube, wire, 15 ft., made by A. A. Barker, Cambridge, UK, 1969.

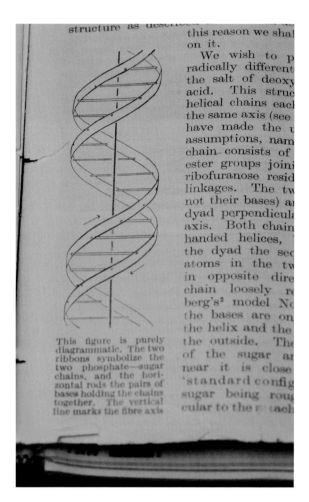

ABOVE: The first published illustration of the double helix. James D. Watson and Francis H. C. Crick, "Molecular Structure of Nucleic Acids: A Structure for Deoxyribose Nucleic Acid," *Nature* 171.25 (April 1953): pp. 737–38. The caption reads: "The figure is purely diagrammatic. The two ribbons symbolize the two phosphate-sugar chains, and the horizontal rods the pairs of bases holding the chains together. The vertical line marks the fibre axis."

OPPOSITE: This sculpture, suspended from the ceiling of the NLM's rotunda, was originally displayed in a 1969 exhibition on the work of Nobel laureate Dr. Marshall W. Nirenberg. It represents the atomic constituents of DNA: hydrogen (white), oxygen (red), nitrogen (blue), carbon (black), and phosphorus (purple). A complete DNA molecule on the scale of this 15-foot-high model would be 142 miles long. Photo: J. D. Talasek.

The paper is only about eight hundred words and the text is almost superfluous. The real content lies in the single unnumbered figure. It is a mere cartoon, platonic in its simplicity, "purely diagrammatic," according to the legend. Two ribbons, side by side and linked by crossbars, wrap sinuously around a thin central axis. Two arrows, one angling up, the other down, suggest polarity for the ribbons. There are no nucleotides, no As, Cs, Gs, or Ts. No hydrogen bonds, phosphates, or pentose rings.

Its meaning is conveyed in a single arrogant sentence, one of the most memorable in biology: "It has not escaped our attention that the specific pairing we have postulated immediately suggests a possible copying mechanism for the genetic material." A with T; C with G: Chargaff's rules. Specifying the copying mechanism of course specifies cell division, which in turn specifies development and evolution. In *The Double Helix: A Personal Account of the Discovery of the Structure of DNA* (1968) James Watson reported Francis Crick as bursting into the Eagle pub, bellowing, "We have found the secret of life!"

The image was just another pretty picture until researchers elsewhere turned that "possible copying mechanism" into the foundation of the science of heredity. It happened gradually. Although well received in the scientific community, the double helix had little impact on the public consciousness until the 1960s. Watson (b. 1928), Crick (1916–2004), and Maurice Wilkins (1916–2004) won the Nobel Prize in 1962, following publication of the "operon" model of the gene and the first cracks in the genetic code.

Crick lived in the Golden Helix, his house in Cambridge, but it was Watson who transmuted the snipped tin plates of their model into gold. After the Nobel, he sat down to write the first textbook of DNA. It was a hit. Then in 1968 he published *The Double Helix*, his memoir of the discovery. The book infuriated his friends, confounded his enemies, made him rich, and made his twisting diagram famous.

The double helix became Watson's logo. When he became director of the laboratory at Cold Spring Harbor he stamped it on the stationery, the sign at the entrance, the spines of the books published by the in-house press. Helical imagery infected the laboratory, from the hilltop bell tower to the statuary in the lobby to the wallpaper and light fixtures.

As medicine went molecular, DNA became its emblem. The double helix became as interesting to sociologists and literary theorists as it is to biologists. Since the fiftieth anniversary of the 1953 article's publication it has been commemorated federally and commercially each April 25 as DNA Day, a day of celebration of all things nucleic—including discounted subscription prices from genomics companies that provide DNA mapping to individual customers.

Where the Bohr atom represents elemental nature, the double helix stands for human nature. It is an icon of identity. In its claims to tell us who we are and how we are made, there is encoded both the power and danger of science. The double helix satisfies graphically, elegantly, the double-edged, near universal desire for determinism—for a single, simple "secret of life."

—NATHANIEL COMFORT

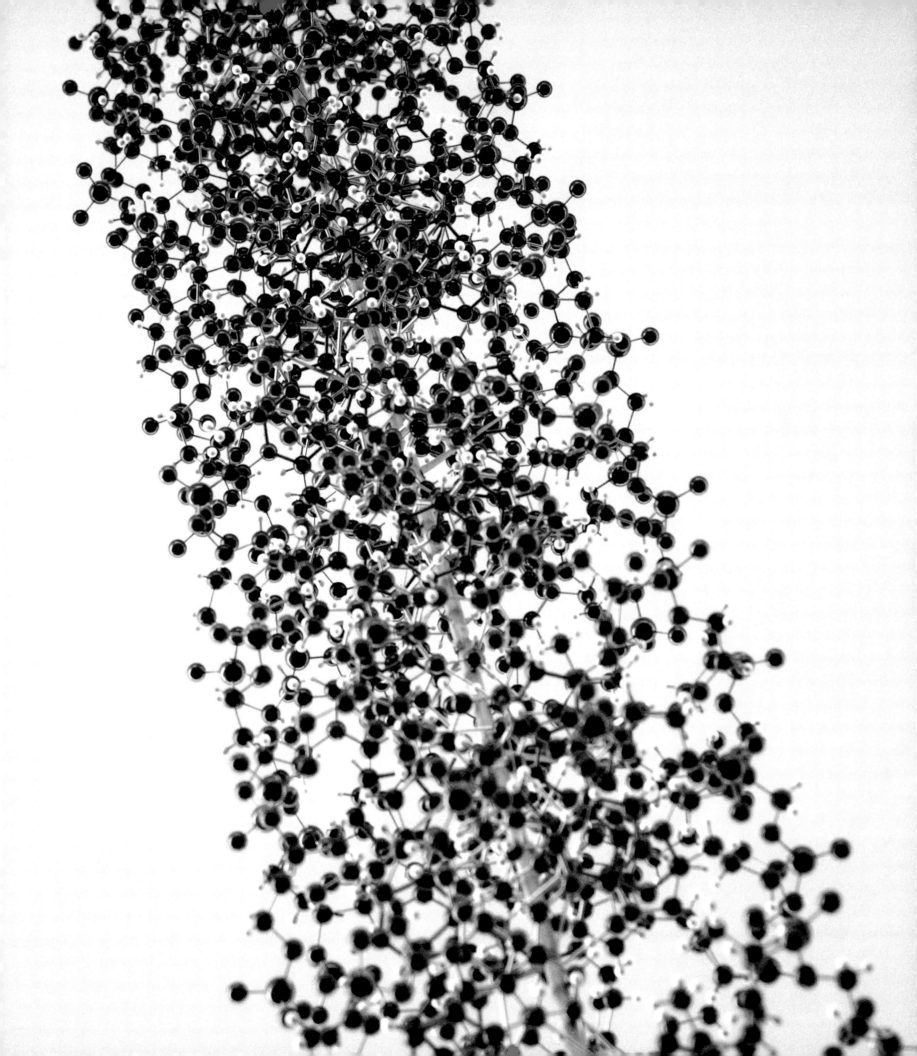

The X-Ray: Or, Photography of the Invisible and Its Value in Surgery (1896)

William J. Morton with Edwin W. Hammer

New York. Printed book, illustrated with wood engravings and halftones, 196 pp. + plates; 5⅓ x 8 in. (13.5 x 20 cm)

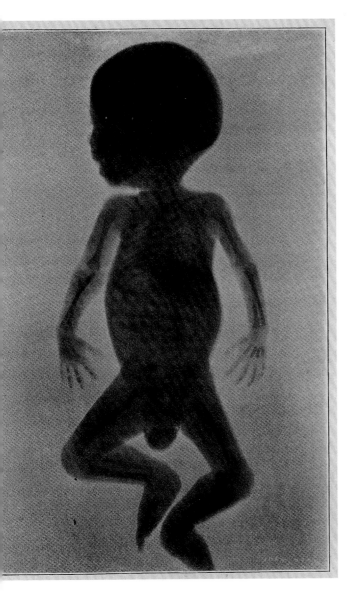

ABOVE: Properly exposed X-ray plates captured clear outlines of the skeleton and also softer tissues, such as the skin, muscles, tendons, and even veins and arteries. But many of the finer details could be lost in the transfer to print. This figure displays the first-ever outline of an infant's liver, within its natural surroundings of flesh and bones. *The X-Ray*, fig. 59

r. William J. Morton (1845–1920) hurried this book into print in September 1896, a mere nine months after Wilhelm Röntgen made public his discovery of the new ray. The news of a strange kind of radiation that defied all standing theories of light and matter—and enabled people to see through opaque objects—had generated worldwide excitement. Almost overnight the mysterious rays and their eerie images began to circulate not only in scientific and medical journals but also in newspaper and magazine articles, advertisements, stories, songs, and cartoons. Physicists rushed to experiment with the new rays that seemed unrefractable and indifferent to electromagnetic fields, while other investigators attempted to use them to capture all kinds of objects previously hidden from the human eye—from hearts and bones to thoughts and souls.

Morton was the professor of "Diseases of the Mind and Nervous System and Electro-Therapeutics" in the New York Post Graduate Medical School and Hospital and one of the first American physicians to experiment with the new rays. His father, the dentist William T. G. Morton (1819–68), in a September 1846 tooth extraction had famously demonstrated the magical powers of anesthesia, a miraculous technology that would revolutionize surgery. Half a century later, it was his son's turn to demonstrate, to the medical profession and the public, a miraculous technology—the magical powers of new rays that could look into the human body without cutting it open.

Written with the help of the electrical engineer Edwin W. Hammer, Morton's little green book describes the electrical apparatus and photographic techniques essential to X-ray photography. It quickly became popular among doctors, surgeons, dentists, and others who were contemplating the addition of an X-ray apparatus to their laboratory or office. The complex relations between the electrical apparatus and the properties of the rays it emitted were far from understood in 1896. If the rays were too "soft," they barely passed through the skin; if too "hard," they passed through the thickest bones and produced little contrast on the photographic plate. The only reliable way to calibrate the rays' penetrating power was for the operator to inspect his own hand against the fluoroscope screen (opposite). No precautions were taken against radiation exposure: no one suspected the dangers involved. Morton did note that, after prolonged X-ray sessions, his eyes often got sore and his eyelids were often inflamed. Many X-ray pioneers would die of painful debilitating cancers before the danger was recognized and protective measures taken.

Rapid improvements in the infant technology soon allowed for ever shorter exposures and increasingly better imaging. Mastering X-ray technology was not enough, though. Medical practitioners would need more experience and training before they became competent to reliably read the exotic images and distinguish between normal and pathological appearances. It took more than two decades for the medical professions to fully adopt the new visual technology and combine it with traditional diagnostic methods: interviewing, listening with the stethoscope, and touching the body.

—TAL GOLAN

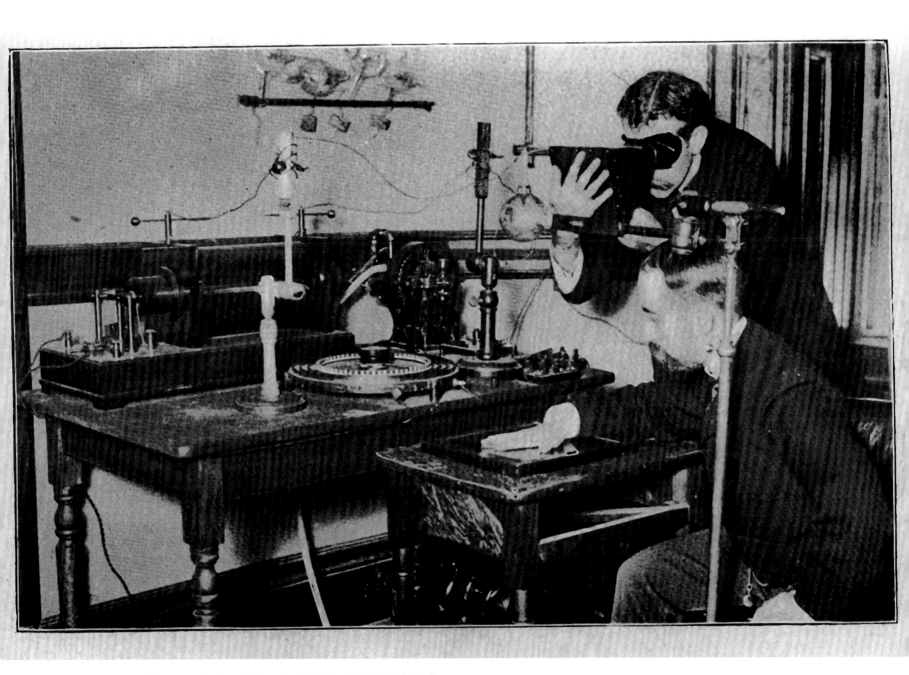

ABOVE: The apparatus in early X-ray photography: a huge induction coil (on the table against the wall) provides high voltage to drive the rays in a partially evacuated gas tube; behind it, in the back corner, a motor-operated interrupter repeatedly breaks the direct current supply to create magnetic-field changes for induction. The large flat disk in front of the table is the power control, made of an adjustable resistor. A rack on the wall holds spare gas tubes. The complicated interactions between the electrical characteristics of the tube, its gas pressure, and the properties of the rays it emitted were not well understood. Much of the operator's expertise lay in knowing his tubes by heart and choosing the right one for the task. The X-Ray, fig. 54

OVERLEAF: Selected photographs from The X-Ray, figs. 66, 67, 53, 51, 73, 60, 63, 68

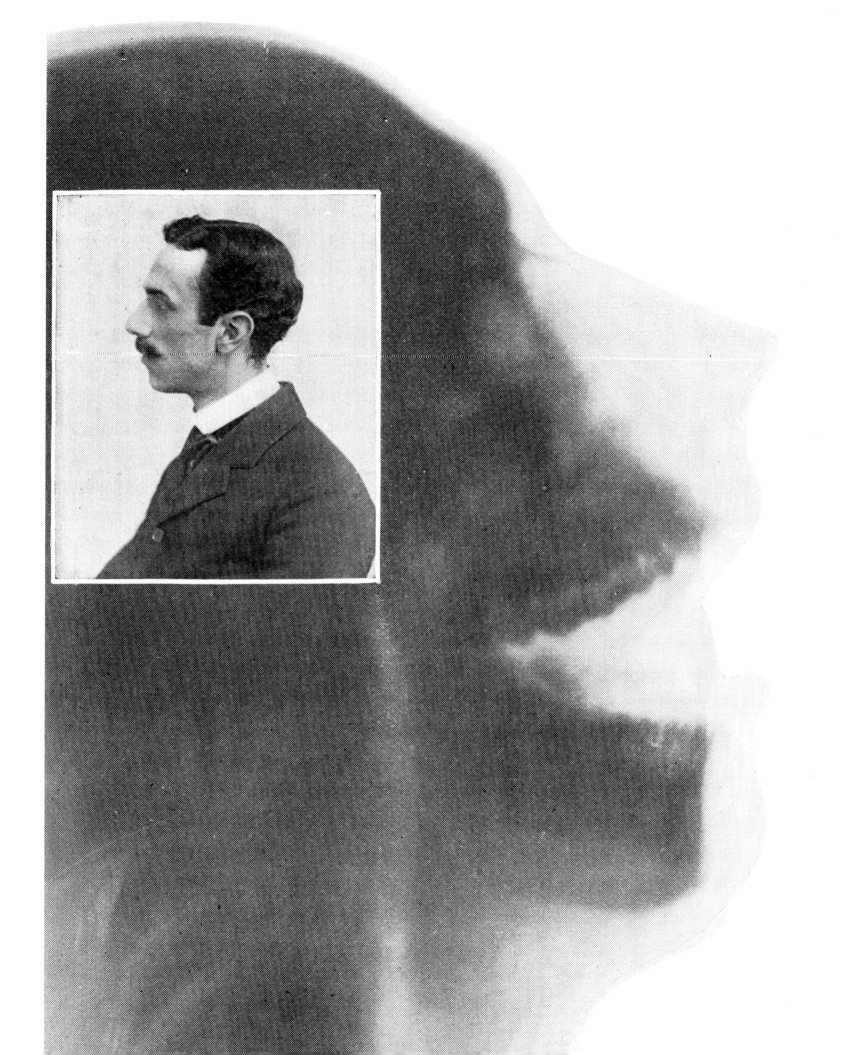

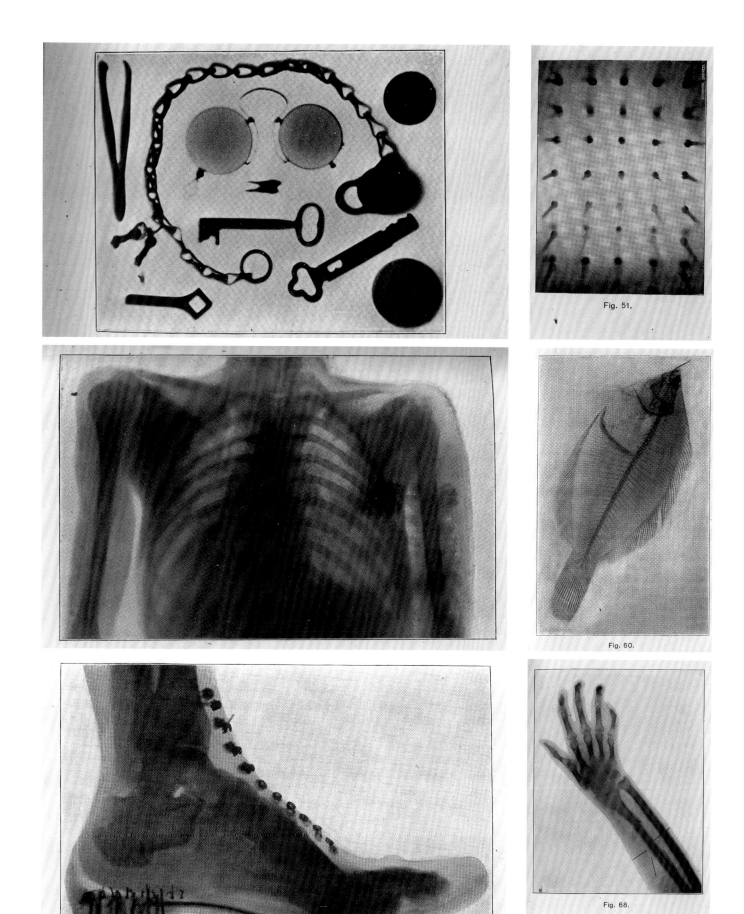

Fig. 51.

Fig. 60.

Fig. 68.

The Doctors: A Satire in Four Seizures (1922)
Elbert Hubbard

East Aurora, NY. 1st ed., 1909; printed book with two-color linocut illustrations on textured paper, embossed leather cover, 108 pp.; 5½ x 8 in. (13.8 x 20.3 cm)

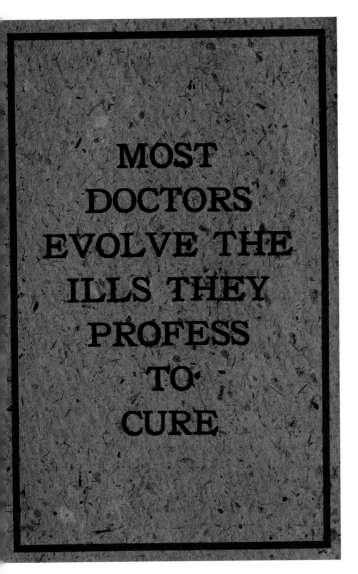

ABOVE: An aphorism from *The Doctors*

OPPOSITE: Illustrations in the volume were printed in two colors on textured paper. The figure of the greedy, lustful, deceitful, manipulative doctor presented in *The Doctors* looks very much like anti-Semitic caricatures of the Jew, which were appearing with increasing frequency in the central European press of the day.

Elbert Hubbard (1856–1915), Arts and Crafts guru and follower of the British reformer William Morris (1834–96), is best known for writing the inspirational self-help essay "Message to Garcia" (1899). In the early 1900s his books could be found in many middle-class homes. He was an opponent of formal education and the professions in general, which he saw as destroying self-worth and poisoning individual initiative. *The Doctors*, his "satire in four seizures," is similar in tone to other contemporary critiques of medicine, such as Mary Baker Eddy's Christian Science.

The plot is familiar: Mrs. X is sent unconscious and in chains to the State Hospital by her husband, the Reverend Cecil Kelrusey, whose family is distraught that he has married an "actress." Seizing their young child, he tries to have his wife declared incompetent. The story echoes that of Mrs. Elizabeth Packard, which made headlines in the 1860s when her husband, the Reverend Theophilus Packard, had her committed to the Illinois State Hospital for disagreeing with his theology. Freed after a widely publicized court case, Mrs. Packard went on to found the Anti–Insane Asylum Society and wrote *Marital Power Exemplified, or Three Years' Imprisonment for Religious Belief* (1866), which provided Hubbard with many of the details for his satire.

In Hubbard's play the doctors treat Mrs. X with fashionable techniques such as the "rest cure" (presented here as a torture in which the patient is strapped to a bed for weeks at a time, causing her to lapse into despair). The physicians are based on prominent "alienists" of the day: the asylum superintendent is Dr. Agnew Weir (S. Weir Mitchell invented the rest cure); his assistant is Dr. Jean Charlcot (Jean-Martin Charcot was a proponent of the hysteria diagnosis). With the help of asylum workmen Mrs. X outsmarts her doctors and becomes a force for good in the lives of the other patients, introducing "healthy" activities such as gardening and exercise. Eventually she converts Dr. Weir to the cause, is granted a divorce, reclaims her child, and marries the doctor, who decides to run the asylum on modern principles—healthy food, light gymnastics, fresh air—which sound a lot like those of J. H. Kellogg's Battle Creek Sanitarium. Drugs and invasive therapies are out. The other doctors quit in disgust.

Hubbard, as was his wont, intersperses the pages of the play with artfully illustrated aphorisms: "The Three Learned Professions [medicine, law, religion] surely need our sympathy, since they know so many things that are not so." "Is the World all wrong? Reform yourself." "Breathe more, eat less and think well of everybody especially doctors." Seemingly an early example of anti-psychiatry, *The Doctors* is more prone to preach the dogma of the "self-made man," a phrase coined by Frederick Douglass (1817/8–95) and propagated in the novels of Horatio Alger (1832–99). Hubbard is as critical of patients as he is of institutions: "Fool patients evolve fool doctors." Writing for a middle-class audience in the heyday of muckraking progressive journalism, Hubbard planted his critique in the pages of a beautifully wrought, leather-bound, letterpress gift book.

—SANDER L. GILMAN

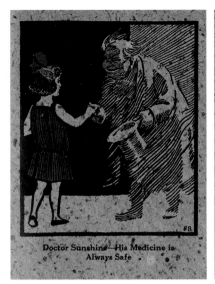

Doctor Sunshine—His Medicine is Always Safe

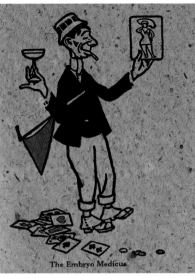

The Embryo Medicus

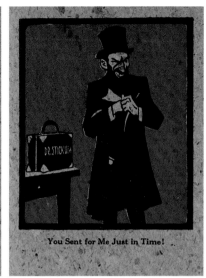

You Sent for Me Just in Time!

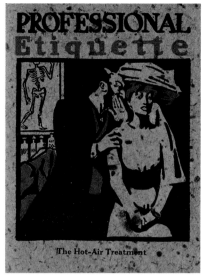

PROFESSIONAL Etiquette

The Hot-Air Treatment

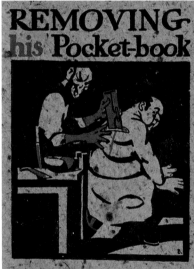

REMOVING his Pocket-book

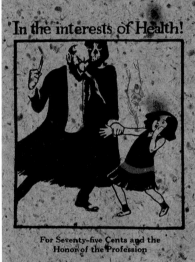

In the interests of Health!

For Seventy-five Cents and the Honor of the Profession

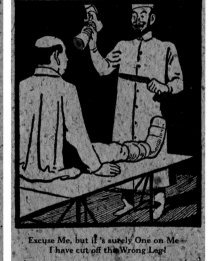

Excuse Me, but it's surely One on Me— I have cut off the Wrong Leg!

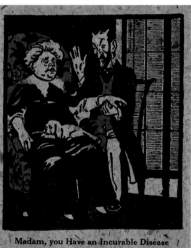

Madam, you Have an Incurable Disease

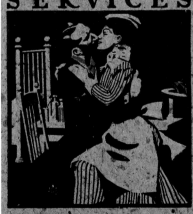

PROFESSIONAL SERVICES

Defiance of the Microbes, or His Most Innocent Experiment

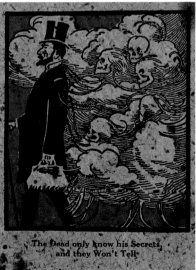

The Dead only know his Secrets, and they Won't Tell

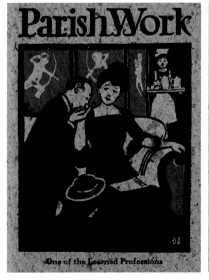

Parish Work

One of the Learned Professions

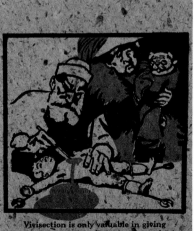

Vivisection is only valuable in giving facility in cutting into the human subject —Dr. J. H. Tilden

The Dance of Death (1744)
Jacques-Antony Chovin

Todten-Tanz / Danse des Morts. Basel, Switzerland.
Printed book with copper-plate engravings, text in German and French, 132 pp.; height 8 in. (20.3 cm)

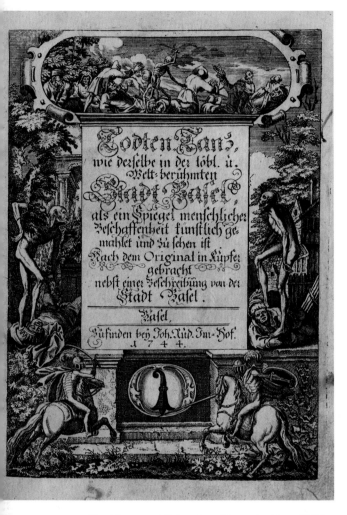

ABOVE: The title page of *Todten-Tanz / Danse des Morts* (1744) refers the reader to the Basel mural on which the plates were based.

OPPOSITE: Selected pages: top left, Death dances with the queen; center, Death dances with a painter; top right, Death dances with an itinerant hawker of wares; bottom left, Death dances with the pope; bottom right, Death dances with a moneylender.

This collection of copper-plate engravings, published in 1744 by the engraver Jacques-Antony Chovin (1720–76) of Basel, features the naked, decaying figure of Death dragging women and men to the dance floor. All of the types of Renaissance society are represented: rich and poor, noble and lowborn, religious and apostate, beautiful and ugly, young and old, educated and ignorant. No one appears to be looking forward to this last pas de deux. But there is no choice: Death is in the mood for dancing, as the accompanying poetry (in French and German) makes clear.

Todten-Tanz / Danse des Morts is an allegory on the universality of death: we all must die. This is perhaps an unpleasant thing to contemplate. Why then did Chovin, a specialist in engraving maps and globes, choose to publish on the theme? A popular subject in the late Middle Ages, by the eighteenth century the fragility of life and inevitability of its ending had lost much of its appeal as "enlightened" readers strove for a life of reason. Indeed, it seems probable that Chovin had no deep commitment to the *danse macabre*. The copper plates were not even his own; he merely reengraved an older set of plates made in 1649 by the famous Basel-born engraver Matthäus Merian (1593–1650). Merian's preface, reprinted in Chovin's 1744 publication, further reveals that Merian did not create the death scenes but faithfully reproduced them from a churchyard mural. Dating to the plague of the mid-fifteenth century and some sixty meters (nearly two hundred feet) long, the mural had been commissioned by the city council to commemorate the many residents killed by the deadly calamity. The mural survived the iconoclastic controversy of the Reformation and became one of the city's main tourist attractions. For Merian to publicize such a famous feature of his beloved hometown fitted well with his business interests; he was well known for his *Theatrum Europaeum* (1635) and *Topographia Germaniae* (1642–54, 16 vols.), collections of hundreds of prints of city scenes, maps, and topographies of German- and non-German-speaking regions. He had published maps of Basel in 1615, and his preface explains it was then that he began his first sketches for the *Todten-Tanz* (seventeenth-century German for "Dance of Death").

By the time Chovin came to reengrave Merian's plates the mural had fallen into disrepair. New aesthetic values, together with incomprehension and even disdain for medieval religiosity, led some citizens of Basel to call for its demolition (which was finally accomplished in 1805). Hence Chovin's new edition of *Todten-Tanz* was more a reminder of Basel's former most famous landmark than of human mortality. And it was a reminder too of the quaintly morbid and "unenlightened" obsessions of Europeans in centuries past: not a memento mori at all. Chovin, like Merian before him, kept an attentive eye on the market. By the eighteenth century the educated European traveler no longer conversed in German but in fashionable French *à la mode*. To accommodate his trendy readers, Chovin translated Merian's German poetry, and *Todten-Tanz* became *Danse des Morts*.

—CLAUDIA STEIN

Left column top:

Tod zur Königin.

FRau Königin eur Freud ist aus,
  Springen mit mir ins Todten-Haus,
Euch hilfft kein Schöne, Gold noch Geld,
Ich spring mit euch in jene Welt.

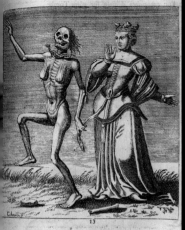

13

Antwort der Königin.

O Weh und Ach, O weh und immer,
Wo bleibt jetzund mein Frauenzimmer,
Mit denen ich hat Freuden viel:
O Tod thu g'mach, mit mir nicht eil.
B 3

Left column bottom:

Tod zum Babst.

KOmm heiliger Vatter werther Mann,
Ein Vor-Tanz müst ihr mir mit han:
Der Ablaß euch nicht hilfft davon,
Das zweyfach Creutz und dreyfach Cron.

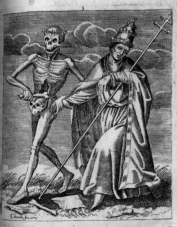

Antwort des Pabsts.

HEilig war ich auf Erd genannt,
Ohn GOtt der höchst führt ich mein Stand:
Der Ablaß thät mir gar wohl lohnen,
Nun will der Tod mein nicht verschonen.
A 3

Center:

Tod zum Mahler.

HAns Hug Klauber laß Mahlen stohn,
  Wir wöllen auch jetztmahls davon:
Dein Kunst, Müh, Arbeit hilfft dich nit,
Wann es geht dir wie ander Leut:
Hast du schon greulich g'macht mein Leib,
Wirst auch so g'stalt mit Kind und Weib:
Hab GOTT vor augen allezeit,
Wirff Bensel hin samt dem Richtscheit.

79

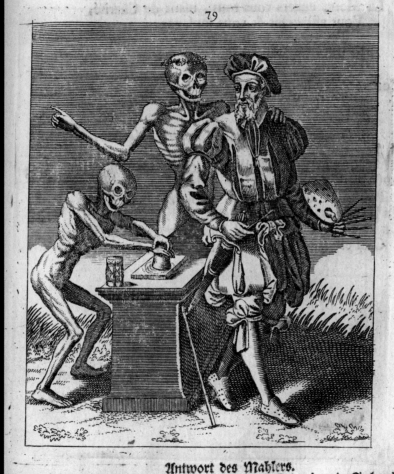

Antwort des Mahlers.

MEin GOtt du wöllest mir beystohn,   Und der Tod mir mein Seel austreibt,
Dieweil ich auch muß jetzt davon: Verhoff doch, mein Gedächtniß bleibt,
Mein Seel befehl ich in dein Händ,   So lang man diß Werck haltet schon:
Wann die Stund kommt zu meinem End   Behüt euch GOtt, ich fahr davon.

Right column top:

Tod zum Krämer.

WOhl her, Krämer du Groscheneyer,
Du Leutbscheisser und Gassenschreyer:
Du must jetztmals mit mir davon,
Dein Humpelkram ein andern lon.

65

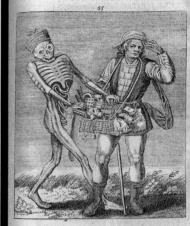

Antwort des Krämers.

ICh bin gezogen durch die Welt,
  Und hab gelöst allerley Geld:
Viel Thaler, Müntz, Kronen und Gulden,
O Mord, wer zahlt mir jetzt die Schulden.
I

Right column bottom:

Tod zum Wucherer.

DEin Gold und Geld seh ich nicht an,
  Du Wucherer und gottlos Mann:
Christus hat dich das nicht gelehrt,
Ein schwartzer Tod ist dein Gefehrt.

51

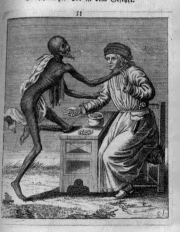

Antwort des Wucherers.

ICh fragt viel nach Christi Lehr:
  Mein Wucher der trug mir vielmehr:
Jetzt bleibt der Leiden all dahinten,
Was hilfft mein Schaben und mein Schinden.
G 2

ACKNOWLEDGMENTS

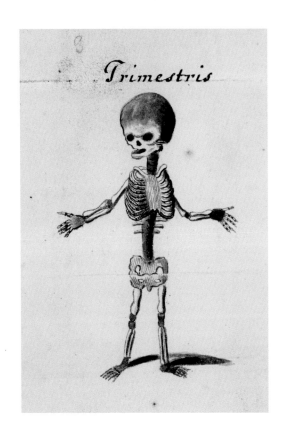

The making of a volume such as this requires the hard work, care, and special expertise of many people. The editors of *Hidden Treasures* want to particularly acknowledge the help of Doug Atkins, Ba Ba Chang, Dr. Milton Corn, Kristi Wright Davenport, Elizabeth Fee, Erin Goldstein, Stephen Greenberg, Holly Herro, Margaret Kaiser, Donald Kennison, Kelli Langley, Dr. Donald A. B. Lindberg, Michael North, Karen Pitts, Emmett Powell, Jeffrey Reznick, Crystal Smith, Ken Swezey (Blast Books), Sandy Taylor, Paul Theerman, and Déshaun Williams. Additional photography was done by Joanna Ebenstein (Morbid Anatomy Library), Hank Grasso (Office of NIH History), and Ginny Roth (History of Medicine Division, Images and Archives).

We also want to thank Jay Aldam and Kim Bradway (The Studley Press), Simon Chaplin (Wellcome Library), Joe Charuhas, Walter Cybulski, Todd Danielson, Marie Dauenheimer (medical illustrator), Dora Deegbe, Cathy Dorsey, Nancy Dosch, Linda Draper (Museum of Optometry, St. Louis), Laurie DuQuette, Sarah Eilers, Laura Hartman, Robin Hope, Sheldon Kotzin, Wendy Kramer (San Francisco Public Library), James Labosier, Joan E. Lynaugh (University of Pennsylvania School of Nursing), Melanie Modlin, Christie Moffatt, Willem J. Mulder (independent scholar), Thanh Nguyen, Phil Osborne, Niki Papavramidou (University of Thessalonika), Gregory Pike, Kathy Powderly (SUNY, Downstate Medical Center), John Rees, Michael Rhode (National Museum of Health and Medicine), Suzanne Salinetti (The Studley Press), Fran Sandridge, Aris Sarafianos (University of Ioannina), William Schupbach (Wellcome Library), Jerry Sheehan, Akihito Suzuki (Keio University, Tokyo), and Sheng Tarn.

CONTRIBUTORS

EVA ÅHRÉN, a Swedish historian of science and medicine, has been a postdoctoral fellow at Yale University; curator and head of research at the Nobel Museum, Stockholm; and research fellow at Uppsala University. The author of *Death, Modernity, and the Body: Sweden 1870–1940*, she has focused her research mainly on nineteenth- and twentieth-century anatomy. Åhrén holds a fellowship in the History Office of the National Institutes of Health and is working on turn-of-the-century bacteriology in the United States.

BRIDIE ANDREWS holds a doctorate in the history of medicine from the University of Cambridge and is affiliated with Bentley University. She has co-edited two volumes on the history of modern medicine in non-Western environments and is completing a monograph on the history of Chinese–Western medical exchanges in China.

ALEXANDER BAY teaches East Asian history at Chapman University. A Japan specialist, he focuses on the history of science and medicine across the premodern/modern divide as well as during the interwar years. He is completing a manuscript entitled *Making a National Disease: Beriberi, Medicine and Power in Modern Japan* and writing a short history of hemorrhoids in Japan. His next book-length project concerns Hansen's disease in Japan.

ZOE BELOFF is an artist and Associate Professor at Queens College, CUNY, in the departments of Media Studies and Art. She works with a range of media. Her projects grow out of historical research, investigating a space where technology intersects with the unconscious. Her work has been exhibited internationally at venues including the Whitney Museum, MoMA, Pacific Film Archives, and the Pompidou Center.

TIMOTHY BILLINGS is Professor of English Literature at Middlebury College. He is the editor and translator of Matteo Ricci's Chinese essay *On Friendship* and of Victor Segalen's French and Chinese poems, *Stèles*, which received the Modern Language Association's Aldo and Jeanne Scaglione Prize for translation. He holds advanced degrees from Cornell University and the School of Oriental and African Studies at the University of London.

SHEILA S. BLAIR and JONATHAN M. BLOOM, a wife-and-husband team of art historians who share the Norma Jean Calderwood Professorship of Islamic and Asian Art at Boston College and the Hamid bin Khalifa Endowed Chair of Islamic Art at Virginia Commonwealth University, write on all aspects of Islamic art and architecture. Their latest work is the three-volume *Grove Encyclopedia of Islamic Art and Architecture*.

RON BROGLIO is author of *On the Surface: Thinking with Animals and Art* and *Technologies of the Picturesque*. His research focuses on how philosophy and aesthetics can advance a rethinking of the relationship between humans and the environment. He is Assistant Professor of English and Senior Scholar of the Global Institute of Sustainability at Arizona State University.

MIKITA BROTTMAN is a British scholar, psychoanalyst, author, and cultural critic known for her psychological readings of the dark and pathological elements of contemporary culture. Her articles and case studies have appeared in *Film Quarterly, American Journal of Psychoanalysis, New Literary History*, and *American Imago*. The author of books on the horror film, critical theory, reading, psychoanalysis, and the work of the American folklorist Gershon Legman, she teaches at the Maryland Institute College of Art.

LIPING BU is Professor of History at Alma College. She has published extensively on public health and international cultural relations. Working with health images, she has created several online exhibits at the National Library of Medicine. Her recent book is *Science, Public Health, and the State in Modern Asia*. She is writing a book on public health and modernization in twentieth-century China.

DAVID CANTOR is Deputy Director of the Office of History, National Institutes of Health, Bethesda, Maryland. His scholarly work focuses on the twentieth-century history of medicine. He is the editor of *Reinventing Hippocrates* and *Cancer in the Twentieth Century* and co-editor with Christian Bonah and Matthias Dörries of *Meat, Medicine, and Human Health in the Twentieth Century*.

MARY CAPPELLO's four books of literary nonfiction include a *Los Angeles Times*–bestselling book-length essay on awkwardness, *Awkward: A Detour*; a critical memoir on cancer, *Called Back*, that won a ForeWord Book of the Year Award and an Independent Publisher's Prize; and the lyric biography *Swallow: Foreign Bodies,*

Their Ingestion, Inspiration and the Curious Doctor Who Extracted Them. She is Professor of English at the University of Rhode Island.

ANDREA CARLINO teaches the history of medicine at the University of Geneva and has taught, as visiting professor, at the Ecole Normale Supérieure in Paris and the University of Western Australia. He is the author of *Books of the Body, Paper Bodies* and, with Michel Jeanneret, *Vulgariser la médecine*. He currently works on the relationship between medicine, natural philosophy, and the humanities in early modern Europe.

NATHANIEL COMFORT is Associate Professor of the History of Medicine at Johns Hopkins University. His books include *The Tangled Field: Barbara McClintock's Search for the Patterns of Genetic Control* and *The Panda's Black Box: Opening Up the Intelligent Design Debate.* His essays have appeared in the *New York Times, Natural History,* and *The Believer* and on National Public Radio. His next book will be a history of medical genetics, tentatively entitled *The Science of Human Perfection.*

HAROLD J. COOK is John F. Nickoll Professor of History at Brown University and from 2000 to 2009 was Director of the Wellcome Trust Centre for the History of Medicine at University College London. He has published extensively on early modern science and medicine, his most recent book being *Matters of Exchange: Commerce, Medicine, and Science in the Dutch Golden Age.*

PIA F. CUNEO, Professor of Art History at the University of Arizona, specializes in northern Renaissance art. Her current research, focusing on illustrated horsemanship manuals, examines the nexus between the production and consumption of books, the practice and evaluation of horsemanship, and social, political, and professional identities in early modern Germany.

OLAF CZAJA of Leipzig University focuses his research on Tibetan history, art, and medicine, particularly the textual tradition of Tibetan medicine. He has pursued Tibetan, Indian, and Mongolian studies in Bonn and Kathmandu and received a doctorate in Tibetan studies at Leipzig University with a thesis on the political history of a Tibetan ruling house.

LUKE DEMAITRE is Visiting Professor of History in the Center for Biomedical Ethics and Humanities at the University of Virginia. He has published widely on the role of the first universities in medical teaching and practice. His most recent book is *Leprosy in Premodern Medicine: A Malady of the Whole Body,* and he is preparing a book-length study, *The Medieval Physician's Manual,* for publication in 2012.

MARK DERY is a cultural critic. His books include *The Pyrotechnic Insanitarium: American Culture on the Brink; Escape Velocity: Cyberculture at the End of the Century;* and *Flame Wars: The Discourse of Cyberculture.* He has been a professor of journalism at New York University, a Chancellor's Distinguished Fellow at the University of California Irvine, and Visiting Scholar at the American Academy in Rome. He is at work on a biography of the artist Edward Gorey.

SHAUNA DEVINE is a historian of science and medicine and is Visiting Research Fellow at the Schulich School of Medicine, Department of Medical History, University of Western Ontario. Her forthcoming book, *Dissecting the Civil War Body: Science in the Practice of Medicine, 1861–1865,* examines the development of scientific medicine during the American Civil War and the impact of the war's events on American medicine. She is researching projects on the Civil War South and human experimentation in Civil War hospitals.

ELIZABETH FEE, Senior Historian at the History of Medicine Division of the National Library of Medicine, has taught at Princeton and Johns Hopkins universities. From 1995 to 2011, she was Chief of the History of Medicine Division. The author of *Science and the "Woman Question,"* she has written many articles and co-edited many volumes on the history of medicine and public health.

MECHTHILD FEND is Lecturer at the History of Art Department at University College London. She specializes in French eighteenth- and nineteenth-century visual culture and art theory; major research interests include the history and representation of the body and the historically changing relationships between art and science. She has worked and published in particular on skin as a scientific object and an object of representation. She is finishing a book, *Fleshing out Surfaces: Skin in French Art and Medicine, 1650–1850.*

PAULA FINDLEN is Ubaldo Pierotti Professor of Italian History at Stanford University. Her publications, in addition to many essays on science and culture in the early modern world, include *Possessing Nature: Museums, Collecting, and Scientific Culture in Early Modern Italy; Athanasius Kircher: The Last Man Who Knew Everything;* and with Pamela Smith, ed., *Merchants and Marvels: Commerce, Science, and Art in Early Modern Europe.*

MARY E. FISSELL is Professor in the Department of the History of Medicine at Johns Hopkins University. Her scholarly work focuses on how ordinary people in early modern England understood health, healing, and the natural world; her most recent book is *Vernacular Bodies: The Politics of Motherhood in Early Modern England*. She is writing a social and cultural history of *Aristotle's Masterpiece*, a long-lived popular medical book.

SANDER L. GILMAN is Distinguished Professor of the Liberal Arts and Sciences as well as Professor of Psychiatry at Emory University. A cultural and literary historian, he is the author of the basic study of the visual stereotyping of the mentally ill, *Seeing the Insane*. For twenty-five years he was a member of the humanities and medical faculties at Cornell University where he held the Goldwin Smith Professorship of Humane Studies. During 1990–91 he served as Visiting Historical Scholar at the National Library of Medicine, Bethesda, Maryland.

ELISABETH GITTER is Emeritus Professor of English at John Jay College, CUNY. A specialist in Victorian literature and culture, she is the author of *The Imprisoned Guest: Samuel Howe and Laura Bridgman, the Original Deaf-Blind Girl*.

TAL GOLAN is Associate Professor of the History of Science and Science Studies at the University of California San Diego. His research has focused on the history of scientific evidence, on the relations between science and law, and on science policy. He is the author of *Laws of Men and Laws of Nature: The History of Scientific Expert Testimony in England and America*.

CHARLES HALLISEY is Yehan Numata Senior Lecturer in Buddhist Literatures at Harvard Divinity School. His academic interests focus on the cultural history of Sri Lanka, especially the history of Buddhism and Sinhala literary cultures.

MARTA HANSON has taught in the Department of the History of Medicine at Johns Hopkins University since 2004. Her book is entitled *Speaking of Epidemics in Chinese Medicine: Disease and the Geographic Imagination in Late Imperial China*. She writes about the history of disease, epidemiology, and public health in China; currents of medical learning, regionalism, and pluralism in Chinese history; and East Asian arts of memory.

MARK HARRISON is Professor of the History of Medicine and Director of the Wellcome Unit for the History of Medicine at the University of Oxford. His publications include *The Medical War:*

British Military Medicine in the First World War; Medicine in an Age of Commerce and Empire: Britain and Its Tropical Colonies, 1660–1830; and *Medicine and Victory: British Military Medicine in the Second World War*.

WILLIAM H. HELFAND, a retired pharmaceutical executive, has published five books, including *Pharmacy: An Illustrated History* (with David Cowen), *The Picture of Health*, and *Quack, Quack, Quack*, the catalogue of recent exhibitions at the Grolier Club and the Philadelphia Museum of Art. A former president of the Grolier Club and the Library Company, in 2003 he received the Lifetime Achievement Award of the American Association of the History of Medicine.

STEVEN HELLER, author and editor of more than 130 books on graphic design, satiric art, and popular culture, is co-founder and co-chair of the MFA Designer as Author program at the School of Visual Arts, New York. He is also co-founder of the MFA in Design Criticism, MFA in Interaction Design, MFA Social Documentary Film, and MPS Branding programs. He writes the "Visuals" column for the *Book Review* and "Graphic Content" for the *T-Style/ The Moment* blog. His website is www.hellerbooks.com.

KATHY HIGH is a media artist from New York working with biology and art. She produces videos, sculptures, and installations that have been exhibited in galleries and museums nationally and internationally. In 2010 she was awarded a fellowship from the John Simon Guggenheim Memorial Foundation. High is Associate Professor of Video and New Media in the Department of Arts at Rensselaer Polytechnic Institute, a department specializing in integrated electronic arts practices.

MAMI HIROSE is President of Asano Laboratories, Inc., and Senior Consultant for Mori Art Museum in Tokyo. She has curated and coordinated numerous exhibitions, including *Zenga—Return from America* (2000, Shoto Museum of Art), *Laughter in Japanese Art* (2007, Mori Art Museum), *Medicine and Art* (2009, Mori Art Museum), and *Roppongi Art Night* (2010). Currently, she is curating *Laughter in Japanese Art* for Maison de la culture du Japon (Paris) and *Hakuin* for Bunkamura (Tokyo).

LUDMILLA JORDANOVA is Professor of Modern History at King's College, London. She has a long-standing interest in medicine and visual culture from 1600 onward and has published on Charles Bell. She is the author of *Sexual Visions*, *Nature Displayed*, and *Defining Features*, each of which explores the visual dimensions

of medicine, including the role of gender in representation. Her next book is *The Look of the Past: Visual and Material Evidence in History Practice.*

LAUREN KASSELL is Senior Lecturer in the Department of History and Philosophy of Science and a Fellow of Pembroke College at the University of Cambridge. She has published on the history of astrology, alchemy, medicine, and magic in early modern England and is directing a project to prepare a digital edition of the fifty thousand medical cases recorded by the astrologers Simon Forman and Richard Napier.

MARK KESSELL inflects his artwork with the strong biological and scientific focus of his previous career as a medical doctor. Much of his work is directed toward a deeper understanding of what it means to be human. He uses a variety of media including daguerreotypes, photography, installation, animation, and sound. Kessell has exhibited at the Philadelphia Museum of Art, George Eastman House, International Center of Photography, Museum of Fine Arts of Houston, and Princeton University.

NIKOLAI KREMENTSOV is Associate Professor at the Institute for the History and Philosophy of Science and Technology at the University of Toronto. He is the author of several books, including *Stalinist Science*; *The Cure: A Story of Cancer and Politics from the Annals of the Cold War*; *International Science between the World Wars: The Case of Genetics*; and *A Martian Stranded on Earth: Alexander Bogdanov, Blood Transfusions, and Proletarian Science.*

SHIGEHISA KURIYAMA is Reischauer Institute Professor of Cultural History at Harvard University and author of *The Expressiveness of the Body and the Divergence of Greek and Chinese Medicine*. His primary area of research is the comparative history of medicine and the body in East Asia and Europe.

HANNAH LANDECKER is Associate Professor at the University of California Los Angeles, in the Department of Sociology and the Center for Society and Genetics. She is the author of *Culturing Life: How Cells Became Technologies*. Her current research interests include the use of moving images in life science and the history and social study of metabolic sciences.

SUSAN E. LEDERER is Robert Turell Professor in History of Medicine and Bioethics at the University of Wisconsin School of Medicine and Public Health. Her books include *Subjected to Science: Human Experimentation in America before the Second World War*;

Frankenstein: Penetrating the Secrets of Nature; and *Flesh and Blood: A Cultural History of Transplantation and Transfusion in Twentieth-Century America.*

BARRON H. LERNER is Professor of Medicine and Public Health at the Columbia College of Physicians and Surgeons and the Mailman School of Public Health. His books include *The Breast Cancer Wars: Hope, Fear and the Pursuit of a Cure in Twentieth-Century America*; *When Illness Goes Public: Celebrity Patients and How We Look at Medicine*; and *One for the Road: Drunk Driving Since 1900*. He is also a practicing internist.

LAURA LINDGREN (designer and publisher) designs art and photography books and exhibition catalogues for publishers and museums. She is also co-publisher of Blast Books in New York, and she is the editor, designer, and publisher of *Mütter Museum* and *Mütter Museum Historic Medical Photographs*, and *Dissection: Photographs of a Rite of Passage in American Medicine 1880–1930*, among others. Her websites are www.lindgrendesign.com and www.blastbooks.com.

MELISSA LO holds a SMArchS degree from MIT's History, Theory and Criticism of Architecture and Art program, where she wrote her master's thesis on Bourgery's *Traité*. She is a doctoral candidate in the history of science at Harvard University. Her dissertation analyzes the images that manifested and transformed Cartesian physics from 1630 to 1690.

MARK S. MICALE is Professor of History, University of Illinois at Champaign-Urbana. His research focuses on comparative European intellectual and cultural history, 1700 to the present; the history of science and medicine (especially psychiatry, psychoanalysis, and neuroscience); French history, 1789 to the present; and historical and theoretical gender studies. He has written *Hysterical Men: The Hidden History of Male Nervous Illness* and *Approaching Hysteria: Disease and Its Interpretations.*

MAREN MÖHRING is Lecturer of Modern and Contemporary History at the University of Cologne. She received her doctorate from Ludwig-Maximilians University with a study on German naturism. She has been awarded fellowships (NEH/GHI Fellowship at the German Historical Institute in Washington, DC; Feodor Lynen Fellowship of the Humboldt Foundation at the University of Zurich) to work on a book on foreign cuisines in West Germany.

SHEENA M. MORRISON is a doctoral candidate in the History and Ethics of Public Health and Medicine Program at Columbia University. She holds a master's degree in public health from Hunter College, CUNY. A practicing historian, she has worked as a contractor for the National Library of Medicine.

ALLISON MURI is Assistant Professor at the University of Saskatchewan. Her research interests include digital media studies and the history of cyberculture in early modern science, medicine, and technologies of communication. In *The Enlightenment Cyborg: A History of Communications and Control in the Human Machine, 1660–1830* she examines the history of mechanically steered, or "cyber," humans in the works of seventeenth- and eighteenth-century thinkers.

MIKE "SPORT" MURPHY is a singer and songwriter who has released three albums on the Kill Rock Stars label and has written frequently about popular culture for the *New York Post* and the *New York Daily News*. He lives with his wife and two children on Long Island, where his hobbies include constructing bogus habitat dioramas, cartooning, and hosting monthly gatherings devoted to the tasting of exotic spirits.

MARCIA D. NICHOLS is Assistant Professor in the Center for Learning Innovation at the University of Minnesota Rochester. A recipient of several fellowships, including a Mellon Fellowship for Early American Literature and Material Texts at the McNeil Center for Early American Studies, she has published essays on bawdy travelogues and Charles Brockden Brown's *Wieland*. Her current book project analyzes constructions of gender, sexuality, and identity in British and American midwifery manuals.

MARIANNE NOBLE is Associate Professor at American University in Washington, DC. She is the author of *The Masochistic Pleasures of Sentimental Literature* as well as articles on Dickinson, Stowe, Hawthorne, and Gothic and sentimental literature. She is working on a book entitled *Sympathy and the Quest for Genuine Human Contact in American Romantic Literature.*

MICHAEL J. NORTH is Head of the Rare Books and Early Manuscripts Section in the History of Medicine Division of the National Library of Medicine. He has worked in special collections at Swarthmore College, Georgetown University, the New York Academy of Medicine, and the Grolier Club of New York.

LISA O'SULLIVAN is Senior Curator of Medicine at the Science Museum, London, where she curates the Wellcome medical collections. In 2010–11 she was Postdoctoral Research Fellow in the History Department at the University of Sydney. Her areas of interest include the history of clinical nostalgia, the history of anatomy and anthropology, the sciences of racial difference, and the place of material culture in academic exchange networks.

ALYSSA PICARD is the author of *Making the American Mouth: Dentists and Public Health in the Twentieth Century*. She directs contract campaigns and guides the formation of new non-tenure-track faculty unions for the American Federation of Teachers' Michigan affiliate. Her next book will be a history of postwar labor, political, and popular-culture constructions of middle-class identity in the United States.

ROSAMOND PURCELL is a photographer and writer whose photography books include *Finders Keepers; Eight Collectors* (with Stephen Jay Gould), *Dice: Deception, Fate and Rotten Luck* (with Ricky Jay), and *Landscapes of the Passing Strange: Reflections from Shakespeare* (with Michael Witmore). Her interests include the history of seventeenth-century science and many twentieth-century artists (Dadaist and surrealist in particular), and she is the author of *Owls Head: On the Nature of Lost Things* and *Special Cases: Natural Anomalies and Historical Monsters.*

ANNE MARIE RAFFERTY is Head of the Florence Nightingale School of Nursing and Midwifery, King's College London, and holds degrees from the University of Edinburgh, BSc (Soc Sci) in Nursing Studies, Nottingham University, M.Phil (Surgery), and Oxford University, D.Phil (Modern History). She was awarded the Agnes Dillon Prize for Nursing History from the University of Virginia, the first non-American nurse so honored, and made CBE in the 2009 New Year's Honours.

SITA REDDY is Research Associate at the Smithsonian Institution's Center for Folklife and Cultural Heritage. A sociologist of medicine, with a doctorate from the University of Pennsylvania, she specializes in Asian history, museology, and cultural heritage policy and is working on an exhibition and book on the social iconography of modern yoga.

ELIZABETH REIS is the author of *Bodies in Doubt: An American History of Intersex* and *Damned Women: Sinners and Witches in Puritan New England*. She is Associate Professor of Women's and Gender Studies at the University of Oregon.

BENJAMIN REISS is Professor of English at Emory University. He is the author of *Theaters of Madness: Insane Asylums and Nineteenth-Century American Culture* and *The Showman and the Slave: Race, Death, and Memory in Barnum's America*. He is also a co-editor, with Leonard Cassuto and Clare Eby, of *The Cambridge History of the American Novel*.

R. ROGER REMINGTON is Massimo and Lella Vignelli Distinguished Professor of Design at Rochester Institute of Technology. He is the author of four books on design history, most recently *Design and Science—The Life and Work of Will Burtin*. He received his master's degree from the University of Wisconsin-Madison and his BFA in Graphic Design from Rochester Institute of Technology.

JEFFREY S. REZNICK, PhD, a social and cultural historian of medicine and war, is Chief of the History of Medicine Division of the National Library of Medicine and a fellow of the Royal Historical Society. He is author, most recently, of *John Galsworthy and Disabled Soldiers of the Great War* in the Cultural History of Modern War series of Manchester University Press.

MICHAEL RHODE is Archivist in the U.S. Navy Bureau of Medicine's Office of Medical History and for many years was Chief Archivist of the National Museum of Health and Medicine. He is the editor of *Harvey Pekar: Conversations*, and an editor of the *International Journal of Comic Art*. He is an author of the book *Walter Reed Army Medical Center Centennial: A Pictorial History, 1909–2009* and the exhibit catalogues *Battlefield Surgery 101: From the Civil War to Vietnam* and *"American Angels of Mercy": Dr. Anita Newcomb McGee's Pictorial Record of the Russo-Japanese War, 1904*.

STEPHEN P. RICE is Professor of American Studies at Ramapo College of New Jersey. He is author of *Minding the Machine: Languages of Class in Early Industrial America*. His current research focuses on nineteenth-century commercial wood engraving and visual culture in the United States.

HARRIET RITVO is Arthur J. Conner Professor of History at the Massachusetts Institute of Technology, where she teaches courses on British history, environmental history, the history of natural history, and the history of human-animal relations. Her books include *The Animal Estate: The English and Other Creatures in the Victorian Age*; *The Platypus and the Mermaid, and Other Figments of the Classifying Imagination*; *The Dawn of Green: Manchester, Thirlmere, and Modern Environmentalism*; and *Noble Cows and Hybrid Zebras: Essays on Animals and History*.

CHARLES ROSENBERG is Ernest Monrad Professor in the Department of the History of Science, Harvard University. He has written widely on American medicine and science and has a long-time interest in the place of print in the culture of medicine.

MICHAEL SAPPOL is curator-historian at the History of Medicine Division of the National Library of Medicine and the author of *A Traffic of Dead Bodies: Anatomy and Embodied Social Identity in Nineteenth-Century America* and *Dream Anatomy* and co-editor of *A Cultural History of the Body in the Age of Empire*. His current work focuses on twentieth-century modernist medical illustration and the history of medical film.

EMILIE SAVAGE-SMITH, recently retired as Professor of the History of Islamic Science, University of Oxford, is Senior Research Consultant to the Bodleian Library. She has written extensively on the history of anatomy, surgery, and ophthalmology in the medieval Islamic world and prepared the online catalogue *Islamic Medical Manuscripts at the National Library of Medicine*. Recent publications include *Medieval Islamic Medicine* (with P. Pormann) and *Ibn Hindu: The Key to Medicine and a Guide to Students* (with A. Tibi).

JONATHAN SAWDAY is the Walter J. Ong, SJ, Chair in the Humanities in the Department of English at Saint Louis University. His books include *The Body Emblazoned: Dissection and the Human Body in Renaissance Culture* and *Engines of the Imagination: Renaissance Culture and the Rise of the Machine*. He is a Fellow of the Royal Historical Society, of the English Association, and of the Royal Society for the Arts.

WALTON O. SCHALICK, III, is a practicing pediatric rehabilitation physician as well as a historian of medieval medicine and of modern disability. He is Assistant Professor of Medical History and Bioethics, Orthopedics and Rehabilitation, Pediatrics, History, and History of Science at the University of Wisconsin, where he is also Director of the Disability Studies Cluster. He has published on all of these subjects and has received federal and private funding for his research.

ANTONY SHUGAAR is a writer and translator. He is the author, most recently, of *Coast to Coast: Vintage Travel in North America*; *I Lie for a Living: Greatest Spies of All Time*; and (with Gianni Guadalupi) *Latitude Zero: Tales of the Equator*. He is the translator of *Margherita Dolce Vita* by Stefano Benni and *Everybody's Right* by

Paolo Sorrentino, among other works. He lives in Charlottesville, Virginia, with his wife and daughter.

JONATHAN SMITH is Professor of English and Director of the Science and Technology Studies Program at the University of Michigan-Dearborn. He is the author of *Charles Darwin and Victorian Visual Culture, Fact and Feeling: Baconian Science and the Nineteenth-Century Literary Imagination*, and numerous articles on Victorian literature, science, and culture.

JENNIFER SPINKS is Australian Research Council Postdoctoral Fellow in the School of Historical Studies at the University of Melbourne. She is the author of *Monstrous Births and Visual Culture in Sixteenth-Century Germany* and, with Susan Broomhall, co-author of the forthcoming *Early Modern Women in the Low Countries: Feminizing Sources and Interpretations of the Past*. She is working on a study of "wonder books" in early modern Europe.

CLAUDIA STEIN is Associate Professor in the Department of History, University of Warwick, and Director of the Centre for the History of Medicine. The author of *Negotiating the French Pox in Early Modern Germany*, she is working on a study of the emergence of biopower in eighteenth-century Germany and, with Roger Cooter, on a history of biopolitics and visualization strategies in Germany and Britain, ca. 1880–1930.

ARNE SVENSON (photographer) is the author of *Prisoners* and *Mrs. Ballard's Parrots* and photographer and coauthor (with Ron Warren) of *Sock Monkeys* and *Chewed*. He is currently working on a new book on forensic facial reconstructions, *Unspeaking Likeness*. He lives and works in New York City.

JAMES TAYLOR's *Shocked and Amazed! On & Off the Midway* is the world's only periodical devoted to the history and current status of sideshow, novelty, and variety exhibitions. He has been covering "the other entertainment" for more than two decades and has been featured in assorted media worldwide for his work. He is the co-founder of Baltimore's American Dime Museum and the Palace of Wonders in Washington, DC.

PAUL THEERMAN is Head of the Images and Archives Section of the History of Medicine Division of the National Library of Medicine. Trained as a historian, he has an abiding interest in the cultural history of modern science and medicine. He oversees programs in Archives and Modern Manuscripts, Prints and Photographs, and Historical Audiovisuals and digital projects based on those collections, notably Profiles in Science and Images from the History of Medicine.

CHARLES W. J. WITHERS is Professor of Historical Geography at the University of Edinburgh and a Fellow of the British Academy. He has teaching and research interests in the historical geography of science, the Enlightenment, and the history of cartography. His latest book is *Geography and Science in Britain 1831–1939: A Study of the British Association for the Advancement of Science*.

HIROO YAMAGATA is an infrastructure development consultant as well as a prominent writer and translator. Based in Tokyo, he specializes in interdisciplinary subjects ranging from economics, third world development, the Internet, and free software to architecture, urban planning, art, and literature. He writes a regular column in *GQ Japan* and serves on the book review board at *Asahi Newspaper*.

Index

page 1: Detail, Charles Bell, Drawings of Arteries, ca. 1797, pl. 9, fig. 2
pages 2–3: Dorsal view of walking skeleton, from John Fotherby, *Anatomy*,
England, bound manuscript on paper, ca. 1730. Ink on paper, 74 x 53 cm
pages 4–5: Detail, Axel Key and Gustaf Retzius,
Studies in the Anatomy of the Nervous System and Connective Tissue, 1875–76
page 228: Trimester foetal skeleton, from John Fotherby, *Anatomy*

Library of Congress Cataloging-in-Publication Data
Hidden treasure : the National Library of Medicine / edited by Michael Sappol ;
designed by Laura Lindgren ; photography by Arne Svenson ; National Library
of Medicine. — 1st ed.
    p. ; cm.
    Includes bibliographical references and index.
    ISBN 978-0-922233-42-7 (alk. paper)
    I. Sappol, Michael. II. National Library of Medicine (U.S.)
    [DNLM: 1. National Library of Medicine (U.S.) 2. Libraries, Medical —
United States — Catalogs. 3. Libraries, Medical — United States — Collections.
4. History of Medicine — United States — Catalogs. 5. History of
Medicine — United States — Collections. 6. Library Materials — United
States — Catalogs. 7. Library Materials — United States — Collections. Z 675.M4]
    026'.610973 — dc23   2011039323

Published by Blast Books, Inc.
P. O. Box 51, Cooper Station
New York, NY 10276-0051
www.blastbooks.com

Managing Editor: William Zeisel / QED Associates, LLC

Printed by The Studley Press in the United States
10   9   8   7   6   5   4   3   2   1